Understanding Dementia

For Churchill Livingstone:

Publishing Manager: Mary Law
Project Development Manager: Valerie Dearing
Project Manager: Jane Shanks

Understanding Dementia

Alan Jacques MB BCh DPM FRCPsych
Consultant in Old Age Psychiatry, Royal Edinburgh Hospital, Edinburgh, UK

Graham A. Jackson MB ChB MRCGP MRCPsych
Consultant in Old Age Psychiatry, formerly General Practitioner, Glasgow, UK

THIRD EDITION

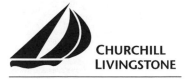

**CHURCHILL
LIVINGSTONE**

Edinburgh London New York Philadelphia St Louis Sydney Toronto 2000

CHURCHILL LIVINGSTONE
An imprint of Harcourt Publishers Limited

© Harcourt Publishers Limited 2000

✷ is a registered trademark of Harcourt Publishers Limited

The right of Alan Jacques and Graham Jackson to be identified as authors of this
work has been asserted by them in accordance with the Copyright, Designs and
Patents Act 1988

First edition   1988
Second edition   1992
Third edition   2000

0 443 05512 2

British Library Cataloguing in Publication Data
A catalogue record for this book is available from the British Library

Library of Congress Cataloging in Publication Data
A catalog record for this book is available from the Library of Congress

Note
Medical knowledge is constantly changing. As new information becomes
available, changes in treatment, procedures, equipment and the use of drugs
become necessary. The authors and the publishers have, as far as it is possible,
taken care to ensure that the information given in this text is accurate and up to
date. However, readers are strongly advised to confirm that the information,
especially with regard to drug usage, complies with the latest legislation and
standards of practice.

The
publisher's
policy is to use
paper manufactured
from sustainable forests

Printed in China

Contents

Preface to the third edition

For this third edition of *Understanding Dementia*, Alan Jacques has been joined by Graham Jackson, who has a particular interest in the treatment of behaviour problems and the use of drug treatments. The chapters on the nature of dementia and on problems of behaviour have been updated and a new chapter on drug treatment has been added. Attitudes to dementia change gradually and more emphasis is placed on the ways in which those with dementia can be involved in decisions about their own care, and how the experience of the earlier stages can be shared. The basic need to understand dementia based on how it affects the person's brain, and how the person and those who care for her react to that disease process, remains central to the book.

Throughout the text we have referred to dementia sufferers as female. This is not intended to be in any way sexist. It is simply a reflection of the fact that the great majority of sufferers are women. We have also tended to call them patients. This is not only because we are doctors, but also is justified since dementia is a serious illness which often causes great distress to sufferers and carers. Purely for convenience, we have referred to professionals as males, even though this does not reflect the realities of care.

We hope that this book will be of help to the wide variety of professionals, volunteers and informal carers who become involved in the care of those who have the misfortune to develop dementia, and that it will encourage a positive approach to that care.

We would particularly like to thank Margaret Mitchell for her assistance in preparing the manuscript for this edition.

1999   Alan Jacques
                                                Graham Jackson

What is dementia?

Dementia is a syndrome which may be caused by a number of different illnesses. It is a progressive failure of many cerebral functions.

Despite growing public awareness of the problem of dementia there are still many people who think that it is a normal part of the ageing process. They assume that any psychological change or eccentricity in old age is evidence of dementia and therefore untreatable. This sort of 'just old age' generalization is now out of date. For, thanks to great advances in research, we are able to define the syndrome of dementia reasonably well, both by saying what it is and by saying what it is not, even if there is still some woolliness at the boundary.

In this chapter we shall look at what dementia is and the illnesses which cause it, by examining the statement above more closely. In the past few years some real progress has been made in understanding its commonest causes. This is a developing area of research, which may eventually lead to effective treatments for a group of devastating illnesses which are becoming increasingly common as more people survive into their 80s and 90s, and which also cause enormous distress in the smaller number of younger people who are affected.

DEFINING DEMENTIA

Dementia is a syndrome

Firstly, what is the evidence that dementia should be seen in terms of illness or disease at all? It is, after all, quite a common condition and could be seen as a variant of old age, at the end of a spectrum of normality, rather like extreme shortness of stature or very high intelligence. Using the word 'illness' implies that a patient's condition is out of the ordinary, not part of her normal life. It implies that there are some detrimental effects which seriously impair the patient's ability to lead a normal life, or may even be fatal.

A *syndrome* is a characteristic pattern of clinical features – the symptoms and signs – which can be caused by one or other of a number of illnesses. Each of these illnesses will have a clear underlying pathology, whether organic or psychological. We should be able to explain how that pathology leads in each illness to the *common clinical features* of the syndrome.

There are various definitions of dementia, but the one we will refer to here is that of the World Health Organization (Box 1.1).

Box 1.1 World Health Organization's definition of dementia

Dementia is a syndrome due to disease of the brain, usually of a chronic or progressive nature, in which there is disturbance of multiple cortical functions, calculation, learning capacity, language and judgement. Consciousness is not clouded. Impairments of cognitive function are commonly accompanied, and occasionally preceded by deterioration in emotional control, social behaviour, or motivation.

An abnormal condition

Dementia is not a part of normal life. Indeed, it is important to note that at all ages, even into the 90s (or the 100s for that matter) dementia is a minority condition (Table 1.1 and Fig. 1.1). The figures quoted summarize a large number of community surveys

Table 1.1 Prevalence of dementia in the community (adapted from EURODEM data, 1995). The figures show the numbers of people who at any one time are suffering definite dementias, mostly moderate to severe cases. This may considerably underestimate the number of mild cases where diagnosis is more difficult.

Age group (years)	Percentage with dementia	Percentage without dementia
30–59	0.1	99.9
60–64	1.0	99.0
65–69	1.4	98.6
70–74	4.1	95.9
75–79	5.7	94.3
80–84	13.0	87.0
85–89	21.6	78.4
90+	32.6	67.4

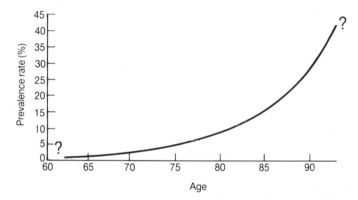

Fig. 1.1 The same figures in graphical form. Note how many people at any age *do not* suffer from dementia.

of elderly people which have looked at the prevalence of dementia. They show that the vast majority of elderly people are not deteriorating mentally. It is not therefore justified to say 'when I am old and demented' as if the one condition followed the other inevitably. Neither is it reasonable to treat 80 or 90 year olds who can still count their own money or do the crossword or keep up to date with the news as if they were in some way special – they are unfortunately merely average, unless of course they could not do these things before!

Dementia is very rare in people under 60 and it increases in prevalence at later ages – the older one is the greater the risk of suffering dementia. One fascinating gap in our knowledge is that we do not know whether this increase in prevalence goes on into extreme old age or slackens off – are 110 year olds very likely to suffer dementia or are they somehow relatively immune? The figures we have suggest that, roughly speaking, the prevalence doubles with each 5-year age group up to the nineties, what is called exponential growth. So it is an illness of old age but not a normal part of it. The difficulty in definition only comes when we try to draw a clear dividing line between what is normal in old age and what is dementia. We will discuss this more fully in Chapter 2.

Detrimental effects

Throughout the book we will be emphasizing how much damage dementia does to the lives of sufferers and those around them. No one can doubt the magnitude and importance of this damage; it poses an enormous challenge to health and social services and to the community as a whole.

In terms of seeing dementia as illness, however, the most significant effect of all is its final outcome – dementia kills (Table 1.2). It was shown about 40 years ago that dementia markedly shortens expectation of life. These patients, who were in long-stay psychiatric wards, were mostly in their 60s and 70s. When this study was repeated in hospitals of the late 1970s, where the average age had risen to over 80, this shortening of life was less apparent. Perhaps better hospital conditions contributed, but it also may be that dementia beginning in a person who is in her 80s is a less malignant disease (see p. 26). This thought should make us pause when we consider that there are now very many

Table 1.2 Life expectancy of dementia sufferers

Group studied	Average expectation of life (years of remaining life)	
General population at birth	Women 78 years	Men 73 years
General population at 65	Women 16 years	Men 12 years
General population at 75	Women 10 years	Men 8 years
Dementia sufferers in the 1950s (mostly in their 60s and 70s)	2–5 years	
Dementia suffers in the 1970s (mostly in their 70s and 80s)	5–10 years	

more people in this older age group (see Table 3.1, p. 85), and that many of them have few available relatives to support them.

A pattern

The main purpose of this book is to show the characteristic pattern of symptoms and signs in dementia. The word 'de-mentia', implying loss of the mind or loss of mental powers, describes the basic process well. Other terms which have been used, such as *chronic brain syndrome* or *chronic cerebral failure*, are no better and no worse. Although we will emphasize how complex the mental decline is in a particular individual, there are clear common features in all patients. These are due to progressive damage to widespread areas of the brain, and are different in pattern and degree from the normal changes of old age. Certain symptoms may be more common in dementia due to particular illnesses. There have been a number of attempts to distinguish separate subtypes of dementia, such as 'subcortical dementia', as will be discussed later in the chapter. However, despite this it can be said that, whatever the cause of the dementia, the basic general pattern of symptoms and signs and the pattern of decline are roughly the same; in other words, it is a syndrome.

Illnesses which cause dementia

The second part of this chapter will describe some of the many illnesses which can cause the syndrome of dementia. Some of these illnesses have other characteristic symptoms in addition to those of dementia, but in each of them we will be able to see how the characteristic pathology of the illness leads to gradually progressive cerebral failure.

So there are some good reasons for thinking of dementia in terms of illness – its minority occurrence, its damaging effects, its causes and their characteristic pathologies. Thinking this way has stimulated research and encouraged attempts at treatment. It has helped make dementia respectable.

Dementia is progressive cerebral failure

From normal to death

Before the dementing process began the victim was, of course, her normal self, and this 'normal' is the baseline from which we measure how much she has changed. At the end of the illness the patient is dying. What actually causes death in simple dementia is not clear. Presumably, as more and more functions decline, the brain's ability to adjust to changes in the environment (for example, by heat regulation, control of the heart and breathing or resistance to infections) eventually deteriorates to such an extent that life can no longer be supported. These final stages leave the patient bereft of mental powers, unable to understand, communicate or reason, needing everything done for her, incontinent and chairbound.

But between the normal self and this terminal vegetable-like existence lie years of usually gradual deterioration. The commonest illnesses which cause dementia are quite likely to last for 5, 10 or even 15 years. During this long period the patient is dement*ing*, not dement*ed*. We should try to emphasize the gradually progressive nature of dementia by using the former term.

Presenting complaints

Within the basic syndrome of dementia there is considerable variation in the rate of the decline from person to person, and in a particular individual different brain functions may fail at different rates. This is obvious even at the beginning of the process, for there is a variety of ways in which dementia declares itself – the presenting complaints (Table 1.3).

Most people are aware that memory loss is an important feature of the condition and this is, indeed, often the first

Table 1.3 Common presenting complaints in dementia

Losses	Memory impairment
	Decline in self-care
	Decline in management of one's affairs
	Decline in work performance
Change in behaviour	Uncharacteristic behaviour
	Social withdrawal
	Personality change
	Mood change
	Paranoid ideas
Delirium which fails to clear	Due to illness
	Due to a change of environment

complaint. But, in looking back, relatives may recall other more subtle changes in personality, personal habits or motivation, which started perhaps several months before the decline in memory. Sometimes it is an uncharacteristic way of behaving (e.g. hoarding, wandering, shoplifting, disinhibited behaviour) that shows that something is wrong, sometimes it is an episode of delirium. But, unfortunately, early referral for diagnosis, assessment and help or referral when the decline is steadily and quietly progressing are not usual. In many cases the insidious onset, the common attitude that it is 'just old age' and the assumption that nothing can be done conspire to keep relatives from complaining. The patient herself may not be aware of the changes, may try to cover them up out of embarrassment or may share her relatives' unhelpful attitudes, so that she does not complain either. Many doctors are also reluctant to diagnose dementia. This is often because they think that nothing can be done, but in fact lack of a diagnosis usually leads to lack of appropriate help. One of the most important reasons for an early diagnosis is to access that appropriate help (see Chapter 11).

In many cases it is actually very difficult to date the onset of dementia. Indeed, we must assume from what pathologists have found that the damage to the brain in a case of, say, dementia of Alzheimer type has been going on for several years before it has any perceptible effect. This is because the brain can function quite normally if it has only been mildly damaged – there is a *cerebral reserve*. As the damage progresses, eventually the brain can no longer compensate, the reserve is used up and the person shows the beginnings of mental impairment. The stage before dementia reveals itself will clearly become very important when we have treatments which can slow or prevent the progress of the disease.

Crises

Because of the gradual onset of most dementias and the various other reasons why people do not ask for help in the early stages, it is still too often the case that a sufferer will first be brought to the attention of helping agencies when there is a crisis, and 'something must be done' (Table 1.4). Indeed, the dementia may have been progressing for several years before one of these crises

Table 1.4 Crises in dementia

Crises of behaviour	Gas left on
	Water taps left on
	Lost in the street
	Disinhibited behaviour
	Shoplifting
Crises of care	Death of carer
	Illness of carer
	Relative arrives on holiday
	Relative goes on holiday
	Home help goes
Medical crises	Drug mistake or overdose
	Physical illness
	Delirium
	Strokes in multi-infarct dementia

occurs. In vascular dementia, a common cause of dementia, the patient's state may suddenly take a turn for the worse because of a small stroke, and so medical crises are a bit more common.

However, the usual crises of dementia are about quite extraneous events, as Table 1.4 shows. Not only are they of different origins but they may lead to calls for help from different agencies. In crises of behaviour it may be the police, the housing department or social services who are called; in crises of care it may be the social workers or primary health care team; in crises of health the primary health care team or hospital. To make matters worse, a health problem is sometimes referred to social services, a crisis of care to the police, and so on.

Management of the decline

Of course crises cannot be totally avoided, but one of the vital tasks facing the professions and voluntary organizations who deal with dementia is to shift the focus away from crisis management on to managing the slow decline. It is this decline which *is* dementia and which causes the main burden of care, 24 hours a day, 7 days a week for several years. This shift will be achieved when we persuade relatives to make that early referral, when proper diagnosis and assessment is seen as a worthwhile effort by general practitioners and other professionals and when this assessment takes into account the multiple problems of dementia, needing multiple solutions.

When a crisis does occur, it should not necessarily be seen as a reason to rush an old lady into long-term care, but rather as a reason for a cool and sensitive review, by all involved acting together, of those multiple problems and of the care being given. Surprisingly often, the crisis can be survived and better care organized for the future.

Ribot's law

This cooler look at the problems facing a patient whose entire brain is failing requires some understanding of the course of dementia. A generalization called Ribot's law is helpful, though only as a generalization. This law states that the advanced co-ordinating and connecting functions of the brain, which develop relatively late in life, are the first to deteriorate when widespread damage occurs. When we look at the most specific and basic functions of the cerebrum, for example hearing or sight which have very direct and definable representations in small areas of the cerebral cortex (Fig. 1.2) and which develop very early in life, we find them unaffected at least in the early stages of most dementia, as Ribot's law suggests.

These more primitive, basic functions of the brain will be affected later in the course of dementia, so that physical decline follows mental decline. Thus we would expect that, as a rule, urinary incontinence would begin to be a problem at a later stage than decline in memory, and that faecal incontinence would develop later than urinary incontinence. If this general sequence

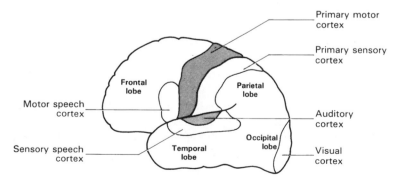

Fig. 1.2 The surface of the cerebral hemispheres from the side, showing some specific funtional areas.

is not followed and the patient is, say, incontinent at an early stage of dementia or incontinent of faeces while still continent of urine, then we should think again.

There is actually, of course, a lot of variability in the course of dementia. When a symptom does not fit the usual pattern of decline we may merely be seeing that variability. But it could be that there is a quite separate diagnosis as well as the dementia; the early incontinence could be due to a urinary tract infection, the early faecal incontinence due to constipation, for example. The other, treatable illness is in danger of being missed if we think that anything that looks like a sign of dementia *must* be dementia, without trying to fit it into the overall pattern.

Dementia affects many cerebral functions

One of the shocks which awaits the relatives of a dementia sufferer is that what they thought of as a simple memory problem becomes a much more general one, with effects on every aspect of that person's life. Slowly all her mental faculties decline – her intelligence, imagination, judgement, self control, her ability to attend, concentrate and be motivated, her orientation, communication and behaviour, her habits and old memories, her ability to learn, her emotional life. Her whole personality disintegrates while her physical powers and health may remain quite normal until late in the illness. Relatives need to be warned early about all these changes, so that they can be prepared and know how to look for help.

From the professional's point of view there is also a problem. It is relatively easy to assess certain brain functions – intelligence, memory, constructional skill – and test them reliably. The areas of the brain where these functions are carried out can be quite well identified and pathologists can show damage in these areas in people who have died of dementia. It is, however, rather more difficult to measure behavioural changes or to localize them in the brain. It is almost impossible to measure judgement or imagination. We are in danger of concentrating in dementia on the measurable, useful though the tests are, and forgetting the more subtle general changes, which are much more important in the day-to-day life of the sufferer.

In fact, to understand the basic process of dementia, we need simply to think of all that the more advanced parts of our brains do, as that is the list of functions which are likely to decline. It is the whole personality, all that was ever learned, the basic controlling and organizing functions of the cerebrum, which are affected. We will detail these changes in Chapters 4 and 5.

General damage and patchy damage

We will see that, as research clarifies the illnesses of dementia and their effects, it is becoming evident that dementia does not usually damage absolutely all the functions of the brain; as our definition says, it affects many different functions.

Dementia of Alzheimer type does not damage every bit of the cerebral cortex equally (p. 18); there is even more patchy, though widespread, damage in vascular dementia (p. 30) and researchers are on the lookout for other patterns of damage which might be specific to other causes of dementia. Nevertheless, when we look at the more general functions, such as intelligence, thinking and understanding, what has been called the *law of mass action* seems to apply in dementia. This states that when there is widespread damage to the cerebrum, even if it is patchy, there is proportionate damage to these general functions. So a lot of little injuries, even if they are patchy, act as if they were one large general injury.

CAUSES OF DEMENTIA

Any syndrome may have a number of different causes. If we see the syndrome of dementia as a gradual decline in the function of the cerebrum, then to understand its causes we must look at all the reasons for gradually increasing cerebral damage (Table 1.5).

PRESENILE AND SENILE DEMENTIA

In the past, the syndrome of dementia was subdivided into a presenile and a senile type, with the dividing line drawn at an age of onset somewhere around 65 years (Table 1.6). There is no doubt that this division into subsyndromes had some value; the relative frequency of the various causes of dementia differs between the two age groups and there are different effects on the

Table 1.5 Causes of dementia

Illness	Type of damage	Treatment available	Potential treatment
Dementia of Alzheimer type (DAT)	Plaques, tangles, transmitter defects, abnormal amyloid deposition	+ (?)	Anticholinesterases, nerve growth factor
Vascular dementia	Multiple infarcts, stroke, small vessel disease	+ (?)	Aspirin, lower blood pressure, lower cholesterol
Lewy body dementia	Lewy bodies, transmitter defects	+ (?)	Anticholinesterases
Parkinson's disease	Lewy bodies especially in basal ganglia	−	Antiparkinsonian drugs do not help dementia
Frontal lobe dementia	Various, including Pick's	−	
Normal pressure hydrocephalus	Obstructed cerebrospinal fluid flow due to previous damage, e.g. subarachnoid haemorrhage, meningitis	+	Surgery (shunt)
Punch-drunk syndrome	Repeated head injury	+ (?)	Stop the damage
Slow-growing brain tumour	Pressure causes destruction of brain	+	Surgery
Aluminium and other metals	Direct toxic effect	+	Remove the poison
Wilson's disease	Toxicity of copper	+	Penicillamine
Alcohol abuse	Toxic effect and thiamine deficiency	+	Abstinence, thiamine treatment
Huntington's chorea	Genetic abnormality	−	Screening available
Syphilis (GPI)	Infective	+	Antibiotics
AIDS	Infective, secondary infection	+	Anti-AIDS drugs
CJD	Infective (?)	−	
Vitamin (e.g. B_{12}) deficiencies	Toxic (?)	+	Replacement
Hypothyroidism	Toxic (?)	+	Replacement
Parathyroid disorders	Calcium metabolism altered	+	Medical or surgical

family and social life of a person of working age and an elderly retired person. However, as a consequence of the subdivision, younger, 'presenile' patients may have been referred more often to neurologists for expert diagnosis and possible treatment, but got little practical help, while the older, 'senile' patients were seen as suffering from the ordinary problems of old age and referred, if at all, to one or other of a wide variety of agencies, to find the solution to the crisis of the moment. The result has been a clearer definition of the dementia syndrome in younger patients, with an emphasis on its more neurological manifestations, and considerable vagueness in describing 'senile dementia'.

There are now good reasons for questioning the presenile/senile subdivision. In the first instance, when examined closely, the pattern of symptoms and decline is actually very similar in patients who develop dementia in their 50s or early 60s and those who develop it in their late 60s and 70s, even if the social effects are different. Attempts to distinguish the genetics of the two conditions have brought confusing results but the case for a break at 65 is, at the least, unproven. Most crucial is the fact that is has been impossible to distinguish any major differences between the pathological or chemical changes in the brains of the two groups (but see p. 26 for other ideas about a dividing line).

It is, however, important to emphasize the special needs of younger sufferers. The term *early onset* dementia is a good one; but this term – referring to the age at which the dementia starts – must be clearly distinguished from *early* dementia, which refers to the first stages of the illness, whatever the age of onset.

'Senile'

The distinction between presenile and senile dementia was further muddled by the use of the term 'senile dementia' to describe an *illness* which is the most common cause of senile dementia the *syndrome* (Table 1.6)! It is thus unclear, when a person is described as suffering from 'senile dementia', whether it is merely being stated that they are over 65 and have dementia (the syndrome), or whether they are suffering from the specific disease which we now call senile dementia of Alzheimer type.

Table 1.6 Old and new terms in dementia

Syndrome	Subsyndrome	Causal illnesses	New terms for the illnesses
Dementia Chronic brain syndrome	Presenile dementia	Alzheimer's disease	Dementia of Alzheimer type (DAT)
Chronic cerebral failure etc.		Arteriosclerotic dementia	Multi-infarct dementia (MID) or vascular dementia
		Other causes in Table 1.5	
	Senile dementia	Senile dementia	DAT or senile dementia of Alzheimer type (SDAT)
		Arteriosclerotic dementia	MID or vascular dementia
		Other causes in Table 1.5	

The word 'senile' has in any case been much misused in common speech, often vaguely and sometimes pejoratively. It can mean old, more likely to happen in older people, physically decrepit, mentally infirm or just plain unwanted. In the absence of clarity we would be better to avoid its use altogether. We will drop the presenile/senile distinction, look at dementia as a whole and examine the underlying diseases.

At all ages the commonest causes are *dementia of Alzheimer type* and *vascular dementias*. We will first describe these conditions and then look at the relatively uncommon causes.

DEMENTIA OF ALZHEIMER TYPE (DAT)

When Alois Alzheimer first described this illness in 1907, the population structure and pattern of mental illness were very different from today. In Britain and other similar countries the proportion of the population aged over 65 was around 5% (today the figure is over 15%), and the proportion over 75 was very much smaller; so small indeed that it was not even measured in the census, a statistical anomaly whose present-day importance was only fully recognized in the mid-1970s.

In asylums 90 years ago, inmates included two important groups who would have been described as 'demented'. Firstly, there were sufferers from chronic *schizophrenia*, or *dementia praecox* – the dementia of adolescence. The decline in drive and emotion and the typical social withdrawal of the schizophrenic were seen as a form of dementia. However, pathologists failed to show any significant damage in the brains of schizophrenics at postmortem and the changes began to be seen as purely functional, not organic. This, by the way, is the origin of the much misused word *'functional'* in relation to psychiatric illnesses – it means 'not organic'. In a functional illness there seemed to be a disorder of the function of the brain without any disorder of the organic structure, such as could be seen by a pathologist. It is interesting that in the last few years the debate on the distinction between organic and functional disorder has reopened, with many claiming that there is, after all, brain damage of some sort in chronic schizophrenia, though not a dementia like DAT. In practice, it would be best to avoid this use of the word 'functional' altogether, since it has no clear meaning today.

The second group of asylum inmates, possibly up to one-third of the total, would be suffering from a true dementia, but very few would have had Alzheimer's disease. The most common cause of their dementia was probably the late effects of syphilis – general paralysis of the insane (GPI, see p. 39).

One of the most important episodes in the transformation of psychiatry from a humanitarian custody of the insane in asylums to a medical speciality was the linking of GPI to infection with syphilis, the finding of the bacterium which causes syphilis in the brains of GPI patients and the subsequent beginnings of effective treatment for a previously incurable illness.

Alzheimer, then, was picking out from among these dementia sufferers another small group of patients who were suffering profound dementia not due to syphilis and with different pathological changes. He was describing 'presenile' patients, but it quite soon became obvious that many senile dementia cases were largely indistinguishable from his presenile cases. It was only with the development of specialized neurochemical tests and electron microscopy in the last two decades, leading to more detailed pathological studies, that the identity of the two conditions was confirmed. In Alzheimer's day there would anyway have been few senile cases in the asylums. The relatively small numbers of very old people and the large numbers of potentially supporting relatives, coupled with few expectations of treatment, kept sufferers in their own homes with their own families. This situation is still the case in most non-Western cultures, that is, in most of the world.

Pathology

We are now able to define the pathology of Alzheimer's dementia quite clearly (Table 1.7), although distinction from normal ageing in the early stages remains a problem.

Shrinkage

The cerebral hemispheres shrink and lose weight (Fig. 1.3). This change is more easily definable in younger sufferers and can be easily displayed by brain scanning using computed tomography (CT scanning). However, in older patients and in normal, undemented old people, brain size is more variable and demonstrating whether the shrinkage of DAT is present or not is less reliable and so less helpful in diagnosis.

Site of the damage

The cause of the shrinkage lies mainly in the cerebral cortex, the convoluted grey matter covering the cerebrum which contains many millions of nerve cells or neurones – though the white matter, which consists mostly of nerve fibres, or axons, which

Table 1.7 The pathology of dementia of Alzheimer type

Site of demage	Type of damage
Cerebral hemispheres especially temporal, parietal and frontal lobes	Shrinkage Enlarged ventricles
Grey matter of these areas	Shrinkage and cell loss or damage Senile plaques
In some subcortical nuclei	Similar changes
In the plaques	Dead cells, amyloid
Within the neurones in the affected areas	Neurofibrillary tangles Loss of enzymes which help make the neurotransmitters, especially ACh
At the nerve endings	Lack of neurotransmitters, so that messages are not passed

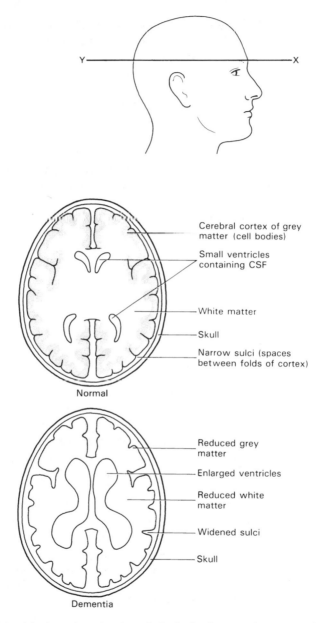

Fig. 1.3 A horizontal section through the brain of a normal person, and a similar section through the brain of a sufferer from severe dementia. CT scan and MRI scan pictures resemble these and can provide evidence of dementia.

make the multitudinous connections between different parts of the brain, also shrinks. It is still not absolutely clear to what extent it is the death of nerve cells, or their damage and shrinkage, or changes around the cells which cause the general shrinking of cerebral grey matter in DAT, for measuring the number of cells in the cortex is difficult.

A variety of studies show that, in DAT, damage is concentrated in certain areas of the brain, especially the temporal lobes, which include the hippocampal region, an area specifically involved in recent memory, the parietal lobes, involved with spatial orientation among other functions, and the frontal lobes, the area involved in self control (Fig. 1.2). In these areas, and most especially in the hippocampus, cell deaths have been demonstrated. We will see how this pattern of damage is reflected in the main clinical features of DAT in Chapters 4 and 5.

Plaques and tangles

More significant than the actual death of cells may be the widespread evidence that neurones, and especially their endings and connections, are degenerating. The characteristic pathological finding under the microscope in Alzheimer's dementia is of *argentophil* or *senile plaques* and *neurofibrillary tangles*. Plaques show up with silver stains under the microscope (as the name 'argentophil' suggests) and contain degenerating nerve endings and a variety of the substance amyloid which is often found in connection with inflammatory changes or degeneration. The number of plaques is greatest in the areas of brain where there is most shrinkage, and the number of plaques is proportional to the degree of intellectual decline in a dementia sufferer. Plaques are also present in smaller numbers in the brains of many undemented older people. Plaques contain beta amyloid, a protein which appears to be dealt with in an abnormal way in people with DAT. It is becoming increasingly likely that abnormal amyloid metabolism is involved in the development of DAT, no matter the underlying cause, i.e. it is the common end-stage of various pathways in its development.

The tangles also relate in number and site to the damage of dementia. Normal old people usually only develop a few tangles in the hippocampus. It is still not absolutely clear where the tangles come from, but one likely possibility is that they are the remains of damaged parts of neurones, for they lie within the cells.

The existence of plaques and tangles implies that there is a reduction in the number and health of nerve cell connections throughout the areas that are damaged.

Neurotransmitter deficits

Further important evidence comes from the chemical study of the neurotransmitter substances which convey the signal that there has been an electrical change in one neurone to another (Fig. 1.4). In the brain there are a number of these transmitter substances and each cell usually transmits one specific transmitter chemical. The transmitter causes an electrical change in a second neurone, making it either more or less likely to

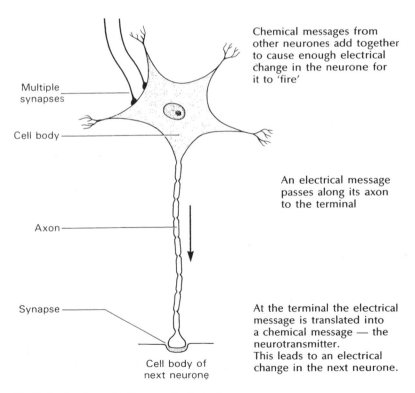

Multiple synapses

Cell body

Axon

Synapse

Cell body of next neurone

Chemical messages from other neurones add together to cause enough electrical change in the neurone for it to 'fire'

An electrical message passes along its axon to the terminal

At the terminal the electrical message is translated into a chemical message — the neurotransmitter. This leads to an electrical change in the next neurone.

Fig. 1.4   A schematic diagram of a typical neurone.

release *its* chemical transmitter. The entire functioning of the brain depends on millions upon millions of these messages between neurones.

Acetylcholine. The enzymes which are involved in the creation of transmitters and their breakdown show whether a particular sort of nerve cell is working or not. It was shown about 20 years ago that the enzymes related to the neruotransmitter acetylcholine (ACh) were greatly reduced in the brains of DAT sufferers, particularly in the most affected areas such as the hippocampus. It was already known that drugs which interfere with acetylcholine can cause delirium as a side-effect or in overdose ('anticholinergic' substances include many antidepressants and some antiparkinsonian drugs). There has also been evidence that substances which stimulate or simulate the action of acetylcholine in the brain ('cholinergic' substances) may actually improve memory temporarily in non-demented people. There is even an old wives' tale that fish, which is rich in choline, the precursor of acetylcholine, is 'brain food'. It began to look as if DAT was a specific disorder of acetylcholine-producing nerve cells and their connections. We could guess that if the acetylcholine nerve cells die or degenerate they would fail to pass electrical and chemical messages, so interfering with the general functioning of the cerebrum.

Multiple deficits. This simple theory of DAT as a failure of acetylcholine nerve cells soon had to be modified because of further research. This showed that other transmitters as well as acetylcholine are affected in DAT, though not all of them and not to the same extent. The transmitters noradrenaline (NA) and 5-hydroxytryptamine (5-HT) show decline in a similar sort of way to acetylcholine, though to a lesser degree, the transmitter gamma-aminobutyric acid (GABA) also declines somewhat, and the substance somatostatin, which is probably a transmitter, is reduced. So there must be damage to the nerve cells which transmit these chemicals too.

Subcortical nuclei. The next step is to try to find the origin of the damage to these groups of cerebral nerve cells. The axons which end in synapses in the cerebral cortex come from nerve cell bodies within the cortex making short connections, from cell bodies far away in the cortex making long connections, or from lower centres of the brain. To trace back the source of damage in DAT we need to look for the cell bodies of ACh-, NA- and 5-HT-

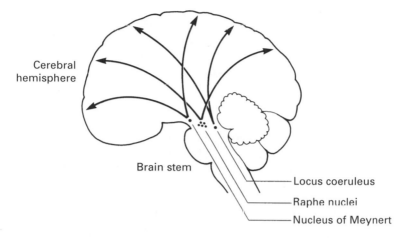

Fig. 1.5   Cell bodies in subcortical nuclei have long axons which end at synapses in widespread areas of the cerebral cortex, the areas which are affected in DAT.

releasing neurones. In fact, many of the cell bodies of ACh-producing neurones lie not in the cortex but deep in the middle of the cerebral hemispheres, in a small nucleus of cell bodies called the nucleus basalis of Meynert. Here there is obvious death of neurones in DAT cases. The same goes for other nuclei in the centre of the brain for two other affected transmitters – the locus coeruleus for NA, and the raphe nuclei for 5-HT. (Fig. 1.5).

Possible causes of DAT

So DAT, which originally was seen merely as a shrinkage of the brain, is now seen as a disorder of a few particular types of neurone and especially of those that produce acetylcholine. It could be a disorder of particular cell bodies in subcortical nuclei, resulting in a failure of transmission at the ends of their axons and at synapses widespread throughout the cortex, resulting in the pathological changes in the cortex and the consequent decline in cerebral function. Or it could be that the basic damage is to the nerve endings where the plaques are (this seems more likely at present). Whatever the site, we now need to look for what is causing the damage to these particular types of neurone. A number of possibilities have been considered.

Is DAT inherited?

This is a question being increasingly asked by families of those with DAT. Though answering this question would not at first sight appear to be too difficult, there are many problems in working out genetic factors. First, it is difficult to diagnose DAT with certainty. There are many overlapping features with the other causes of dementia, and indeed with normality. Secondly, dementia occurs in the later part of life, so many potential sufferers die of quite unconnected illnesses before they could develop dementia; it is impossible to know whether it would have developed if they had survived.

There is nevertheless strong evidence that there is a genetic contribution to the development of DAT. As long ago as 1963 it was suggested that the presence of DAT in a first degree relative (parent, brother, sister or child) increased someone's risk of developing DAT by a factor of four. Most recent research has suggested a two-fold increase. Twin studies have also pointed to an increased risk in an identical twin of a sufferer, though the fact that this risk is not 100% implies that factors other than genetic contribution are involved.

In some rare families there is a clear pattern of inheritance, and dementia may even be passed on as a dominant condition (as in Huntington's chorea – see p. 38). In most of these DAT families dementia is of early onset; the age of onset tends to 'run true' in these families, i.e. tends to be the same in successive generations.

One stimulus to look more closely at genetic factors came from the surprising finding that sufferers from Down's syndrome, if they survived to middle age, invariably developed the typical pathological changes of DAT, and similar neurotransmitter changes.

Down's syndrome has long been recognized as being due to an abnormality of chromosome 21. The gene for beta amyloid protein, involved in amyloid deposition in the brains of Alzheimer sufferers, has also been found to be on chromosome 21. Could an abnormal gene on chromosome 21 be implicated in DAT? In fact, although an abnormal gene has been found in some families with early onset DAT, this has turned out to be a rare occurrence. Since then various other abnormalities have been found in the uncommon familial varieties of DAT, including abnormalities of chromosome 1, chromosome 14 and chromosome 19.

Thus, there is not only one pathway in the development of Alzheimer's disease. Much further work is required to assess the way in which these various gene abnormalities eventually lead to the pathological changes of DAT. Is there a common pathway at all, or is what we term DAT a collection of illnesses with a similar end result?

Apolipoprotein E (ApoE)

ApoE is a protein which is involved in the transport and metabolism of fats in the body. It is also found in the membranes of neurones. It occurs in three major forms – ApoE2, ApoE3, and ApoE4 – these being the products of three variants of a gene on chromosome 19. Each person has two of these forms present, one inherited from each parent; 60% of the population have E3/3, 23% have E3/4 and 12% E3/2. These are the commonest combinations.

There is some evidence that ApoE4 is associated with an increased risk of DAT, and that those who have two ApoE4s have a very high incidence of DAT. ApoE4 is also associated with other diseases such as heart disease and with vascular dementia, Creutzfeldt-Jakob disease and motor neurone disease. It would also appear that the presence of ApoE2 has a protective effect, reducing the risk.

There is no case at present for screening for ApoE status. If more accurate identification of people at risk of DAT were to be carried out, there would be major ethical problems. Unlike other genetic conditions where screening is possible, those who will subsequently develop DAT have a long period of 'normal life' before the illness starts. In the absence of effective treatments, there is nothing to be gained by knowing whether or not one might develop dementia in the future, and indeed being tested might lead one into problems with depression and, on a more practical level, with getting life insurance. Testing those with suspected DAT, however, could increase the accuracy of diagnosis. Further research is continuing in this field.

Chemical damage

A variety of poisons is known to damage the nervous system. There has been speculation that aluminium might be involved in the genesis of DAT, and some years ago we were being advised to get rid of aluminium cooking utensils. Patients receiving renal dialysis were noted to be at high risk of developing dementia. When this was looked at, it was found to be due to the concentration of aluminum in water, the concentration being increased with the large quantities of water being used in dialysis (this has now changed with the use of specific dialysis fluids). In experimental work, rabbits fed with large amounts of aluminum were found to develop tangles, similar to, but not identical with, those found in patients with DAT. The third piece of suggestive evidence is that a high concentration of aluminium was thought to be present in the core of the senile plaques found in the brains of DAT sufferers.

These factors appeared to be strong evidence of aluminium involvement. However, on the other hand, there is no evidence of increased incidence of DAT in areas where there is a higher concentration of aluminium in the water – this would appear to undermine the theory of aluminium being a causal factor.

Other chemical substances might well be involved in the development of Alzheimer's. Older neurones build up potentially toxic chemicals, which might be damaging to the nerve cells. Lead had been implicated and there has been some publicity about lead levels in the brains of children living near motorways. However, no definite association with cognitive impairment has been found. The concentration of *free radicals* (ionized atoms in the brain) has been shown to increase with age, and this has also been implicated in the development of DAT.

Nerve growth factors

A further possibility to explain why nerve cells degenerate is that they lack factors which help them grow again when they are damaged, or which keep them healthy. These are called nerve growth factors and research is going on to see whether they are important in the damage to ACh neurones in DAT, or whether they might even be used as treatments (p. 189).

Infection

A cell may also be damaged by the invasion of infection which may interfere with function. There are a group of diseases now recognized as being caused by small particles called prions; these appear to enter a cell and in some way cause it to produce more prions. The most widely known of these diseases is Creutzfeldt-Jakob disease (CJD) (p. 40). There has been speculation that DAT may be caused by an infectious agent, but nothing has (so far) been identified, and the idea of DAT being infectious appears unlikely.

Recent research has suggested that exposure to relatively common bacteria or viruses in earlier life may increase the risk of developing DAT. The numbers involved in this research are too small to draw any definite conclusion, but it may be a pointer to further investigations.

Head injury (see p. 37)

Conclusion

DAT appears to be due to damage to particular types of nerve cells in the brain. It is likely that several different disease processes produce the same end result – the death of cells. Whatever the cause, we can see that DAT is commoner in older people, is associated with Down's syndrome and can be strongly hereditary in some rare cases.

Protective effects

ApoE2 has already been described as a probable protective genetic factor for DAT. There is some research which has shown that a higher education level has a protective effect on the development of DAT. People who have reached a higher education level appear to have a later age of onset if they do develop it. The reasons for this are not clear; it may be because of what is called 'cerebral reserve' (p. 7) – greater thinking capacities may protect functioning. There is also (less strong) evidence that changing career later in life may be protective. Women who have taken hormone replacement therapy (HRT) have been shown to have a later age of onset of DAT. This finding might be artificial. Women on HRT tend to be (on average) of higher social class and to have a greater awareness of health issues than other women. Factors other than HRT may therefore be the reason for this later onset; these include better diet and more exercise. But HRT may protect neurones from damage.

One often-quoted study showed that smokers seemed less likely to develop DAT. The theory here is attractive. Nicotine is a neurotransmitter acting at the acetylcholine receptor site, and it could be that any protective effect is mediated in this way. Other studies, however, have not confirmed the reduced incidence of DAT. Any effect may have been an effect of 'selective mortality' in the positive study; smokers tend to die earlier, so many do not reach the age at which DAT would exhibit itself. In any case, though there may be some effect on the incidence of DAT, smokers are likely to have a higher risk of developing vascular dementia.

Treatment of DAT

Research into the causes of DAT has expanded very rapidly in the past few years. There are three reasons; first, the rapid increase in the number of dementing people because of population changes; second, the growing feeling that dementia should be looked on as an illness, not just old age; third, the chemical findings which have led researchers to believe that an effective treatment might now be found (see Chapter 6).

This is an exciting time to be working with dementia. Research is progressing in many different directions, and already there is some, albeit limited, evidence of benefit to some sufferers. The development of treatment to date has made only small strides forward. Even though we still await any progress in finding a treatment which prevents the brain damage in DAT, the research and development of these drugs is helping to raise the profile of dementia with doctors and with politicians, and helps to remove the 'nothing can de done' pessimism which has so often delayed access to other supports.

'Young-old' and 'old-old' DAT

Before leaving the subject of DAT it is worth noting a further direction in which research is heading. Although the distinction between senile and presenile DAT now seems pointless, a dividing line at a greater age is emerging (Table 1.8). This later division was first suggested by the term 'benign senescence', used to describe 'old-old' people who, in their 80s and 90s, begin to develop a less profound memory disorder than younger DAT sufferers, with less widespread effects on general brain function,

Table 1.8 A comparison of 'young-old' and 'old-old' DAT

	Younger patients (onset below 75 years)	Older patients (onset above 75 years)
Life expectancy	Shortened	Less shortened or normal
Damage to cerebral cortex cells	More widespread More severe	More localized Less severe
Neurotransmitter losses	More transmitters affected More widespread	Mainly acetylcholine loss More like normal old age changes
Genetics	Some families with clear dominant inheritance and chromosome 21 abnormality	Less clear genetic link found (ApoE)

and who surprisingly have a more normal lifespan than younger patients. It was next suggested that those younger patients, with an age of onset mostly in their 60s, tended to suffer more damage to their parietal lobes (see Fig. 1.2). This suggestion has been at least partly confirmed by CT scanning and the pathological changes. The neurotransmitter evidence adds further support – in older DAT patients, with dementia starting in the 80s and 90s, the transmitter loss is less widespread over the brain and is more confined to the acetylcholine neurones. In fact, this old-age DAT bears a much closer resemblance to changes in the brains of normal older people of the same age, who usually have some degree of acetylcholine loss, than does the multiple transmitter loss in younger patients. So it may be that we should divide DAT into two varieties: a more malignant, early onset 'young-old' dementia and a more benign, 'old-old' dementia. The implications of this for health and social services are enormous. Not only is dementia a commoner problem among the expanding numbers of very old people, but it may be that these older patients, who are mainly women, have a more normal lifespan than younger patients.

Down's syndrome and DAT

Most Down's syndrome patients who reach the age of 35 have developed pathological changes similar to those in

DAT sufferers. Some of these patients will develop DAT, however, in spite of the presence of pathology, many do *not* develop the condition itself, perhaps because of ApoE status.

The issues regarding care and management of these people who have both learning difficulties and dementia are very different from those of older people with dementia; changes in mental function are of course related to previous functioning as well as to the effects of DAT. In general, it is probably best that they continue to be looked after by the carers who have been involved with them all of their lives, with advice if necessary from the specialist dementia services.

VASCULAR DEMENTIA (VAD)

DAT is generally thought to be the cause of dementia in 50–60% of sufferers. The next most common cause is vascular dementia, accounting for 20–30%. Many of the remainder suffer from a mixed dementia. VaD is primarily due to disease of the arteries. These patients usually show evidence of vascular disease elsewhere in the body, such as heart disease, poor circulation to the legs, or high blood pressure. VaD is the current preferred term for 'arteriosclerotic' dementia. There are several different types of vascular dementia. In the commonest type pathologists have shown that the brain has developed multiple small areas of damage. Under the microscope these areas contain nerve cells which are seen to be dead or degenerating. The local blood supply has been impaired. Sometimes there is blockage of a blood vessel; this may be due to blood clots originating in the damaged walls of the bigger arteries in the head and neck, or indeed in the heart itself. These clots are called emboli. Sometimes the blockage develops locally by thrombosis and sometimes by bleeding from arteriosclerotic vessels in the brain itself.

The area of dead brain tissue caused by such a blockage is called an infarct – hence the term 'multi-infarct dementia' (MID). However, the demonstration of infarcts in itself is not necessary for a diagnosis of VaD. Damage to the brain cells in vascular dementia is also due to disruption to various neurotransmitters, most notably a transmitter known as NDMA. It is not fully clear how this occurs, but identification of these pathways may be helpful in developing treatment of VaD.

The course of VaD

Understanding the pathology of VaD helps us to understand how a patient with this condition deteriorates. Some idea of the clinical features can be seen on the Hachinski score (Table 1.9) developed to help distinguish MID from other types of dementia (though this scale is sometimes inappropriately used to *diagnose* VaD). The score is criticized for giving too much emphasis to stroke, i.e. a patient who has had a stroke will score as having multi-infarct disease, even if any dementia the patient is suffering is due to other causes.

The law of mass action usually applies

In general terms the total volume of cerebral damage, i.e. the total area of cerebral infarction, is proportional to the degree of intellectual impairment. It has been said that at least 100 cubic centimetres of the brain must be damaged before dementia will develop, though this now appears in some doubt.

Irregular course

The fact that cerebral damage occurs repeatedly over a number of years is reflected in the course of the dementia. Most of the

Table 1.9 Hachinski's score for the diagnosis of MID (adapted from Hachinski V C et al 1975 Archives of Neurology 32: 632)

Abrupt onset	2
Stepwise deterioration	1
Fluctuating course	2
Nocturnal confusion	1
Relative preservation of personality	1
Depression	1
Somatic complaints	1
Emotional lability	1
History of hypertension	1
History of stroke	2
Evidence of arteriosclerosis elsewhere	1
Focal neurological signs	2
Focal neurological symptoms	2
Total score possible	**18**

A score of more than 7 is said to favour the diagnosis of multi-infarct dementia changes are subtle, and merge into one another. The result is generally a steady decline as in DAT. From time to time, however, a more major incident may occur; there is a sudden decline, often followed by a period of improvement, not quite to the previous level of functioning. During an acute episode, just as with strokes in general, the suddenness of the change and the disruption and swelling (oedema) around the infarct can lead to a more generalized, though temporary, disruption of brain function (delirium or acute confusion, p. 56). The patient becomes noticeably more disorientated with 'clouding of consciousness'. This acute confusion may begin to clear quite quickly, as can happen with the physical after-effects of stroke such as a paralysis or speech problem. Sometimes the delirium after a stroke can persist for weeks before it clears. Only then can we begin to see how much permanent damage there is. A brief stroke episode, recovering within 24 hours and with no evidence of permanent damage, is called a *transient ischaemic attack* (TIA). This may be a warning of an impending stroke.

In contrast to these sudden changes, VaD patients may also go through *plateau* periods where their functional abilities remain fairly static, or may even improve, these periods lasting for weeks or even months.

Patchy damage

Though it is widespread, the damage in VaD is patchy throughout the brain. It may hit areas serving very specific functions, the result being that the patient may suffer temporarily or permanently an impairment of speech, paralysis of one side of the body, or partial blindness (hemianopia). Most damage, however, will occur in the association or connecting areas of the brain. The quite extensive areas of cortex not damaged by stroke can go on working relatively normally, though of course the connections between these and other areas may have been damaged. The result is that some general functions, such as personality, or insight, or the ability to respond emotionally, may not decline as much as, say, memory and speech; alternatively memory function may be quite good and other functions may be badly affected.

VaD may therefore be much more distressing to the patient than DAT, where the patient's ability to respond is usually blunted and insight lost along with the general decline. Those with VaD are more likely, as a result, to be distressed by the experience of dementia, or show aggression or agitation related to frustration, particularly where communication difficulties are a prominent feature.

Despite the patchiness and irregular progression of VaD, the overall course of the illness is downwards and the decline may be just as steady and generalized as in DAT. At any stage this course is likely to be complicated by disorders of the other arteries in the body, such as a heart attack, blood pressure-related problems or of course a more major stroke. The cause of death in VaD is therefore likely to be one of these events rather than the more gradual fading away of DAT.

Causes of VaD

The cause of generalized arteriosclerosis is not yet fully understood. It is not clear why a particular tiny vessel should block at a particular time and cause an area of brain to infarct and the cells around it to die.

There is an association between smoking and diet in all types of vascular disease. It is likely that lipid abnormalities such as elevated cholesterol have a part to play. Genetic factors are also involved in these causes, but more specifically a number of rare familial vascular dementias have been identified, in particular CADASIL (cerebral autosomal dominant arteriopathy with subcortical infarcts and leukoencephalopathy). The gene responsible for this disorder has been located on chromosome 19. CADASIL tends to affect middle-aged adults with none of the usual known vascular risk factors. They have recurrent transient ischaemic attacks and strokes, and eventually develop dementia.

Drugs for VaD

There have been many attempts to use drugs to improve cerebral circulation. Such drugs (e.g. Co-dergocrine mesylate) are unlikely to help in VaD, other than possibly during the immediate aftermath of a stroke, where a local thrombosis or bleed has caused an infarct. Here the blood supply to the rest of the brain appears to continue to function well or, if reduced, recovers quickly. In the area of the infarct, some of the damage is permanent, the cells are dead and cannot be revived. Although it has long been thought that the damage to the neurones is due to loss of the blood supply leading to hypoxia, it is likely that some damage is due to neurotoxins or to loss of neurotransmitters; research is proceeding along these lines. It may be possible to develop drugs which are 'neuroprotective' to prevent or lessen the damage to cells after a stroke.

In practice it is surprisingly difficult to show whether or not drugs are effective, since fluctuation and variability in VaD make assessment of the results a complicated matter. As yet, however, there has been no definite proof that any particular drug delays the process of dementia.

Aspirin and other drugs have been used to reduce the risk of other cardiovascular events such as myocardial infarction, stroke and transient ischaemic attacks by lessening the chance of clots developing. There is some evidence of effectiveness in VaD. This more hopeful approach may lead to development of preventative drugs.

There is an association between the presence of high blood pressure and VaD; gentle control of blood pressure with drugs such as thiazide diuretics may well slow the progress of the dementia.

We often see lists of potentially treatable causes of dementia. It is surprising that VaD is not usually included in this, as potentially there are many different ways of reducing the risk of developing it, or of slowing the progress of this common form of dementia.

VaD and DAT

Despite the differences in pathological changes and the supposed difference in their courses, it is very often quite difficult to tell a case of vascular dementia from one of Alzheimer-type dementia. Indeed, surveys suggests that even with the most sophisticated tests and scans doctors often mistake one for the other. Furthermore, pathological studies seem to show that there are many mixed cases with both diagnoses. It is almost impossible to be sure in what proportion the two conditions occur, since it is very difficult to find a representative sample of people who die of dementia and have a postmortem examination. One estimate suggests that there are about 60 DAT cases to 20 VaD cases to 20 mixed.

It is curious that there should be so many mixed cases. Perhaps some are actually pure cases of DAT where amyloid has damaged the blood vessels and led to strokes, or perhaps mild changes of the two conditions can add together in some way to increase the likelihood of obvious dementia occurring – the so-called *threshold effect*.

For practical purposes we are at present only able to distinguish very definite, classical VaD cases from very definite DAT cases, with considerable vagueness in between. At present the main value in making the distinction is to tell patients or relatives either that in VaD the decline is likely to be erratic, with strokes and other evidence of arteriosclerosis, or that in DAT it is likely to be more gradual.

It is more important to make an accurate distinction for the purposes of research, where is it essential to study as pure as possible a sample of DAT and VaD patients. As treatments become available to alter the course of dementia it is becoming increasingly vital to be able to make a proper diagnosis, for we would not want to give drugs with possible side-effects to the wrong patient. The Hachinski score (Table 1.9) is one not very successful attempt to make the distinction. As scanning techniques and genetic testing get better we will be able to improve on this.

Other vascular dementias

There are many different types of vascular illness that can lead to all sorts of variations in the course and pattern of dementia. Included in this list are MID, single strokes affecting crucial subcortical areas of the brain, amyloid angiopathy in DAT, Binswanger's disease and lacunar dementia (see p. 42). Scanning techniques are improving constantly, allowing better understanding of these conditions and letting us assess their importance.

OTHER CAUSES OF DEMENTIA
Dementia of Lewy body type (DLBT)

Lewy bodies are tiny spots found within the damaged nerve cells in the substantia nigra (a small nucleus of cells at the top of the brain stem) of patients suffering from Parkinson's disease. In the last few years Lewy bodies have also been identified in the cortex of patients with a specific pattern of dementia. This form of dementia is now referred to as dementia of Lewy body type (DLBT). Typically, patients experience bizarre visual hallucinations, for example of silent visitors in their house who can suddenly appear and disappear. The mental impairment tends to fluctuate (often dramatically) and extrapyramidal symptoms (p. 192), such as muscular rigidity and slowness of movement, are common. Of particular importance is the fact that these patients may react badly to even small doses of common antipsychotic drugs, and indeed there is even a danger of death as a result of their use. The frequent occurrence of hallucinations could tempt doctors to use these drugs more. With the death of cells in the basal ganglia there is a reduction in the neurotransmitter dopamine, and this causes the extrapyramidal symptoms. However, the cognitive impairment is thought to be due to a reduction in acetylcholine (as in DAT) and there is evidence in affected patients of cell death in the nucleus of Meynert.

In DLBT the deterioration often affects visio-spatial skills more than memory skills, particularly in the early stages of the condition. In general, patients with DLBT tend to deteriorate more rapidly than these with DAT. There is still dispute as to the exact nature of DLBT. Some authorities feel that it is a variant of DAT, others that it is a separate illness. It certainly appears to have a different course from that of DAT.

The features of DLBT can be seen in Box 1.2. There may be a spectrum of disease with DAT at one end, Parkinson's disease at the other and DLBT somewhere in the middle.

Box 1.2 Features of Lewy body dementia

- Visual or auditory hallucinations (or both), usually with secondary paranoid ideas.
- Mild spontaneous extrapyramidal features (i.e. features of Parkinson's disease) or undue sensitivity to neuroleptic drugs.
- Repeated unexplained falls or transient changes in the level of consciousness.
- Despite a fluctuating pattern the features persist over weeks or months, unlike delirium which rarely persists as long.
- Underlying physical illness must be excluded as a cause of fluctuating cognitive state, as must evidence of cerebrovascular damage.

Parkinson's disease

We have discussed Lewy body dementia and its connections with Parkinson's disease above. However, patients with Parkinson's disease (PD) itself are known to be at higher risk of dementia, and perhaps 20% of sufferers are so affected. The symptoms of Parkinson's disease are due to a reduction in the neurotransmitter dopamine, and this is what causes the typical symptoms. The dementia which PD patients develop, however, is thought to be due to a reduction in acetylcholine, and there is evidence in affected patients of cell death in the nucleus of Meynert. So the dementia of PD is quite like that of DAT, though it is probably not identical.

Transmitter defects as we have seen are also found in DAT, in Huntington's chorea (see below) and in dementia of other types.

Frontal lobe dementia (FLD)

DAT affects various parts of the brain. Memory impairment is mostly due to involvement of the temporal lobe. Less commonly, dementia can be due to prominent frontal lobe damage. It is often unclear whether this is a variant of DAT or a separate form of dementia. FLD has been said to be a cause of 10% of cases of dementia. The effects of specific frontal lobe damage have been recognized since 1868 when a railway worker (Phineas Gage) blew a tamping iron bar through the frontal lobe of his brain. Surprisingly, he survived, and his doctors were able to observe the changes in him. Most notably he became disinhibited, with frequent outbursts of swearing and rage. He was described as 'not Gage'. His personality had totally changed.

In those with FLD the main effect is a progressive decline in self control and deterioration in personality without marked memory or intellectual loss. The ability to plan and make judgements, the so-called higher executive function, is located in the frontal lobe, so these skills may also be affected. Sexual and social disinhibition can be particularly distressing to relatives and to other carers. Since sufferers usually have no insight, they may do uncharacteristically unwise or even immoral things without any apparent concern (see Chapter 5). Pick's disease is one form of FLD in which typical inclusion bodies are found in the damaged neurones of the frontal lobe. However, these bodies are only found in a small percentage of those with FLD, and it is unclear what (if any) significance they have.

Unlike DAT, FLD tends to develop in people in late middle age, and there appears to be a greater genetic component than in DAT.

Other causes

There are many other potential causes of a gradual decline and they are all much less common (see Table 1.5). No more than 5% of older people with dementia suffer from these rarer diseases, though they may be relatively more common in younger patients. It has been suggested that the dementia of as many as 15% of patients under the age of 70 has a remediable cause. Diagnostic investigation is therefore more important in younger patients, and in some cases leads to effective treatment.

Physical damage

Normal pressure hydrocephalus

Though this is an uncommon condition, it is relatively more common amongst younger dementia sufferers. The flow of cerebrospinal fluid inside the brain is partially or intermittently blocked. This may occur spontaneously, or may occur after brain injury, meningitis or neurosurgery. These events may have occurred some time before, even many decades. As a result of this blockage, the ventricles of the brain expand. The brain substance enclosed within the rigid skull is thus damaged and gradually shrinks. There is a classic *triad* of symptoms – dementia, lack of coordination in walking and incontinence.

It is always important to keep this condition in mind, especially if walking problems or incontinence occur very early in the course of dementia. Referral to a neurologist allows cerebrospinal fluid pressure studies to be carried out. If the diagnosis is confirmed, a special tube or *shunt* can be inserted to remove the excess fluid, as in the treatment of congenital hydrocephalus seen in babies. Sadly, surgery rarely causes much improvement in the dementia. However, further deterioration can be prevented and the physical symptoms may improve, if the condition is diagnosed at an early enough stage.

Repeated head injury

If a person suffers repeated injuries to the brain, the law of mass action eventually operates and generalized impairment of the brain's function can occur, often together with other neurological abnormalities such as parkinsonism. This is well recognized amongst boxers, the *punch drunk syndrome* or *dementia pugilistica*, to give it its technical term. Impairment may only develop some time after the boxer retires, suggesting that other factors such as ageing may add to the damage to make the patient *cross the threshold* for dementia. There has been a suggestion that footballers may also be at increased risk of dementia, possibly from repeated heading of the heavy, often water soaked, leather balls used in the past.

There is some evidence that a history of head injury may increase the risk of DAT, though the connection is not yet proven. It could be at least partly the result of selective memory. Relatives may have discussed at length among themselves why someone has developed dementia, and previous head injuries come back to their memories. But it may be that head injuries stimulate the production of harmful beta amyloid.

Slow-growing tumours of the brain

Secondary tumours arising from a primary cancer elsewhere in the body, or a primary tumour of the coverings of the brain (a meningioma), which may grow very slowly, can lead to gradual mental impairment as they gradually take up more space within the skull. These are, therefore, potentially treatable causes of the dementia syndrome. It is important that we keep this cause in mind in all patients, particularly where there are unusual or 'localizing' features.

Toxic damage

One of the most potent insidious poisons which can cause brain damage is lead, and there has been much public debate on the effect lead in petrol might have on children. We have already discussed aluminum toxicity in dialysis patients (p. 23). Certain poisons can also reach toxic levels in the brain because of a failure to excrete them from the body. For example, copper levels are not controlled in the bodies of patients suffering from Wilson's disease, and they may therefore develop dementia at a young age. Wilson's disease is a genetic condition whose effects on the brain can be avoided with treatment with the drug Penicillamine.

Alcoholism

Chronic alcoholics often develop a specific recent memory loss called *Korsakoff's syndrome* (p. 69). This is progressive if the patient continues to drink. If he or she stops drinking, the damage becomes static or, as after a head injury or stroke, some recovery of function may be possible over months or even years. Since it does not affect the overall function of the cerebrum, Korsakoff's syndrome is not strictly speaking a dementia. Like DAT, Korsakoff's syndrome is now thought to be due to damage to acetylcholine systems, but in a much smaller area at the base of the brain.

In addition to this syndrome, however, there is now evidence that some alcohol abusers develop a more generalized shrinking of the brain which shows up on CT scanning. It is likely that this shrinkage is a sign of a developing general dementia ('alcoholic dementia'), but it is also possible that this dementia is reversible if the sufferer stops drinking.

Genetic disorders

Many forms of dementia are likely to have at least some hereditary component. In DAT and VaD, family history certainly has some part to play in the development of the illness, and some variants are hereditary. There is a strong genetic component in FLD. Genetic factors are also important in Wilson's disease, in Creutzfeldt-Jakob disease and in Gerstmann-Straussler syndrome (p. 40).

Huntington's chorea

This form of dementia is perhaps the most devastating form for families because of its mode of inheritance, its age of onset, and its clinical features. It usually develops earlier in life, often in the 30s and 40s. In some families it may start even earlier, as early as the teens, and in some other families in the 70s or even later. The dementia is combined with, and often preceded by, the development of jerking, dancing, uncontrollable movements of the limbs and body, called *chorea*, the Greek word for dance. The disease tends to progress slowly, and lasts many years. Disorders of personality or psychiatric disorders such as depression or paranoia often precede the development of the illness. Sufferers of Huntington's chorea usually retain insight until very late in the progress; this is not only very distressing for themselves, but also for family carers. Patients and their families will have seen other family members going through the same thing.

As well as the widespread cortical and subcortical damage of dementia, there is also local damage to a group of nerve cells deep in the centre of the brain, called the *caudate nucleus*. It is this damage which leads to the typical involuntary movements. As in DAT and in PD there is a defect of neurotransmitter systems. In Huntington's chorea the transmitter involved is gamma-aminobutyric acid (GABA).

Inheritance in Huntington's chorea is by a dominant gene which always results in illness if it is present, i.e. it is 'fully expressed'. There is no difference in risk between the sexes. If either parent suffers from the condition, each child has 50% risk of developing it. As it may well develop later in life, a potential sufferer may have had children before the disease exhibits itself.

The abnormal gene has now been identified on the short arm of chromosome 4. On the normal chromosome there are a number of repeat sequences of certain amino acids of the DNA, usually 9–30 in number. In Huntington's chorea there are usually over 40. The number of extra repeats is related to the age of onset; the more repeats, the earlier the onset is.

The recognition of the abnormal gene now allows the possibility of pre-illness and indeed prenatal diagnosis. The fact that the disease develops later in life however, with a normal and productive life prior to this, makes for major ethical issues around testing, both for the individual and for society. Similar difficulties will become apparent if screening ever becomes available for the other forms of dementia. This will be discussed later (p. 207).

Infections

General paralysis of the insane (GPI)

Historically, this is the most important type of dementia, being the end-stage of the 'scourge of Europe', syphilis, an untreatable condition until early this century. It usually starts 5–15 years after the initial infection if that was untreated. As well as the dementia, patients show other neurological signs. Despite treatment now being available for syphilis, occasional cases still occur and it is worth looking out for since, even at the late stage at which it occurs, GPI is treatable if an antibiotic is given before the brain damage has become too severe.

AIDS dementia complex

The HIV virus which causes AIDS is known to enter the brain, and in some sufferers can cause a dementia. This dementia may advance rapidly so that the sufferer dies in about a year, or more slowly, like DAT. Drugs such as Zidovudine, which can affect the HIV virus, have been shown to slow the progress of the dementia, so it is at least potentially treatable. However, it is sometimes difficult to distinguish this HIV-caused dementia from the many possible infections in the brain which can occur in full-blown AIDS, and which can cause severe confusion and need other treatments.

It is important to put the phenomenon of AIDS dementia in perspective. This is a relatively new illness and a very devastating one, since it is commonest in youngish people who do not expect to suffer debilitating illnesses, far less to die of dementia. Early reports of a high rate of AIDS-related dementia suggested that there would be a rapidly increasing number of patients with this condition.

However, the studies concerned were carried out in special centres, and it is now apparent that the number of cases who develop full AIDS dementia without full-blown AIDS is small. Dementia is usually, though not invariably, an end-stage phenomenon, so care for the person is not likely to concentrate on any thinking problems but rather will deal with the devastating physical problems often associated with AIDS.

Creutzfeldt-Jakob disease (CJD) and associated disorder

The similarities between bovine spongiform-encephalopathy (BSE) in cows and CJD has led to a great deal of speculation that the disease may have been transmitted through consuming brain, spinal cord or other products from affected animals. A similar condition (scrapie) in sheep is believed to have been transmitted to cows through feeding them material from dead sheep. A new variant of the disease in humans (nvCJD) has developed in the past 10 years, and affects younger people. It now seems likely that nvCJD in people is caused by transmission from BSE-affected cows. This has lead to a greatly increased profile of CJD. However, it remains a very rare disease, affecting perhaps one person in two million. Males for some reason tend to be more often affected than females, and rare familial cases have been described.

CJD tends to be a rapidly progressive disorder and most patients die within 6 months of diagnosis. Muscle wasting, convulsions, myoclonic jerks (jerky movements of muscles often in response to touch), delusions and hallucinations are common features of the illness. Diagnosis is usually suggested by the typical clinical picture combined with a typical abnormal electroencephalogram (EEG) showing a pattern of slow sharp wave discharges.

The illness appears to be caused by small particles of protein called *prions*. Prions appear, unlike viruses, to be non-living particles, unable to replicate themselves. However, they increase in number by inducing cells into which they enter to produce further prions, by interfering with the cell's own genetic material. As well as the link with BSE, there have been well-documented cases of spread via growth hormone prepared from people who have died, via corneal grafts, and via surgical instruments. The prions are resistant to conventional forms of sterilization.

Other prion-related conditions have been described including Gerstmann-Straussler syndrome, a disease not dissimilar to CJD. Another similar dementia (kuru) has long been recognized amongst a tribal group in New Guinea. Here, transmission was found to be due to ritual cannibalism, eating the brains of affected sufferers.

Vitamin deficiencies

Deficiencies of various vitamins such as niacin, B_{12} and folic acid have all been reported as causes of dementia. Shortage of thiamine (vitamin B_1) is implicated in the development of Korsakoff's syndrome (p. 69). However, with the exception of thiamine, replacement of these vitamins has generally been disappointing in terms of improving cognitive function.

Endocrine disorder

Disturbance of the thyroid and parathyroid hormones can lead to dementia. Thyroid deficiency, or hypothyroidism, is common in older people (especially women); hormone replacement does not usually influence the dementia. Of course there will be many people who, by chance, have hypothyroidism and a common form of dementia such as DAT.

Both over- and underactivity of the parathyroid gland, which in turn cause abnormalities of calcium metabolism, can lead to dementia. Overactivity can be due to a benign parathyroid tumour (adenoma) and there have been a few reports of dementia improving, or in some cases deterioration being arrested, following removal of an adenoma. This is, however, a rare cause of dementia.

White matter damage

Multiple sclerosis

This, and indeed any condition which involves widespread patchy damage to the brain, can eventually lead by 'mass action' to a general decline. The dementia of multiple sclerosis is usually fairly mild, and is sometimes first noticed when the patient seems surprisingly unconcerned in the face of his or her progressing disabilities. The damage in multiple sclerosis is caused by 'plaques' (quite different in size and nature from the senile plaques of DAT) which develop in the white matter of the brain; the grey matter is not directly affected.

Binswanger's disease

This is one of the many variants of vascular dementia. It was first described many years ago, but was rediscovered recently when CT scanning showed that in some cases of vascular dementia it was the white matter which was affected, rather than the grey matter of the cerebral cortex. Like other forms of VaD, it is connected with arteriosclerosis and high blood pressure.

Another vascular dementia, which leads to holes or lacunae appearing in subcortical areas has also been recognized and has been named *lacunar dementia*.

Subcortical dementia

In recent years it has become fashionable to lump together a number of different types of dementia in which the white matter, or nuclei such as the caudate nucleus, substantia nigra or other subcortical nuclei, is the main seat of damage. These dementias have been called *subcortical*. They include the dementias of Parkinson's disease, Huntington's chorea, an illness called progressive supranuclear palsy and various vascular conditions including Binswanger's disease and lacunar dementia.

It has been suggested that in these forms of dementia there are particular clinical features which are different from those of the mainly *'cortical'* dementias such as DAT. These features include mental slowness and difficulty with retrieval of memories, despite the sufferer being able to store memories reasonably normally (see p. 124), while in DAT there are more prominent symptoms of cerebral damage, such as language difficulties and parietal lobe signs, as well as a general impairment of memory (see p. 18). However, just as it is often difficult to tell VaD from DAT, so it has proved difficult to tell subcortical dementia from cortical dementia in individual patients.

CONCLUSION

There are many causes of dementia and the list here is far from exhaustive. As yet there are no specific treatments in most cases, and indeed there are no definitive diagnostic features to differentiate the common causes one from another. Postmortem examination is the only positive test. Nevertheless, it is important, particularly in younger patients, to investigate the cause of dementia fully and to look for remediable conditions, and in older patients to keep in mind the rare possibility that something more curative can be achieved. Two illnesses, DAT and VaD, remain the chief causes of the decline and disability of dementia.

2

What is not dementia?

Dementia is cerebral failure – a decline from normal
  Dementia and the normal changes of ageing
    Differentiating from dementia
Dementia is progressive
  Dementia and brain damage
  Treatable or reversible dementia
  Age-associated memory impairment
  Dementia and mental handicap
  Dementia and delirium (acute confusional state)
    Delirium during dementia
    Differentiating from dementia
    Management of delirium

Dementia affects most aspects of mental function
  Dementia and Korsakoff's syndrome
Pseudodementia
  Depressive illness
    Differentiating from dementia
  Other psychiatric disorders
  Mania
  Late paraphrenia
  Personality disorder
  Alcohol and drug dependence
  Pseudodementia in physical illness

Having defined what dementia is, the next step is to define what it is not. In other words, what other illnesses or states of mind can be mistaken for dementia? From our original definition (p. 1) we can see that:

- Any condition in which there is not a significant decline from normal cannot be dementia
- Any condition which is not gradually progressive cannot be dementia
- A decline affecting only one mental function cannot be dementia.

This may seem like stating the obvious, but, as this chapter will show, looking at each of these statements in turn can help to clarify dementia and its boundaries. There are three good reasons for examining these boundaries closely.

Careless diagnosis

In the first place, there has been a tendency to be careless with the word dementia and this carelessness can have serious consequences. If it is *assumed* that an old person's failure to cope at home is due to dementia, without considering other possible causes, she may be wrongly placed in residential or hospital care when in fact she is suffering from a simple physical condition or a different psychiatric disorder which could have easily been treated in her own home, or treated better in a different setting.

Likewise, this carelessness tempts doctors, brought up to consider only a cure as success and seeing that dementia is largely incurable, to dismiss people with dementia from their attention, except as an increasing nuisance. Elderly patients in an acute medical ward who are labelled as 'demented' without adequate diagnosis or assessment of their problems may be put in the corner, as it were, to get a second-class sort of treatment. If dementia is the right diagnosis, then their special needs are likely to be overlooked. If it is the wrong diagnosis, then their actual illness will go undiagnosed and untreated.

There are lesser versions of this hasty labelling. We do it when, as visitors to a residential home or geriatric hospital, we see all the residents in the day room as the same and assume that they are all 'confused elderly'. There is an implication that everybody has the same problem and that problem is dementia. The undemented are treated as demented and all may be poorly treated.

Difficult diagnosis

A second reason for spending time on definition is that, with the best will in the world, being sure that a person actually suffers from dementia can be surprisingly difficult. This again has practical implications. We would like as early as possible in the illness to alert the patient and his or her relatives to the problems they will face in the future, and to teach them how best to cope with these problems. On the other hand, the diagnosis of dementia is an ominous one; if it is diagnosed wrongly, unnecessary distress can be caused.

Giving a diagnosis of dementia leads carers to have certain preconceptions, in particular that their relatives will show gradual deterioration to a state of dependency. The carers may grieve, then, for future losses. They may also become over-protective, leading to loss of independence and 'deskilling' of the sufferer, i.e. taking over daily living activities from the person may cause her to lose them.

At the earliest stages there is no test which will clearly distinguish the normal person from the dementing person. Indeed, many who appear to be developing dementia and perform rather badly on tests of memory or intelligence actually seem to improve on later testing, so it can be dangerous to make the diagnosis too early.

In the World Health Organization's diagnostic criteria for dementia (p. 2), a definite diagnosis is only made when the impairments have been present for *at least 6 months.* There is often pressure from carers and others to make an early diagnosis, but in possible early dementia we would do well to keep this 6 month rule in mind to avoid falling into the trap of misdiagnosis.

Research diagnosis

The third reason to attempt a clear, exclusive definition concerns research. If it were possible to draw clear boundaries between what is and what is not dementia, then we could study the dementing group as a whole, comparing it with the rest of the population or with groups of sufferers from other conditions. In this way we could find out much more about the specific causes and effects of dementia.

At present there are quite good diagnostic definitions of dementia, but they only work well when it is past the early stages. This makes research difficult. We are only able to compare groups of patients who are *definitely* dementing against groups who are not dementing. Other research will have to focus on the grey area between dementia and normality and on the grey areas between dementia and other conditions. Are the boundaries vague because suitable tests are not yet available in order to make clear distinctions; are they vague because there is actual overlap between the conditions, so that one merges into the other; or are they vague because there are other, intermediate conditions which complicate the picture?

We will touch on these points further as we now look again at the stages of our definition to examine the *differential diagnosis* of dementia – what it is not.

DEMENTIA IS CEREBRAL FAILURE – A DECLINE FROM NORMAL

DEMENTIA AND THE NORMAL CHANGES OF AGEING

Dementia is not 'just old age'. In the first chapter we have outlined some of the evidence that distinguishes the *pathology* of the illnesses of dementia from *normal* changes in the ageing brain. In practical terms, how can we make this distinction?

Let us first look at what normal psychological changes occur in old age; then we can compare these with the changes of dementia (Table 2.1). This is difficult, however, because one of the chief characteristics of older people as a group is the huge range of their mental and physical capacities. Different individuals seem to age at different rates, and different aspects of each particular person's bodily and mental functions seem to age at different rates. Furthermore, each individual and each function have begun the changes of old age from widely different 'normal' levels in earlier life. So it is quite difficult to decide what is normal and what is abnormal in the ageing mind. Even trying to follow change in one individual over the decades of old age is

Table 2.1   Psychological changes in normal old age and in dementia

	Normal ageing	Dementia
Degree of change	Slowing	More severe and increasing
	Cautiousness	Variable
	Reduced ability to solve new problems	More severe and increasing
	Disengagement?	Variable
	Mildly impaired memory?	More severe and increasing
	Mildly impaired intelligence?	More severe and increasing
Extent of damage	Difficulty in word finding, but no dysphasia, dyspraxia, agnosia	Dysphasia, dyspraxia, agnosia often found
Rate of change	Very slow change over many years	More rapid though gradual changes

difficult, for many factors complicate the interpretation of tests of intelligence, memory and other brain functions.

Slowing

Some changes are clear and almost universal. The most striking one is that both physical and mental activity slow down. Indeed, this change will be obvious to anybody who is over the age of 40, though it probably begins as early as our 20s. It becomes more and more obvious as we enter old age.

This slowing in reactions affects our ability to perform any test which requires speed, for example, many intelligence tests. It is a source of frustration to many older people, who miss the ability to be quick off the mark, and an annoyance to quicker younger people, who become impatient with their elders. One of the first lessons which anybody caring for an old person has to learn is that they must slow down to a speed that allows the older person to work with them. When older people complain that they are becoming 'confused', they are sometimes referring to this slowness in their interactions with younger people, and the resulting feeling of being rushed.

An exaggeration of the mental slowing of old age is a prominent feature of dementia (p. 133), and is said to be very obvious in the subcortical dementias. It is possible to measure reaction time to a variety of stimuli and show that this is greatly delayed in moderately or severely demented patients, but, as with other mental changes in dementia, it is extremely difficult to define the boundary between normal slowing and this *excessive* and *progressive* slowing.

Rigidity and disengagement

Another frequently noted change of old age is an increasing abhorrence of the new-fangled. Although it is true that some old people are as adventurous (or as fickle) as adolescents exploring their life, their emotions and their relationships for the first time, for many old age is a time of regularity, order and sameness. To some extent this may come about because both young people and old people expect it to be so. But there does seem to be a natural biological change towards rigidity. The ageing brain may not be as able to adjust to new patterns of experience; it may not be as flexible as in young people. The result is that older people tend to be more cautious when new things occur, tend to have difficulty learning new concepts and activities and tend to prefer a routine existence.

The older person may well feel quite comfortable doing very little for long periods. In the past this 'disengagement' from activity has had its advantages. The elder has been a stable focus for family life. Distance from the hurly-burly, coupled with a lifetime's experience, could allow elders to be wiser than their rash young relatives. With greater social mobility and an increase in the numbers of old people, this traditional role has been challenged. Older people are nowadays not so likely to be in a stable social position for the rest of their lives. They may need to make quite major and dramatic decisions about where they live, or need to develop new relationships and interests which must last for many years of retirement or widowhood.

The normal mental changes of old age do not help in these crises and many an old person clings to the limited life that they have, instead of facing up to the need to be adventurous and explore in order to obtain satisfaction in life. In dementia there is a gross and progressive exaggeration of this rigidity and difficulty with new situations (p. 153).

Intellectual functions

When it comes to memory, intellect and all the other higher mental functions which decline so obviously in dementia, it is surprisingly uncertain how much change occurs during normal old age. As we have indicated, many people interpret the slowness of old age as a decline in intellect. Moreover, when intelligence tests are given in the right circumstances, allowing for the older person's slowness and cautiousness, they show remarkably little general decline until very old age. There is argument about memory impairment too. Probably some of the complex aspects of processing memories do decline in old age, but never as severely as in dementia.

It is strange, then, that nearly one-half of a surveyed group of people over 75 complained of memory impairment, whereas we know that probably well over 80% of them are mentally entirely normal (see Table 1.1, p. 3). The statistic is stranger still when we consider that if there *were* dementia sufferers in the group some of them might well not realize that their memory was impaired, and so would *not* complain.

Who are the 25% or more who complained of memory impairment but were not in fact impaired? Some must have been noticing the normal changes of old age and were worried by them. Some may have been suffering from other illnesses or the effects of drugs which made them feel mentally dulled or actually confused. Some may have been feeling distressed for other reasons, but interpreted their distress as mental impairment.

Cohort effect

In dealing with older people, most specialists see 65 as their 'cut-off' age. However, there is an enormous age range within this group, with more and more people living to their tenth decade and indeed beyond. The life experiences of someone born in the 1930s and the experiences of someone born last century are dramatically different; the length of time spent in education, their diet, work, and many other aspects of life can be vastly different. These differences may result in changes in social attitudes, in abilities, and in different responses to tests, so-called 'cohort effects'. We must keep this in mind when assessing older people.

Differentiating from dementia

What then can we say to an older person who thinks that she may be losing her memory, that is, developing dementia; or to her family who are worried that she is declining mentally?

Likelihood of dementia

First, we need to ask carefully why they are worried at this particular time, because quite separate events or concerns may be on their minds. Then we can look at the statistics and see that the chances of dementia occurring in a particular individual are actually quite low, maybe one in four or five if they survive into their 80s. This statistic is, of course, of little reassurance to an individual. If the concern has arisen because one of the person's own parents or a brother or sister suffered dementia we can look at the genetic statistics, but once again these are of little individual help. We can say that, on average, the hereditary component to dementia has some effect, but the risk is still small, though it is bigger than if there had not been a close relative who suffered dementia and is very significant indeed in the rare genetic cases.

Pattern and degree of change

It is important to look at how the complaint has developed over time. Dementia is a new development, failure at a much greater rate than anything that could be the result of normal ageing. If we can get a history of how well the patient was functioning previously – her *baseline level* – we can work out the pattern of decline. But, even with a good baseline, change will only be obvious over many months. Nevertheless, this is the best way of ensuring proper diagnosis. Three features of dementia help further in making the distinction.

First, when someone is severely demented there is little doubt about the diagnosis. Although some of the changes resemble normal old age the *degree* of change is far beyond what would normally occur.

Secondly, some of the symptoms of dementia, such as disinhibition, dysphasia, dyspraxia, incontinence, never occur in normal older people (though they may occur in other illnesses that are common in old age). So the *extent* of brain damage is greater in dementia than normal ageing.

Thirdly, the *rate* of change in dementia is far faster than any normal decline there may be in old age. An illness which kills even in 10 years is quite different from the very slow changes of normal ageing.

If the person has not reached the stage where diagnosis is clear, then the correct action is to 'wait and see' (p. 47), a very uncertain position for both her and her family to be in. The uncertainty can be tempered by reassurance that the patient will be reviewed later and that, if necessary, help will then be available. This should not stop us from trying to assess dementia sufferers as early as possible. Early assessment can rule out other causes of the patient's apparent decline and helps to provide the baseline from which it is easier to see at a later stage whether there is indeed a progressive dementia or not.

On the other hand, fixing on a diagnosis of dementia too early is a mistake which can lead to wrong decisions being made on the patient's behalf by overconcerned relatives or doctors. It is best if relatives and patients can tolerate the uncertainty for a while until the diagnosis is clear one way or the other.

DEMENTIA IS PROGRESSIVE

Dementia and brain damage

The decline of dementia can be relatively fast or relatively slow, but in all patients it is progressive; the patient is always on a downward slope. For a particular patient the decline will not always continue at an even rate. Occasionally DAT patients have long static spells (or *plateaux*) in between periods of more rapid decline. The reason for this is not entirely clear; perhaps the brain finds some more reserve for a time. In VaD, the downward course is often modified, as we have seen, where repeated strokes occur throughout the illness. At each of these strokes there may be a sudden deterioration followed by a static period (or plateau), or even a temporary improvement. But there are many such episodes and the general impression, taken over months and years, is still of progressive decline.

Now, if a person has had only one episode of brain damage, say one stroke, or a head injury, the damage is once and for all and will not progress further. Indeed, although the damaged brain's *structure* cannot be repaired in the way a skin wound repairs, the brain can reorganize its connections to some extent so that over a few months, or sometimes 1 or 2 years, some recovery of *function* is possible and improvement occurs. Eventually that recovery is as complete as it can be. From then on, for the rest of that person's life, there will be a residual degree of brain damage which is *static*. Box 2.1 gives a list of some of the possible causes of non-progressive brain damage.

The 'law of mass action' (p. 11) applies here as in dementia. The greater the volume of brain damaged or destroyed, the greater the loss of general functions such as intelligence, long-term memory, abstract thinking and reasoning. So there might be justification in describing a severely but now statically brain-damaged patient as demented, but if she is not progressively declining mentally, she is not dementing. Using the term dementia at all here can be misleading. If we use the term *chronic*

Box 2.1   Some causes of chronic (non-progressive) brain damage

Head injury
Brain surgery
Cerebrovascular accident
　Stroke
　Embolus
　Intracerebral haemorrhage
　Subarachnoid haemorrhage
Encephalitis
Meningitis

---

brain damage, implying a permanent condition, we describe exactly what has happened and can expect the characteristic slow improvement in the first months after the injury.

Unfortunately, there is a tendency for doctors to use the term dementia to cover both types of general brain damage, and so 'confusion' is possible. This confusion can be avoided if we talk of 'progressive' dementia or make a guess at which type of dementia a patient suffers from ('probably Alzheimer-type', for example).

Furthermore, there are intermediate cases between dementia proper and what we have called chronic brain damage. If a person suffers a *few* strokes, but with long intervals between them, then during those long intervals his progress will follow the rules of brain damage. But each ensuing stroke adds to the previous damage so that overall his impairment gets worse and worse. Neither term is quite appropriate here, and either will do.

Treatable or reversible dementia

Some illnesses follow the course of dementia only as long as their particular cause is present (see Table 1.5, p. 12) and so are intermediate between brain damage and dementia in another way. The punch-drunk boxer may stop getting worse or may even recover a little over the next few years if he stops boxing (but not always – see p. 37) Likewise, surgery for hydrocephalus or a brain tumour can halt the progress of dementia. The patient with syphilis who develops GPI continues to decline mentally till antibiotic treatment is given and then may recover well if the damage has not been too severe.

As we learn how to treat DAT, VaD or the other rarer causes, they also will be added to the list of partly or wholly reversible dementias. It is therefore quite reasonable for the present to describe patients who have treatable causes as dementing while the cause continues progressively to damage their brains, and then as chronically brain-damaged if, after the cause is removed, the damage becomes static.

Age-associated memory impairment

This refers to a 'normal' decline in memory of old age. By definition cognitive problems are confined to memory; other aspects of thinking are unimpaired. Age-associated memory impairment is relatively benign (the older term was benign senescent forgetfulness) and non-progressive. There is some argument about whether it is an early dementia or whether it is a separate entity. To use 'non-progression' as a criterion means that a definite diagnosis can only be made retrospectively after a long time has passed.

A common reason for referral to specialist services for assessment is a subjective feeling of memory difficulties, not borne out by testing. Follow-up of these patients over a number of years has shown that a relatively high percentage subsequently go on to develop dementia. This implies that our current tests are not sensitive enough to differentiate what minor degrees of 'normal' forgetfulness are or are not dementia. The existence of this concept is in danger of giving false reassurance in a suitation where uncertainty is the correct response.

Dementia and mental handicap

When dementia begins, the sufferer's brain has been in its adult developed state for many years. In mental handicap, however, the brain is damaged at a stage when it is still maturing and developing. There are some parallels between the brain damage/dementia distinction and the two principal types of mental handicap.

In the first type an episode of brain damage before or around the time of birth leaves a static amount of residual impairment. The brain still has some capacity to mature and develop, though now limited by the damage. The child does develop mentally but lags behind other children. This, then, is a form of chronic brain damage. The other type of mental handicap is more like dementia. For example, some metabolic disorders lead to the deposition of more and more of a toxic chemical in the brain, causing progressive impairment. This counteracts the process of maturation, so that the child declines and dies.

In recent years there has been a growth in the number of mentally handicapped people who survive into old age. There can be some difficulty in distinguishing whether an already mentally impaired person is simply continuing with their lifelong disability or has begun to develop dementia. Again, the clues are in the change from normal, its degree, extent and rate.

A particular problem arises from the new phenomenon of people with Down's syndrome surviving to middle age, only to develop DAT (p. 27). We need to consider how the ways we have learnt to help elderly dementia sufferers can be applied and modified for a special group.

DEMENTIA AND DELIRIUM (ACUTE CONFUSIONAL STATE)

If dementia can be seen as a *gradual* failure of the workings of the brain, then delirium is *rapid* failure. Like dementia, delirium is a *syndrome*, a characteristic pattern of symptoms and signs. It can be caused by anything which rapidly damages the brain as a whole – direct damage to the brain by injury or disease, general illnesses which disturb brain function, or poisons and drugs which affect the brain (Table 2.2).

Reversibility

The importance of recognizing delirium comes from the fact that, if the disease or damage that is causing it can be treated or stops spontaneously, the confusion will clear. Delirium is not progressive unless the cause is progressive. On the other hand, if the cause is very severe or very progressive, it will take the patient past the stage of delirium to coma or even death. Delirium is therefore a medical problem, requiring accurate diagnosis and treatment of its cause as a matter of urgency, with hope of recovery.

Table 2.2 Some causes of delirium

Direct damage to brain	Head injury Cerebrovascular accident (thrombosis, embolus or haemorrhage) Subdural haemorrhage after injury Epileptic fit (post-ictal) Postoperative Infection (meningitis, encephalitis) Sudden change in a brain tumour
General disorders which disturb brain function	Constipation (reason unclear) Infection (especially chest or urinary tract) Cardiac failure and other heart disorders Kidney failure (raised blood urea) Liver failure Respiratory failure (raised carbon dioxide) Vitamin deficiency (lack of thiamine – vitamin B_1 – in alcoholics) Endocrine disorders (especially hypoglycaemia in diabetics)
Drugs	Tranquillizers including alcohol Antidepressants Antiparkinsonian drugs Digoxin and other cardiac drugs Cimetidine (for peptic ulcers) Anticholinergic drugs and many others
Drug withdrawal	Alcohol (delirium tremens – DTs) Benzodiazepines (including diazepam and lorazepam) Barbiturates Antidepressants

Delirium due to any cause is more likely to occur in young children, the elderly and dementia sufferers

Terminology

The word delirium is, unfortunately, not agreed by everyone to be the best term for this acute mental impairment. It is an old word which has been revived in recent years. Nor are the terms *acute confusional state* or *toxic confusional state* any better, for the word 'confusion' can be used to mean muddled thinking, disorientation, clouding of consciousness or the whole syndrome of delirium, and is even regularly used to mean dementia (as in 'the confused elderly'). It should be avoided where possible, or only used to mean 'the syndrome of acute confusion'. Rather better would be to use other terms such as *acute cerebral failure*, *acute brain failure* or *acute brain syndrome*, which are gaining in popularity. The name in any case is less important than understanding the syndrome.

The word 'acute' is a bit more helpful. In medicine acute always means rapid in onset and usually brief in duration. It describes the course of delirium well.

Course

Figure 2.1 shows the course of delirium after damage to the brain. It may take hours, or even days, to develop after the cause begins. Sometimes there is a *retrograde amnesia*, the patient losing memories from shortly before the time the delirium started. Thus she may not recall the fall, or taking the extra pills, or the beginnings of a chest infection, which caused the delirium. Delirium reaches a maximum level if the cause is not progressive and the patient will begin to recover after the cause is removed.

However, this recovery can be delayed for quite a long time, particularly in very elderly people or people who suffer from dementia. A patient who develops delirium after a stroke may likewise remain confused for weeks and then recover (in contrast, *physical recovery* after a stroke usually begins quite soon or not at all). So we can hope that a patient will make a quick recovery from delirium, but should not be surprised if it takes longer. Delirium lasting up to several weeks is not uncommon.

Outcome

How much the patient eventually recovers from delirium depends on two factors. First, what was the patient like before the delirium started? If she was not suffering from dementia we can hope that she will return to normal. Sometimes, however, it is a patient who is already suffering from dementia who develops delirium (Fig. 2.1), and her best possible recovery will be to her previous level of dementia.

The other factor is whether or not the damage to the brain is permanent (Fig. 2.2). If it is extensive enough or prolonged enough then, after the acute phase, there will be some degree of *residual brain damage*. The patient will not return to her previous normal but will be left with intellectual or other deficits of brain function, which then follow the course of brain damage (p. 53).

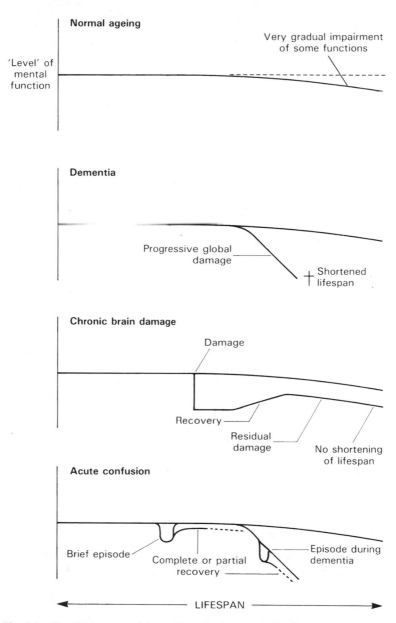

Fig. 2.1 The time course of dementia, chronic brain damage and delirium, compared to normal ageing.

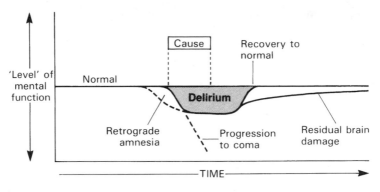

Fig. 2.2 The course of delirium.

Delirium tremens (DTs)

This occurs when an alcoholic cuts down or stops his or her intake of alcohol rapidly. It may last for several weeks before recovery. Full blown delirium is relatively uncommon in alcohol withdrawal, but some of the features, for example visual hallucinations and confusion, are quite common. The main risk in alcohol withdrawal is of grand mal (major) seizures; the risk of these can be reduced by using a benzodiazepine drug such as Chlordiazepoxide, but the risk can be exacerbated by drugs which lower seizure threshold, notably phenothiazines such as Thioridazine or Chlorpromazine.

It is also important that thiamine (vitamin B_1) be used as part of the treatment, in the hope of speeding recovery and preventing further deterioration, such as the development of Korsakoff's syndrome (p. 69).

Delirium during dementia

Delirium is particularly common among dementia sufferers. This is partly because so many of them are very elderly and are therefore prone to develop all sorts of other illnesses and drug reactions which can temporarily interfere with the workings of the brain. Self-neglect and forgetfulness will increase the chances of such problems occurring. Perhaps we also notice delirium more in dementing people because they are so often in care. But, in addition, they have often no other way of complaining. Instead of the limited retrograde amnesia mentioned above, a dementing person may have no memory at all of the recent past. Furthermore, she may not be fully aware of where a pain is and may have difficulty describing other symptoms (p. 114).

The result is that, especially for more severely demented people, just as for children before they can talk, the only evidence that they are ill is either that they look ill or that they become delirious. This makes it doubly important that families and staff caring for dementing people know a little about delirium and are on the lookout for any rapid change that occurs. Doctors need to know that when such a change happens it means that something medical is wrong and that if they can diagnose and treat the cause the patient is likely to recover to her previous level.

Differentiating from dementia

The importance of being able to tell the difference between dementia and delirium, or being able to tell when a dementing person develops delirium on top of dementia, is clear. How can we do this (Table 2.3)?

Time-scale

Dementia is slowly progressive. Delirium is acute, beginning as a rapid change over minutes, hours or days, not months or years.

Table 2.3 Differentiating delirium and dementia

	Delirium	Dementia
Course	Rapid onset	Slowly progressive
Cause	Acute medical cause	Slowly progressive cause
Clinical features	Clouding of consciousness Sleep disturbance	Clear consciousness Normal sleep, but 'clock' may be wrong
	Irregular variability	Tends to be worse towards evening, otherwise stable
	Restlessness and unease	Settled apart from aimless wandering or searching
	Visual hallucinations	Hallucinations uncommon and not usually disturbing
	Emotional lability and distress	Poverty of mood commoner, some are labile

Because of retrograde amnesia and the general disruption of memory and thinking that are part of delirium the patient is not always able to describe this rapid change. We must *always* try to get information from a relative or someone else who has seen the patient regularly over the last few months.

Cause

Often the evidence of a cause is obvious – an infection, the physical effects of a stroke, a head injury – often it will not be so obvious. The commonest missed causes of all are constipation and urinary tract infections, but many of the other causes in Table 2.2 are difficult to detect and the patient may not be able to make the appropriate complaint. Things are further complicated by the fact that in some people a very minor cause may lead to quite severe delirium; in others there may be more than one cause (e.g. an infection and alcohol abuse, or heart failure and the tablets given to treat it); while in yet others a potential cause of delirium may not actually be causing delirium (e.g. the dementing person who is unaffected mentally by a chest infection). Finding a cause is therefore very important but is not the only step in diagnosis.

Clinical features

There are many similarities between the effects of slowly progressive brain failure (dementia) and acute brain failure (delirium). In both conditions the basic ability of the brain to make complicated connections is impaired. In both, therefore, the sufferer will not be able to organize thinking properly, will become disorientated and will be impaired in her ability to lay down, store or recall memories. All her higher mental functions will be affected. But even when the time-scale is unclear, and even when a cause is not obvious, it is possible to make a good guess that mental impairment is acute rather than chronic from the symptoms and signs that go with the impairment (Table 2.3). Acute damage to the brain seems to affect its workings in a different way to chronic damage. The main difference relates to consciousness.

Consciousness. Our level of consciousness, that is, how aware we are, how able to focus attention, how awake, is controlled largely by a switching mechanism deep in the middle of the brain, called the *reticular activating system*. It is this mechanism which wakes us or puts us to sleep, and which switches the brain into active attention when, for example, someone calls our name. In delirium this system appears to be damaged, usually temporarily. If severely damaged, unconsciousness results. So delirium can sometimes present as a sort of 'semi-coma'. The patient is drowsy or dopey, she cannot fix her attention and her thinking becomes muddled.

Sleep. The switching mechanism of sleep, which is also part of the reticular system, is often disturbed in delirium. The patient may sleep for a longer or a shorter period than usual, or never. She may be awake by night and asleep by day. Her sleep may be lighter than normal or disturbed by dreams and nightmares. She may be unclear as to what is real and what is a dream. The dementing patient, on the other hand, is usually clear mentally, in the sense that she is alert and fully awake when awake, and normally asleep when asleep. However, if she happens to go to bed early, she may rise after her normal length of sleep, ready for action at 1 a.m. Many older people do not require as much sleep as younger people and 4 or 6 hours may be quite a 'normal' sleep, inconvenient as it is for family, neighbours or staff. The person with dementia has simply got the timing of her internal clock wrong, not the mechanism of sleep.

Variability. A striking feature of these impairments of consciousness is their variability. Both dementing and delirious people tend to become more disorientated during the evening and night (p. 173). The reason for this is not clear. Much of it is probably due to sensory deprivation – at night there are fewer visual and sound clues to help us find our bearings – but fatigue or other effects on the daily rhythms of the body may play a part. In delirium, however, there is often a much more irregular and unpredictable variation. From hour to hour or from minute to minute, even within the course of a sentence, the patient may move from drowsiness to alertness, from disorientation to complete orientation, from muddled to clear thinking. This type of variability is unusual in a dementing person. Presumably, it is caused by varying damage to the consciousness switch of the reticular system.

Restlessness. Also affected by this variability is another common feature of delirium – restlessness. By restlessness is meant an inability to settle both physically and mentally (a frequent accompaniment of physical illness even without actual delirium). The dementing person is not usually restless in this sense of suffering listlessness and unease. That may come as a surprise to those who work with dementing people in care, but it should be recalled that the majority of sufferers are quietly living at home or are settled in care. Most of the restlessness which does occur in dementia appears aimless, or is understandable as a search for familiar surroundings (p. 172). The restlessness of delirium is more like the result of physical discomfort or of mental distress.

Visual perception. Yet another feature of delirium (and one which in itself can lead to restlessness) is disturbance of visual perception. The patient misinterprets what she actually sees (visual *illusions*) or sees things that are not there at all (visual *hallucinations*). Thus, she may see faces distorted, or strange colours, or faces in an empty window – all very bewildering or frightening experiences. Illusions and hallucinations are sometimes experienced in other senses, for example, hearing (auditory) or smell (olfactory), but visual disturbances are by far the commonest. The reason for these disturbances is not clear. Perhaps there is impairment of another function of the reticular system, namely that of filtering out irrelevant information, which is part of the process of focusing attention (see p. 117).

Hallucinations can also occur in dementia, but they are not usually so vivid or disturbing, indeed they may seem like enjoyable visitors for a lonely sufferer. They may be partially caused by eye problems which the patient has as well as his dementia. They are also particularly common in those with Lewy body type dementia (p. 33).

Lability. Finally, the delirious patient's emotions are likely to be disturbed. As can be imagined, hallucinations and illusions upset the patient and may lead her to believe that someone is out to harm her – she believes that the devil is in the house, or that the nurses are having noisy parties in her ward and are singing rude songs about her, or that the police are after her. It is natural in these circumstance to feel fearful or angry. Furthermore, the experience of disorientation is bewildering and frightening in itself.

But as well as this the patient's *control* of her emotions may be lost, so that she finds herself suddenly losing her temper, or suddenly in tears, or suddenly laughing for no very clear reason, and just as quickly regaining control again. Her emotions may fluctuate like this (emotional *lability*) throughout the period of delirium, or for a time she may get 'stuck' in a particular emotion, be it depression or anger or fear.

On the other hand, in dementia, although lability is not uncommon (p. 161), most sufferers show a more obvious decline or 'poverty' of emotion (p. 134).

Partial symptoms

All these clinical features are very common in people who are delirious, but they are not all always present. For a start, the variability of delirium means that the person may appear clear at one time of the day and very confused at another. This can lead to problems in convincing doctors or senior care staff that the patient is acutely ill at all. A woman who is apparently clear for 90% of the day but for short periods at night becomes drowsy, hallucinating and restless is suffering from delirium, even if she can apparently answer all questions of orientation and memory perfectly during her clear spells (in reality it is likely that she will show patchy loss of memory and slight difficulty with complicated thinking most of the time, but these defects can be very difficult to pick up). But it is not just this variability which leads to difficulty in diagnosing delirium. Only one or two of the characteristic signs may be evident in a particular patient. A patient with dementia may show no other change except that one day she begins to experience hallucinations, another merely develops sleep disturbance, yet these changes are enough evidence to suspect delirium, call for the doctor, and ask what the cause is.

An everyday condition

Most of us have experienced some degree of delirium at some time. The 'flu victim who feels a bit dopey and restless during the day and sleepless by night is suffering mild delirium, due to the effects of the 'flu virus on brain function. And the person recovering from even a mild head injury or an operation who cannot think clearly for a while and asks what time it is (disorientation in time), where he is (disorientation in place) and what has been happening (memory impairment) is showing signs of delirium.

Management of delirium

Find the cause and treat it

Delirium is thus a very common condition. Knowing its course, its distinguishing features and its possible causes, it should be possible for most people who help in looking after elderly people to differentiate someone suffering delirium from someone with dementia. The logical next step should be obvious. The cause of the delirium should be diagnosed as soon as possible (Table 2.2). The commonest causes are constipation, chest and urinary infections and drug side-effects or prescribing mistakes. Causes which are often missed include: falls causing head injury and concussion; haemorrhage in the tissues covering the brain following a head injury (subdural haematoma), which can lead to a prolonged and often very variable confusion; fits; and delirium tremens, for we should always remember that alcohol abuse can occur in 80 year olds as well as in 30 year olds!

It is seldom necessary to look too far for the cause of delirium, since 'common things are common', but delirium does demand medical assessment. Sadly, some of the causes in themselves are not treatable, the commonest of these being a stroke (though active management of the stroke may help to minimize any future damage). During the course of a vascular dementia, short or prolonged episodes of delirium may occur after each of a series of strokes. Despite the fact that such episodes are untreatable in themselves, they nevertheless need medical assessment.

Some aggravating features are commonly found in older people. These include the presence of dementia, relative sensory deprivation (loneliness, deafness or poor sight) and other contributing problems such as medication and chronic disease.

Help with disorientation and hallucinations

Much of what will be said later about the management of disorientation and memory impairment in dementia (see Chapter 4) applies equally to people who are delirious. Special support at night is important, for that is when the disorientation is likely to be at its worst. It is generally found that darkness increases disorientation and encourages hallucinations. A lighted room, with familiar objects and people around, is better.

If a patient experiences hallucinations and realizes that they are imaginary, it is important to reassure her that she is not 'going mad', but that they will disappear when she is physically better. If she believes the hallucinations to be real, then it is of no value to get into an argument about their existence. It is more helpful to reassure her that she is actually seeing these things, but that they will eventually go away, while in the meantime everything is being done to help get rid of them.

Help with distress

Delirious patients are susceptible to the 'emotional temperature' around them and may misinterpret this in the same way that they misinterpret what they see and hear. A calm atmosphere, with the situation explained slowly, clearly and repeatedly, will help to prevent the patient from misunderstanding what is happening, and so lessen her distress. The worst possible place for a delirious patient is, unfortunately, the casualty department of a busy hospital, or a busy medical ward, for the bustle invites agitation and misinterpretation of one's surroundings. The best place is her own home.

Indeed some elderly people, and especially elderly dementing people, develop a sort of delirium just because of a move from one place to another, *delirium of translocation*. This may amount to a temporary disorientation when familiar surroundings are missed, or it may be a full-blown delirious state. We should therefore be wary of moving elderly people around too much, especially if they are physically ill or suffering from dementia. The move itself can cause as much trouble as the reason for the move. Unfortunately, it is not possible to predict exactly who will be affected in this way by a move and who will be unaffected.

Drugs

Calmness, reassurance and orientation can be very helpful, but even so, for some patients the combination of restlessness, emotional lability, bewildering disorientation, muddled thinking and frightening hallucinations is such that they are very disturbed, either frightened or angry. Drug treatment is therefore occasionally necessary, but it should always be borne in mind that among the list of causes of delirium are the very drugs which might be used to treat it (see Table 2.2). The commonly used tranquillizer thioridazine seems to be particularly likely to make delirium worse, in some cases.

If anything is necessary, a night sedative may be used to help ease the worst time of disorientation and lessen fatigue. By day, the smallest dose of tranquillizer that is necessary to prevent severe distress or aggression, or nothing at all, should be used. The only exceptions to this are for delirium tremens and during withdrawal from other tranquillizers such as diazepam or barbiturate drugs. In these conditions epileptic fits may occur along with the delirium and it is often necessary to give an antiepileptic tranquillizer, such as chlordiazepoxide, to prevent the fits.

Avoid long-term decisions

When a dementing patient or, even more especially, an undemented person develops delirium, it is the wrong time to make major long-term decisions. Too often the acutely delirious person lands in a general hospital bed because carers at home or in a residential home feel that they cannot cope. Once in the hospital the disorientation caused by the move and the anxieties of carers lead to the inevitable decision that the patient cannot return home, even if there is little or no residual brain damage. Where delirious patients have been admitted to hospital from home, more are subsequently discharged to nursing home care than is the case with similar patients who have not had delirium at the time of admission.

It is quite understandable that the carers should feel unable to cope during the disturbed period. They need outside support on an acute basis – a rapid response to an acute illness – and the patient requires adequate medical attention, diagnosis and treatment. General practitioners may need to be able to call on specialist hospital services, who will see the patient at home or at the outpatient clinic, so that they can feel supported if they wish to treat the delirious patient at home.

If supportive home-care services and adequate medical back-up were available we could hope that this short-term disorder could be managed without too much disruption to the person's life and that, as a consequence, long-term decisions could be made more sensibly after the delirium is over. If the patient has indeed suffered permanent brain damage new decisions *will* have to be made about her future support and care. If, however, she has returned to normal it is simply a time to reassess the preexisting level of support.

Prognosis

There is a significant mortality associated with severe forms of delirium; as many as 1 in 4 patients with a full blown delirious state do not survive. Some survivors will fail to recover completely to their previous level of function. A significant number will have subsequent mental impairment and reduced independence. Inevitably, therefore, many will require enhanced care when they return home, or will face major decisions about moving into permanent care. Fortunately, however, most delirium is mild, and people will regain their previous function on recovery.

DEMENTIA AFFECTS MOST ASPECTS OF MENTAL FUNCTION

Dementia and Korsakoff's syndrome

The fact that the dementias affect nerve cells and their connections over wide areas of the cerebral cortex means that widespread functions of the cortex are affected. Korsakoff's syndrome is also a progressive disorder but it only affects a small area of the brain, including the recent memory system of the hippocampal region. It is not, therefore, a true dementia.

Recent memory loss and confabulation

Korsakoff's syndrome occurs mostly in people who have been dependent on alcohol for many years, probably as a result of very localized brain damage caused by deficiency of the vitamin thiamine (vitamin B_1). This deficiency is caused by two factors: heavy drinking is often associated with poor diet, so not enough thiamine is taken in; and thiamine is used up in the way alcohol is broken down in the body. There are other rarer causes of Korsakoff's syndrome; these are also probably due to vitamin B_1 deficiency. They include persistent vomiting in pregnancy, anorexia nervosa, and starvation from various causes. The condition has been described in ex-prisoners of war. Since it only affects the one area of the brain, connected with the hippocampus and involving acetylcholine-producing neurones, the chief result of the damage is an impairment of recent memory. The sufferer often tries to compensate by confabulation (making up answers to cover gaps in the memory), which may be either conscious or automatic. Such confabulation is not, however, confined to Korsakoff patients and may not be so deliberate as was once thought. It can occur in anyone who loses their memory, though it may be more elaborate in an alcoholic who has been used to telling tales about his or her drinking for many years.

Recovery

Korsakoff's syndrome is progressive if the patient goes on drinking, but its progress halts if he or she stops. It then follows the natural history of brain damage (p. 53) as long as the patient remains abstinent. Most doctors give thiamine supplements for some time in the hope that this will also help. The response to this is variable, but some patients may continue to improve for 6 months or even longer.

Dementia

Apart from the decline in memory most of the rest of the Korsakoff patient's brain is functioning normally. Personality, intellect and old memories from before the damage started are all pretty well intact; so patients cannot be said to suffer dementia. However, they usually lack insight into the memory loss, and are often apathetic and repetitive. Some have signs and symptoms suggestive of frontal lobe problems. Indeed, there may turn out to be quite an overlap between Korsakoff's syndrome and alcoholic dementia (p. 38), but until we know more about the latter condition, it is better to keep the distinction between them.

The fact that Korsakoff's syndrome affects relatively young people, that the deficits are limited and that some recovery may occur leads to great difficulties in finding appropriate care for sufferers. In the past such patients were in the back wards of mental hospitals. Nowadays they are usually, equally inappropriately, found in general medical wards, acute or rehabilitation psychiatric wards, or in residential or nursing homes for older people. There is an urgent need for a proper specialist service for a small group of men and women in middle age who need help with their memory impairment, advice and help on drinking, time to recover and potentially a new start in life thereafter. Unfortunately, many professionals do not see people with Korsakoff's as an attractive group to work with.

PSEUDODEMENTIA

The conditions mentioned so far differ from dementia in important ways. We now come to a condition which may be difficult to distinguish from dementia, but in which there is no actual organic brain damage – pseudodementia. We already have a list of causes of reversible or treatable dementia (Table 1.5, p. 12). These conditions have sometimes been labelled 'pseudodementias', but it is more accurate to stick to the term 'reversible dementia' where we think that the symptoms and signs of an *actual* dementia are caused by an illness which is slowly damaging the brain but which can be treated. We would then only use term pseudodementia to refer to the situation where the symptoms and signs of dementia are present but there is no evidence of damage to the brain; the patient behaves *as if* she were dementing but she is not in fact dementing. There is one principal cause of this pseudodementia – depressive illness.

DEPRESSIVE ILLNESS

Severe depression is quite a common condition among elderly people, probably nearly as common as it is in people of middle age. We are not referring to the often mild, understandable depression which can follow one or other of the many losses which older people experience (and remember that dementia can be one of those losses – see p. 221). We are referring instead to those depressions whose severity is quite out of proportion to any precipitating loss (indeed, there is sometimes no obvious precipitant at all).

All the patient's activities and interests succumb to a slowing down and an all-pervading gloom. Usually the beginning of such a depression is fairly clear and the main complaints are the feeling of depression, a preoccupation with self-blame, guilt or hypochondriacal ideas, loss of interest (including loss of interest in food with consequent weight-loss), loss of concentration, poor sleep with early wakening and a general slowing which is both physical and mental. Sometimes in depression, however, this mental slowing, together with poor concentration, loss of interest, social withdrawal and self-neglect, produces a state of detachment from the surrounding world which looks just like dementia. The patient appears to be disorientated, cannot concentrate and so cannot remember, and seems to have lost the ability to care for herself. On all the usual tests of intelligence, memory and orientation she may perform as if she were dementing. She may even believe that she is dementing – a variant of the hypochondriasis that is so often part of depression in older people. Perhaps some pseudodementia in depressive illness is caused by the patient acting out this belief, as if to prove his worst fears. If the onset of the illness has been slow, then it can be very easy to agree with her and conclude that she suffers from dementia.

Differentiating from dementia

It is vital to distinguish patients with depressive pseudodementia from those who are truly dementing, for they can usually be treated either by antidepressant drugs or by electroconvulsive therapy (ECT), and will make a good recovery after rehabilitation back to their normal activities. Among the many apparent dementia sufferers, how are we to pick out this particular group (Table 2.4)?

Past history

In the first place, depression tends to be a recurrent condition so it would be quite likely for someone with a depressive pseudodementia to have suffered an episode of severe depression in the past. There are other complicated links between dementia and depression (see below) and a past history of depression in a dementing patient is not unusual. In patients

Table 2.4   Pseudodementia due to depression and true dementia

	Pseudodementia	True dementia
Past history	Depression	None usually
Course	Rapid onset	Very gradual onset
Symptoms	Depressed mood	Depression may occur in the early stages
	Loss of appetite	Unusual
	Weight loss	Not common, sometimes with normal appetite
	Retardation	Uncommon
	Sleep disturbance and early wakening	Uncommon
	Depressive thinking	Rare
	Islands of normality	Rare and only when stimulated
	'Insight' may be excessive	Insight usually diminished
Treatment	Antidepressants cure the 'dementia'	Antidepressants do not treat true dementia

whose first episode of depression occurs late in life, there appears to be an increased risk of subsequent dementia.

Family history

Depression often has a genetic component. Thus, in someone with a strong family history of depression, we should give greater consideration to this as a possible diagnosis.

Depression

The person may complain of depression, or look depressed, though we should note that not everybody who suffers from depression calls the illness by that name, and also note that some degree of depression is quite common in the early stages of a true dementia.

She may show the loss of appetite and weight-loss characteristic of severe depression; she or her family may have noted the striking retardation of depression; or she may have depressive or morbid thoughts.

One of the characteristic features of depressive illness is that it tends to be worse in the morning, with early-morning wakening, so that the patient's mood and activity improve as the day goes on (*diurnal variation*). As we will see (p. 173), dementing patients often function worse as the day progresses. A 'demented' patient who consistently livens up and becomes mentally clearer as the day progresses may not be demented at all but may have a treatable depression.

Thoughts of death are much more common in depression than in dementia. The patient may frequently express a wish to die, or may even ask for 'a wee blue pill to put me out of my misery'. Fears of being unable to return home are also common if the person is in hospital.

Delusional ideas, i.e. ideas which are not founded in reality, are common in dementia whether or not it is associated with depression. However, in depression they usually reflect the patient's mood, for example delusions of guilt, of having lost loved ones or of being punished in some way. These are called *mood congruent* delusions.

Hints of normality

There may be hints that the 'dementia' is not as it should be. The patient maintains beneath the depression a normally active mind. So she may, to our surprise, register and recall the memory of one or two recent events which a dementing person would be expected to forget.

Insight

People who suffer from dementia often lose insight into their condition, or their insight is limited (p. 210). In contrast to this, patients with pseudodementia may have apparently complete insight into their 'dementia', or may exaggerate their complaints. It has even been suggested that a good rule of thumb is that if a patient approaches her doctor complaining bitterly of dementia she is most unlikely to have true dementia and is more likely to have depression or delirium.

These observations and information gained from the patient and her family or friends about the history, course and symptoms of the illness will give us the hint that the dementia is 'pseudo' and that antidepressant treatment should be tried. Indeed, sometimes a trial of treatment is the best way to confirm (or deny) the diagnosis.

Special tests

Many attempts have been made to find a test which will distinguish clearly between depression with pseudodementia and true organic dementia. Psychological tests, brain scans, EEG and biochemical tests have all been tried. Unfortunately, none has yet been successful. There is too much overlap between the results, some dementing people scoring high on tests of depression and some depressed people scoring high on tests of dementia. Such overlaps make it impossible to interpret these tests in a particular individual. Indeed, modern scanning tests have suggested that some elderly sufferers from depression may actually have mild brain damage, and it is possible that in some cases pseudodementia is a very early sign that the person will develop dementia in the future.

Recovery

In general, it is worth erring on the side of optimism and starting treatment (though remaining cautious, as many antidepressants are potent causes of delirium – Table 2.2). It can be extremely gratifying to see someone who was thought to be dementing make a complete recovery, particularly if plans had been made for her long-term care. And it is pleasantly surprising when tests which have seemed to show dementia return to normal after treatment.

OTHER PSYCHIATRIC DISORDERS

Other disorders have frequently been mistaken for dementia, but this really should not occur, since the central feature of dementia is not present – the progressive failure of most mental functions. However, so prevalent is the notion that most or all mental illness or oddity in the elderly can be bundled together and called dementia that it is worth mentioning these other illnesses.

Mania

Mania and hypomania (meaning a milder degree of mania) are in many ways the opposite of depression. The patient is elated and speeded up, full of wonderful ideas and the energy to carry them out. In severe cases the patient's thoughts come at such a rate that she loses touch with her surroundings and appears delirious. A first episode of mania occurring in an older person is uncommon. It is more likely to occur in people who have previously had episodes of depression (*manic-depressive* or *bipolar affective disorder*). The patient is her normal self between episodes and these periods of good health may last for months or for many years. The onset of mania is usually quite rapid, over days and weeks, so it should not easily be mistaken for dementia. However, first episode mania *can* occur in this age group and this possibility must be kept in mind.

Late paraphrenia

This is also a relatively uncommon condition. It is similar to the condition of *schizophrenia* in younger patients, and it is one of the types of *paranoid psychosis*.

The patient, almost always an elderly woman, is usually socially isolated and often made more isolated by deafness. She begins to believe that she is surrounded by persecutors, who get at her and at her property in one or more of a variety of ways. They talk behind her back, spy on her, steal from her house, put in noxious fumes or interfere with her body.

Such ladies are likely to withdraw further socially. Her self-care may decline because she feels that the electricity has been tampered with or their food poisoned. Withdrawal and self-neglect, however, are the only similarities between paraphrenia and dementia, for otherwise the paranoid patient is usually in full possession of her mental powers. Indeed, she may feel that she has to be sharper than usual to keep up with the tricks played by her imaginary persecutors.

This condition differs from schizophrenia not only in the age of onset, but also in its progress. The symptoms tend to remain static, often for many years, and patients do not usually develop the personality deterioration seen in schizophrenia.

Some patients who appear to have late paraphrenia subsequently develop dementia. Paranoid symptoms are quite common in dementia (p. 178) and in delirium (p. 64), but in these cases they are just one part of a much wider syndrome.

Personality disorder

This term is usually applied to a life-long characteristic pattern of attitudes to self, relationships to others and ways of reacting to crises and to the world in general (see also p. 202). A personality type only becomes a personality problem or disorder either when the person seeks help because of the consequences of being that type of person, or when it causes problems for others. There have been many descriptions of personality types and personality traits and no exact 'diagnosis' of a particular person's personality type is possible. Each person's make-up is too complicated for that, and so we can only give general descriptions.

Changes with age

As we age the mental changes previously described (p. 48) must affect our personalities. Of course there are many old people who maintain their full personality colour throughout their lives. But for others the tendency towards detachment and less emotional interaction, and the preference for order, regularity and routine which often occurs, seem to lead towards a mellowing of the stronger aspects of personality and a move towards a more introverted or more obsessional personality type (p. 202). These are only very general tendencies, but in practice they mean that there are fewer 'psychopaths' among the elderly than among young people. On the other hand, in some people the mental changes of old age bring an exaggeration of certain personality traits, such as hypochondriasis, meanness, dependence, independence, irritability, suspiciousness and obsessionality, so that they become a sort of caricature of their previous selves.

Personality and dementia

As with the other mental changes of old age these changes can all occur in dementia. A dementing person may stay unchanged in personality well into dementia, may be a quieter version, a 'shadow' of her former self, or may develop exaggerated or even quite new personality traits (see Chapter 7). When we notice a change in an old person's personality we need to ask: is this simply a gradual change with old age; is it the beginning of dementia; or is it another psychiatric disorder, a depression or a paraphrenia, which is causing her to behave in uncharacteristic ways? The answer is often difficult because personality is so difficult to define.

The key again lies in the pattern of the change over time. A very rapid change probably indicates illness, either psychiatric or physical; a slow change over months should raise suspicions of dementia; a very slow change indeed over many years is more likely to be simply old age. The other clue is the nature and extent of the change. A slight exaggeration or a mellowing of personality may be a simple ageing. A dramatic change with new personality traits emerging or a ridiculous caricature of the previous personality is much more likely to be due to dementia or to another psychiatric illness.

Indeed, these new developments from the patient's previous personality should not technically be called personality characteristics at all. They have become symptoms and signs of the illness from which the patient is suffering. If the illness is treatable we can hope that she will return to her previous usual personality. The personality changes of dementia are unfortunately not susceptible to treatment, though eventually they are likely to disappear as the illness progresses and the sufferer loses all those characteristic patterns of behaviour that went to make the person she was.

Self-neglect

Of particular interest is that change in personality sometimes known as the 'Diogenes syndrome' (after the Greek philosopher and teacher of Alexander the Great who, being a cynic about the values of the world, lived in ostentatious squalor, in a tub). In this syndrome an old person seems to lose all interest in her self-care and the care of her house. She lives in appalling squalor, yet is mentally normal in other ways. In a related condition an obsessional elderly person becomes preoccupied, sometimes to an equally ridiculous extent, with hoarding particular objects.

The often extreme squalor may lead to urgent requests that 'something must be done' from neighbours or housing authorities.

Some patients are probably in the early stages of dementia, particularly FLD, some may have suffered a stroke in the frontal region of the brain (see p. 35). But it is also important to rule out the possibility that they have become depressed now or in the past and have neglected themselves because of this, that they have odd paranoid ideas or have suffered from schizophrenia in the past or are physically ill.

The term 'Diogenes syndrome' should be reserved for those cases who do not show clear evidence of dementia or of psychiatric disorder. Those with the true Diogenes syndrome appear to choose to reject normal social habits. They may have been eccentric people for much of their lives. Social isolation may mean that they seem mentally impaired on testing, but this may be a pseudo rather than true dementia.

Even excluding all these other possibilities there do seem to be a number of elderly people whose personalities change in old age, who become eccentric, but do not go on to suffer from dementia. We should realize, however, that it is commoner for self-neglect, or neglect of an old person's house, to be signs of the onset of dementia, depression or a physical disability than of this uncommon condition.

Alcohol and drug dependence

These conditions are much commoner among the elderly than most people think. The mental dullness, self-neglect, memory impairment and periodic episodes of delirium of the addict can easily be mistaken for dementia. The true cause is often missed simply because the right questions are not asked. This is especially so in the case of elderly women, for alcohol problems may actually be more common in them than in younger women.

Small quantities of alcohol and drugs may lead to quite marked impairment in an older person so that, although many long-standing alcoholics drink less when they are older, this smaller amount may still be enough to affect the workings of the brain and to cause withdrawal symptoms if it is stopped. There are also 'new' alcoholics, elderly people who for the first time become dependent on alcohol, sometimes out of loneliness, sometimes to deal with anxiety, bereavement or depression or even with dementia.

Drug dependence, particularly on the benzodiazepine drugs such as diazepam and lorazepam, is also surprisingly common.

It is characterized by dependence on the tablets for day-to-day living, a tendency to increase the dose of the drug and resistance to stopping it so as to avoid withdrawal symptoms. The patient taking these drugs may feel mentally slowed, with poor concentration and lack of interest, apathy or even depression. These features can seem like dementia. Changes in dose of the drug or stopping it altogether can cause a withdrawal syndrome of acute confusion, often with fits, like delirium tremens. More commonly the patient simply feels very anxious and restless, with sleep disturbance.

After a period of days or weeks, the withdrawal symptoms fade and she will feel much clearer mentally than before, self-neglect is less, concentration and interest recover. It is then possible to look at any problems such as loneliness or depression which have led to the dependence in the first place.

PSEUDODEMENTIA IN PHYSICAL ILLNESS

We have already seen two ways in which physical illnesses can affect the brain – by causing delirium and by causing a reversible dementia. In addition, anyone who suffers a physical illness which causes weakness, tiredness or poor concentration may do badly on mental tests and may give an appearance of mild dementia. In effect they have a pseudodementia. The list of possible causes contains many of the conditions on Table 2.2, but any debilitating disease could have this effect. Usually, proper mental testing reveals that the dementia is apparent rather than real, but in any case treatment can be expected to reverse the 'dementia'.

CONCLUSION

In this chapter we have described a number of conditions which resemble or can be mistaken for dementia. There is endless variety in people's personalities and the illnesses they may suffer. It is most important that, at the earliest possible moment, anyone who is showing signs of possible dementia has access to proper medical diagnosis and testing to search for these other conditions. Clear definition of what is and what is not dementia allows us in most cases to rule out or treat other illnesses and then to concentrate on managing the consequences of dementia in those unfortunate people who suffer from it.

3

Who are the dementing and where are they?

HOW MANY SUFFERERS?

Present figures

In Table 1.1 (p. 3) we saw one estimate of the prevalence of definite dementia among different age groups ('definite' can be taken to mean 'moderately or severely demented'). We can work out that:

- there are altogether 5–600 000 definite dementia sufferers of all ages in Britain (total population 55 000 000; population over 65 years 9 000 000) in the 1990s, of whom:
- possibly 15–20 000 are aged between 40 and 65
- 2–250 000 are aged 65–80
- 3–350 000 are over 80
- the greatest number of dementia sufferers of any age are probably those aged about 82.

So dementia is predominantly a problem for the 'old-old'. A city of 500 000 population would contain roughly 5000 moderate and severe sufferers, a town of 50 000 would expect 500, and a village of 500 would expect 5 sufferers. The average general practitioner thus has around 20 dementia sufferers on his list.

Because of the vagueness of definition at the boundary between dementia and normal old age, it is very difficult to be definite about the figures for milder stages. Some investigators estimate that nearly as many again suffer from mild dementia (which will later, of course, become more severe). On the other hand, some investigators have found a much lower prevalence of all grades of dementia. There have been many arguments about the true figure, and the fact is that at present we can only guess.

What is necessary in order to plan and provide adequate services is to know the *needs* of dementia sufferers: how many people need sitting services, or day hospitals, or long-stay beds. These needs are based on assessment of function, not on diagnosis.

Population changes

The other way in which statistics can help us is in planning future services. Here we are on firmer ground. We can be certain that, whatever the true figures are now, they will change considerably over the next 10 years. The proportion of the total population who are in the 65–74 age group is now beginning to fall slowly while the *percentage* of these people who are dementing is probably static, so that the *actual numbers* of dementing people aged 65–74 will be slowly falling. On the other hand, the proportion of the total population who are aged over 75 is rising fast and within that number those over 85 are increasing even faster, so the number of dementia sufferers over 75, and especially over 85, is rising rapidly. The problem of the 'old-old' with dementia is becoming more significant. The reason for these contrary changes in population structure are to be found back in the early years of this century. A 'baby boom' occurred between the 1890s and the beginning of the First World War. Unlike their predecessors, most of these babies survived infancy because of gradually improving standards of housing, sanitation and diet. They are now in their late 80s and 90s. The birth rate has, with ups and downs, been declining ever since that boom. So now, 80 years after the end of the war, the younger age groups, the 'young-old', are getting fewer, and in 10 years time the older groups will be beginning to diminish too.

The number of pensioners will rise by 3% between 1995 and 2005. It is only after 2005 that patterns will change more dramatically, with the 'baby boom' after the Second World War leading to substantially rising numbers and proportions of elderly people.

There are various other changes taking place. The older population of the future will have many advantages over preceding groups. The number who have never married, have never had children or are widowed will be reduced, and more will have residential property and occupational pensions. These changes are likely to have as much bearing on the needs of elderly people as their numbers.

The effect of the population changes (Table 3.1) on the number of dementia sufferers will vary between different parts of the country. We may assume that the increased age of the population will lead to a greater number of those with dementia and a greater number of more highly dependent patients. However, this is not necessarily the case, and the evidence is equivocal. A variety of genetic, environmental and social factors could lead a particular part of the world, or a particular local area, to have

Table 3.1 **A** Population changes in Britain 1901–2001, emphasizing the continuing rise in numbers of those aged over 75 and, even more dramatically, those over 85. **B** Projected population in Britain (adapted from Government Actuary's Department, 1996)

Year	Total population within each group (millions)				
	65–74	75–84	85+	Total >65	%>65
A					
1901	1.22	0.45	0.06	1.73	–
1921	1.9	0.7	0.08	2.68	–
1941	3.1	1.1	0.1	4.3	–
1961	4.0	1.9	0.3	6.2	–
1981	4.93	2.5	0.55	7.98	–
2001	4.5	2.98	1.03	8.51	–
change 1901–2001	+3.22	+2.54	+0.7		
% change	+260%	+600%	+1700%		
change 1981–2001	−0.39	+0.48	+0.48		
% change	−8%	+19%	+87%		
B					
1994	5.2	3.0	1.0	9.2	15.7%
2004	4.9	3.3	1.1	9.3	15.6%
2014	6.0	3.3	1.3	10.7	17.6%
2024	6.5	4.3	1.5	12.3	20.2%
2034	7.9	4.7	2.0	14.7	24.3%

significantly more, or significantly fewer, older people with dementia than expected.

Sex ratio

Many of those born just before the 'baby boom', and also many boys born during that boom, died in the First World War and the subsequent influenza epidemic. So the population of 85–100 year olds contains a very high proportion of women, and an especially high proportion of single women. The fact that men tend anyway to have a shorter lifespan than women means that those women who did marry usually survived, but are now widowed (the average expectation of life at birth is now about 78 years for a woman but only 73 for a man).

So, among dementia sufferers there is a large and increasing number of very old people and, because of the structure of the elderly population, the majority of dementia sufferers are very old women, especially very old women who are widowed or single.

In addition there is some evidence that the *prevalence* rate of DAT (the percentage of a particular age group who are affected at any one time) is greater in older women than in older men, thus increasing further the numbers of very elderly female sufferers. Among younger old people, VaD is relatively more common, though still not as common as DAT, and it may be more prevalent among men than among women.

We can immediately see some of the social problems posed by dementia.

WHO ARE THE CARERS?
Younger sufferers

There will be a significant increase in people aged 45–64 over the next decade, this being the peak age of those providing informal care, but at the same time the number of people at peak earning capacity (those aged 45–59) will increase by 13%. The small number of early-onset dementia sufferers (exact numbers are not known) are likely to have some support at home: they are most likely to be married with growing children; they may also have brothers and sisters; they may have parents or in rare cases even grandparents! The illness is devastating for these supporters, because it is so unexpected, but at least the supporters exist. Young people suffering AIDS dementia may not have partners, and 'buddy' schemes, which provide trained and supported companions, try to fill this gap. People with Down's syndrome who develop DAT in middle age are likely to have a good social support network, established over many years, but the supporters will need to make major adjustments, learn new skills, and cope with a changing, deteriorating condition.

Older women

The older a woman is when she develops dementia the less support she is likely to have. An elderly woman's husband is likely to have predeceased her and she may well live alone. Table 3.2 shows the living conditions of the general population of elderly people at home at different ages. Similar figures for the living conditions of the dementing elderly are difficult to obtain because of the difficulty in knowing how many sufferers there are in total. Some estimates suggest that 40–50% of sufferers who are at home live alone, which is the same proportion as in the non-demented population. We must assume that many very elderly ladies who are in the early stages of dementia live alone.

This is bad enough in itself, but, in addition, if we look for family support for these solitary ladies we are not likely to find much. Children may have moved to other parts of the country or abroad. Children who live nearby will be grown up and working. They are likely to have their own children to look after. Worse still, the patient's children may themselves be elderly. Trying to support a dementing parent can cause great disruption to family and social life.

Table 3.2 Where elderly people live (adapted from Hunt A 1978 The elderly at home. HMSO, London)

6% live in institutions
94% live in private households
Of those in private households, the percentages living alone are as follows:

	Men	Women
65–74	14	34
75–84	20	47
85+	27	50

In western countries one major change which will have a future bearing on the availability of carers is the great increase in the number of single-parent families, because of not having married or through divorce. The main carer of an older person with dementia is often a daughter-in-law. However, in an increasing number of cases there is no in-law, and it remains to be seen whether single men or women will be as willing to provide ongoing care and support.

Brothers and sisters, if they are still alive at all, will be elderly themselves and are likely to have their own health problems. If the patient has never married, she may depend on the goodwill of nieces or nephews. It is not unusual to find a number of elderly spinster and widowed sisters, some or even all suffering from dementia, being looked after by one or two long-suffering nieces, all that remains of the next generation.

Coping with dementia is a heavy burden for these relatives. In addition, elderly patients are of course quite likely to be suffering from a variety of other physical complaints and disabilities as well as the dementia.

Older men

For an elderly man with dementia the situation is likely to be different. Statistically speaking, he is more likely to have married and his wife is much more likely to be alive. Furthermore, the traditional role of the woman has been to look after men's needs, and many an older wife may simply be extending what she was already doing in the way of 'care' before her husband became ill. For a traditional husband, on the other hand, looking after a dementing wife is much more difficult. He is being asked to learn completely new skills in housework, cooking and giving personal care, so that he can take over from his wife as she becomes less and less capable.

The consequences of these population and social factors is that in practical terms there are three groups of elderly dementing people living at home. First, there is the elderly spinster or widow, living along with few available supporters. Second, there is the elderly wife or widow living with her husband or children. Third, there is the elderly man usually living with his wife. The needs of these three groups are often quite different, but we will return to that subject when we deal in Chapter 8 with the problems facing families.

WHO HAS DEMENTIA?

Who, then, are the sufferers? The research that is trying to find the causes of dementia has not yet succeeded in identifying any definite causal factors in either DAT or VaD, except that both are commoner in old age, that VaD is linked to the causes of arteriosclerosis and that there are some genetic factors in DAT.

Other factors (see p. 23 & 25) may increase or reduce the likelihood of developing one of the forms of dementia, but will not predict it in a particular person. Dementia is no respector of persons. No racial type, social class, intelligence level, personality type, occupation or life-style brings immunity. People with dementia will be found fairly evenly spread throughout different populations, with variations dependent mainly on the age structure of the population.

It is of course likely that different sufferers will try to cope with dementia in differing ways, and have different personal strengths and weaknesses, different family supports and different financial resources to deal with the associated problems. And, as we shall see, the problems presented and the outside help available to deal with these problems will also be very varied, even though the basic process of dementia is the same. So the experience of dementia will be unique in each individual case.

Cultural differences

It is very difficult to compare the prevalence of dementia across different cultural groups. Non-western societies in general tend to hold older people in high regard, and it is seen as a family's responsibility to care for its elders. Hence, contact with medical services is likely to be less, and does not occur until a later stage. In addition, there are difficulties in applying the various tests to groups with totally different ethnic backgrounds, leading to differences in diagnosis.

However, there are some known differences in prevalence among various ethnic groups. Vascular dementia appears to be commoner than Alzheimer's disease in Japan, China and Russia. It is not yet clear whether this is a true difference, or a result of regional differences in diagnostic practice. In the USA, African-Americans appear to suffer a higher proportion of vascular and alcohol-related dementias than people of European origin.

One study has shown dramatic differences in prevalence; there is an apparent rarity of dementia in some areas of Nigeria, and the ethnic population appears to be at lower genetic risk of developing Alzheimer's disease than African-Americans. Some protective factors, genetic or otherwise, may be at play here, and there may be opportunities for important research.

WHERE ARE THE SUFFERERS?

Patients at home

Some people find it surprising that any dementia sufferers at all are in their own homes. We can work out very roughly how many are at home by looking first at the percentage of the elderly population who are dementing (Table 1.1, p. 3), then at the percentage of the elderly population who are in care of any sort (Table 3.2) and finally at the proportion of those in care who suffer from dementia (Table 3.3). We can see that the figures in Table 3.3 are much higher than the figures for the general population in Table 1.1. So there is a concentration of dementing people in institutional care, which is not surprising.

What is more surprising is that when we join all these figures together (remembering that they are approximations and come from rather different sources) we can guess that the great majority of sufferers are not in institutions. Surveys have shown that the ratio of dementia sufferers at home to dementia sufferers in institutions is at the very least 4:1 and is more likely to be as high as 7:1. What is more, this proportion must be rising, since

Table 3.3 The proportion of residents in care who suffer from dementia

Type of care	Estimated proportion who suffer dementia
Psychiatric hospital	45–95% of those aged over 65
Geriatric hospital	45–65% of residents
Acute medical wards	5–15% of those aged over 65
Residential care (Part III or Part IV)	30–70% of residents
Private care	35–75% of residents

The figures are from a number of sources, and show the wide range of estimates which have been made the increase in the number of sufferers is probably outstripping the modest increase in the total number of beds available to care for them, and will continue to do so unless there are major changes in attitudes to institutional care (see p. 351).

Community support

So we can see that the needs of dementia sufferers are largely needs for community support. Countries and regions differ in how much they rely on institutional care, and how much on community care. But there can be few places in the world where the majority, or even a large minority, of dementia sufferers are in institutions. And even if we started to provide a lot of new residential, nursing home or hospital beds we would make little inroad into that proportion of those with dementia who are at home.

Looked at from the opposite direction, quite a small relative change in tolerance of dementia by families or communities could put a relatively very large load on institutional care systems. Furthermore, since the number of sufferers is constantly increasing, the chances of institutional care 'catching up' with the problem are very slim indeed. Whether we like it or not the 'community' has to learn to care.

Sheltered housing

People who live in sheltered housing form a rather special group. As a general rule, sheltered housing organizations quite reasonably feel that they cannot accept dementing people as new residents because of their expected decline in self-care and increasing inability to be independent. However, it is inevitable that there are many residents living alone in sheltered housing schemes who are at least mildly demented (estimates suggest about 12% of residents), and some more severely demented residents who are looked after by their spouses.

Psychiatric care

Looking now at those dementing people who are in institutional care of any kind (Table 3.3) we see some major implications for the staff of the various organizations. The figures for psychiatric hospital patients are not too surprising. The elderly in psychiatric hospitals are composed of three groups.

'Graduates', early-onset and brain-damaged patients. The first are those who have grown old in the hospital, having been admitted because of schizophrenia or other illness in early or middle life. These go under the somewhat ridiculous name of 'graduates', though their 'graduation' depends on failure of their treatment and rehabilitation rather than on any success. Included among these graduates will be some patients who have been admitted before the age of 65 because of a 'presenile' dementia, and who have survived the years into 'old age', and some patients with brain damage due to head injury, who may expect a normal lifespan with no further worsening of their mental impairment. Included among the larger group of people with chronic schizophrenia will be some who, separately from any intellectual decline associated with their schizophrenia (see p. 15), develop an 'ordinary' dementia in their old age.

'Functional' patients. The second group is of patients admitted after the age of 65 who suffer from psychiatric illnesses such as depression, mania and paranoid psychosis – the so-called 'functional illnesses'. Very few of these become longer-term hospital patients, partly because many are successfully treated, but also because there are alternative forms of residential care for mildly disabled elderly people which are not available to younger patients. Of course a few of this group develop dementia or are discovered to have it already.

The elderly with dementia. The third group are those who develop dementia in old age and require admission for care. This was for a time the biggest group, and the numbers involved were expanded steadily. However, over the past 20 years the policies of hospital closures and transfer to nursing-home care have caused a great decline in their numbers.

Less than one in ten elderly dementia sufferers ends their days in a psychiatric hospital. Dementia is in no way the sole responsibility of the psychiatric services. Only those who need specialized psychiatric nursing should be in a psychiatric hospital. These are the patients who as part of their dementia have severe behavioural disorders, emotional disturbances or disinhibition (Chapter 5). They are very much a minority of dementia sufferers, and since their particular problems are likely to be temporary their hospital stay should best be looked at as short-stay or medium-stay and not long-stay unless the person is in the terminal stages of the illness.

Medical care

Perhaps the figures for dementia in geriatric hospitals are not surprising either. We have already pointed out that many elderly patients with dementia suffer physical problems as well as their dementia; and at the later stages of a simple dementia the need for physical care is often the predominant problem. Furthermore, in VaD the strokes which are the essential cause of the dementia, or the other consequences of arteriosclerosis (Table 1.9), can leave the patient with major physical nursing needs.

We should expect, then, that there will be a high proportion of dementia sufferers in geriatric wards and an especially high concentration of those with vascular dementia. In general, these should be people who are not disturbed and therefore do not need psychiatric care, and they should not be independent enough to be looked after in a residential home. However, sometimes 'misplacement' can be a problem. Indeed, some geriatricians view people with dementia as inappropriate to their services, which they see as dealing with acute medical problems in old age. This policy is not realistic. People with dementia are as susceptible as any other people of their age to medical problems, perhaps even more so. They deserve equity of treatment from the specialist services, which will need to be able to deal with the special needs of people with dementia, the special difficulties of rehabilitation and ensuring compliance with treatment, and the special services which might be needed.

General medical wards

In general medical wards the figures are also high. Here there will be some patients who have true acute illnesses and also happen to be dementing. But in many parts of the country shortages of geriatric, psychogeriatric and residential care places lead to misplacement and 'bed-blocking' by patients who are no longer acutely physically ill, or who were admitted with no major medical problem in the first place and who cannot return home (p. 374).

The traditional organization of medical wards, to diagnose and treat complicated medical conditions without much need to investigate the patient's home circumstances or organize elaborate rehabilitation programmes, tends to work against the needs of the dementing elderly person. She gets stuck and quickly becomes no more than a name on a waiting list for long-term care.

Homes for the elderly mentally infirm (EMI homes)

Homes specifically for the care of dementing people are available only in some areas of the country. Ideally, these are for people who do not need specialized nursing care but who are a little too disturbed for ordinary residential home care. Where such homes exist they take some of the load away from hospitals, some from ordinary residential care and some from the community.

Residential and nursing homes

Homes vary greatly in their admission policies with regard to dementia. Most local authority residential homes ('Part III homes' in England and Wales, 'Part IV' in Scotland) wish to accept dementia sufferers only if their impairment is mild and they retain some degree of independence in self-care – dressing, washing, toileting and mobility. They also demand an agreement from the prospective resident that she wishes to enter the home. Theoretically, such an agreement could only be made by a mildly demented person with insight into her dementia, who retained enough reasoning power and understanding to come to an informed rational decision (see Chapter 9).

The figures in Table 3.3 tell a different story. A large proportion of residents in residential homes suffer from dementia. Sometimes the dementia will have begun or progressed after admission, but it is likely that more than half of those admitted to residential care are already dementing.

In homes run by voluntary bodies and in private residential and nursing homes the proportion of demented residents will vary depending on their individual policies. Some homes claim to specialize in looking after 'psychogeriatric' patients, some claim that they specifically do not look after this group.

But in fact in many such homes the proportion of dementia sufferers is as high as in local authority homes and sometimes even higher.

Statistical problems

The lack of accurate figures in this area emphasizes a general lack of knowledge of what dementia is and how it may be defined. Some homes will have residents who are very forgetful and are beginning to be less able to look after themselves, but who are nevertheless not thought of as 'confused' or 'demented'. There is an implication that 'demented' only refers to dementia with behaviour problems. The term 'psychogeriatric' is used, rather more accurately, to mean the same thing.

The only proper way to assess dementia is by a combination of intellectual and behaviour testing coupled with a view of the course of the illness (see Chapter 10). Only when we have figures based on such assessments will we know exactly where the dementing of our community are.

There is a further problem. When people go into residential care of any sort they often cross the artificial boundaries of the catchment areas set up by social services departments and health services. These boundaries rarely coincide. Therefore, it has so far been impossible to accurately identify how many people with dementia who originally lived in a particular area are still in their own homes, how many have moved to sheltered housing, how many to residential, nursing-home or EMI-home care and how many are in hospital either for short-term or longer-term care.

WHO GOES WHERE?

When we look at the proportion of dementing people at home and the figures for different types of care, as far as these are available, the question arises, 'why is one particular sufferer at home, another in residential care, another in hospital?'.

Many people in the different sectors of care talk about 'appropriate' residents. We would all like to be able to decide what sort of person should receive our own sort of care. And for planning purposes it would be helpful to be able to ascertain how much need there is in a particular community for the different sorts of care and from that agree on what to provide: how many home helps, how many sheltered home places and how many nursing care places, how many of the various types of hospital beds. Let us look at what happens in practice. Who goes where, and why?

Severity

The most obvious solution would be that those with mild dementia stay at home, those with moderate dementia go to residential-type care, those with severe dementia are in nursing-home or hospital care, perhaps the most severe cases being in geriatric hospitals, since the terminal stage of the illness involves the greatest need for physical nursing care.

The facts are very different. If we look at people in these various settings we find all stages of dementia in all settings, mild and severe at home, mild and severe in hospital, etc. Part of the reason for this is that there is a very humanitarian tendency of carers, whoever they are, and wherever they are, to wish for *continuity of care*. They keep on looking after the dementing person long after they are out of their depth, because they know and like the patient, can learn as they go along how to deal with the new problems that arise and know how disturbing a move can be. But we also have to explain why some severely demented people stay at home and, more particularly, why some of the more mildly demented get admitted.

Type of dementia

We have already mentioned that patients with VaD are more likely to need specific medical attention, because of strokes and the other problems of arteriosclerosis. For this reason these patients are more likely to be in a medical or geriatric ward. Further, the rather sudden changes in level of impairment and the acute confusional states which may accompany the little strokes of MID are likely to cause minor crises which lead to admission (Table 1.4, p. 8). The steadier progress of DAT patients and the fact that they are often in excellent physical health throughout most of their decline mean that they are less likely to need specific medical care. Younger patients of any diagnosis tend to be of more interest to neurologists because of their wider range of alternative diagnoses, such as Huntington's chorea and normal pressure hydrocephalus. This makes investigation more worthwhile and treatment sometimes possible. Organizations which help those infected with HIV are both being forced and choosing to set up support and care systems for AIDS dementia sufferers. But these are only trends. In practice, all types of dementia are found in all types of setting.

Specific problems

The list of 'crises' in Table 1.4 goes a long way towards explaining why it is not only the severely demented who are in care. Any of these crises can occur at any stage in the process of dementia.

Indeed, as we shall see in Chapters 5 and 7, the 'crises of behaviour' are more likely to occur early in the illness, when the patient still retains the ability to react and interact with others, still has the physical ability and motivation to act and still has some imperfect insight into what is happening to her.

Later, as these abilities are gradually lost, the behaviour problems may dissolve, to be replaced by a passive, withdrawn, insightless condition. The result is that some mildly demented people are admitted to long-term care because of one of these crises of behaviour, while quite severely demented patients may remain at home if they have never been particularly disturbed by their dementia and as long as support for their declining abilities can be gradually increased. The mild cases that are admitted because of a temporary disturbance may live on in care for many years after their disturbed period has passed. On the other hand, if a mild dementia sufferer who is disturbed can be maintained at home through the difficult period, by good community management and support, they may avoid the need to go near nursing care until late in the course of the illness.

It is not just crises, however, that lead to a demand for admission. The burden caused by any of a long list of problems (Table 3.4) can gradually lead to a situation where relatives feel they can cope no longer. Chapters 4, 5 and 7 will explain these problems in more detail, and Chapter 8 will deal with the feelings they evoke in the relatives. If we could develop ways of dealing with these problems we could avoid some premature decisions about long-term care and make 'community care' of the dementing a much more tolerable experience for patients and relatives.

Table 3.4 A checklist of the problems which may affect dementia sufferers and their families. The list is not exhaustive!

Problem	Examples
Memory impairment	Forgets appointments, visits, etc. Forgets to change clothes, wash, go to the toilet Forgets to eat, take tablets Loses things
Disorientation	Time – mixes night and day, mixes days of appointments, wears summer clothes in winter, forgets age Place – loses the way around house Person – difficulty recognizing visitors, family, spouse
Needs physical help	Dressing Washing, bathing Toileting Eating Housework Mobility
Risks in the home	Falls Fire from cigarettes, cooker, heating Flooding Letting strangers in Wandering out
Risks outside	Competence, judgement and risks at work Driving, road sense Gets lost
Apathy	Little conversation Lack of interest Poor self-care
Poor communication	Dysphasia
Repetitiveness	Questions or stories Actions
Uncontrolled emotion	Distress Anger or aggression Demands for attention
Uncontrolled behaviour	Restlessness, day or night Vulgar table or toilet habits Undressing Sexual disinhibition Shoplifting
Incontinence	Urine Faeces Urination or defaecation in the wrong place

Table 3.4 *Cont'd*

Problem	Examples
Emotional reactions	Depression Anxiety Frustration and anger Embarrassment and withdrawal
Other reactions	Suspiciousness Hoarding and hiding
Mistaken beliefs	Still at work Parents or spouse still alive Hallucinations
Decision-making	Indecisiveness Easily influenced Refuses help Makes unwise decisions
Burden on family	Disruption of social life Distress, guilt, rejection Family discord

Social factors

Support by families

Perhaps, however, the most important factors determing whether a dementing person stays at home or goes into care are social. Table 3.3 suggests how this occurs. Dementing patients who live alone with few supporters should be the principal users of long-term care. Those who live alone but get regular support are somewhat less likely to need long-term care early in their dementia, while those who live with their supporters may manage for much longer periods. Among this last group the crucial factor is whether or not the relatives are willing to continue caring.

It has been shown that where there was a good and strong relationship with the dementing person before the illness began (a good marriage, or a good parent–child relationship), the relative will be inclined to continue through the difficult early stages of dementia and on to the late stages when more physical care is required. Only quite severe problems will make such families want to give up, unless, of course, a deterioration in their own health makes it impossible for them to continue caring. If there has been a bad or weak relationship before, then there will be a general tendency to want to give up when the problems of caring for the dementing person begin to become a burden.

There are variants of these two patterns. Sometimes a bad relationship is nevertheless a strong one, for example, in the case of a couple who are bound together closely but nevertheless argue constantly, or that of a 'martyr' daughter who takes on an impossible load of caring for a domineering parent. Sometimes the relationship can change as the dementia progresses. Occasionally, for example, a difficult, aggressive husband becomes much more placid and likeable when dementing. Rather more frequently, less desirable characteristics which emerge as part of the dementia spoil a previously harmonious relationship and lead the relatives to the reluctant decision that they must give up caring.

Support for families

So the presence or absence of support and the willingness of the supporters to continue are very important factors. 'Support for the supporters' is also important. Looking after a dementing person is a 24 hour a day job and only the most loyal, patient and good-humoured relative can manage this alone. The job of caring is much easier where there is a large family or an extended family (involving different generations and different degrees of relationship) who can share the time of caring and can support each other.

Such sharing of care is unfortunately the exception rather than the rule in Britain, though more possible in many other countries. Increased social mobility, emigration, small family size, a wish for independence on the part of children and a feeling that a young couple should run their own lives with only their own children to care for, have all led to a decline in mutual family support. And, as already stated (p. 86), it is very often the case that such extensive family support simply cannot exist because the patient is a spinster or a widow with few children.

Our welfare systems have been developed partly to give expert advice and care to people in need of help but partly also to fill the gaps left by the decline in the ability of families and neighbourhoods to support their disabled relatives or neighbours. It remains a matter of debate whether the existence of such welfare systems encourages supporters to give up supporting, or at least try to give up, earlier than they would otherwise, and whether this is 'right' or 'wrong', but that is not the question here.

For dementia victims and their supporters an either/or dichotomy is unhelpful. It is not a case of the relatives either coping entirely by themselves or giving up entirely. There is a large grey area between these extremes. In this grey area the relatives cope better or worse depending on how supported they feel. If other members of the family, friends or neighbours can give this support, that is well and good. If not, then outside support systems, be they health service, social services, voluntary or private organizations, can fill the gap, working in partnership with the regular supporters and sharing care (p. 353). Most developments in geriatric and psychogeriatric care in the past 20 years have been of this supportive or gap-filling nature.

Financial aspects of care

The physical and cognitive aspects of dementia have an important bearing on where the person with dementia lives. As we have seen, the availability of informal carers is also important. However, another factor is the availability of resources, whether from the individual, from families or from society, to finance care.

The criteria for someone needing care in residential settings vary throughout the country. In general terms one might describe a hierarchy of care settings, from living alone to being cared for in a specialist NHS dementia unit (Fig. 3.1).

The difference in funding in different care settings is a major problem for families and politicians alike. NHS care is free to the patient and is available as need arises. Nursing home and

Living alone
↓
Living with relatives
↓
Residential care
↓
Nursing-home care
↓
Psychiatric ward
↓
Specialized dementia ward

Fig. 3.1 Hierarchy of care settings.

residential care, on the other hand, is means-tested. If a patient has any income or savings, or capital invested in their own home, this is taken into account but the figures are constantly changing. At present, if a person has under £10 000 available, care is 'totally free'. If above £16 000 they must be self-funded. Between these figures a proportion of any cost must be met. Obviously this means that those who have saved and thus are better off, have to pay more for care than their peers. This contradicts the Thatcherite concept of 'wealth cascading down the generations' and means that descendants feel (not without some justification) that they are being 'cheated' out of their rightful inheritance.

The 'greying' of the population is making this an increasing problem. So too is the encouragement (from the early 1980s on) given to people to buy their own (council) homes, meaning that more and more older people have some 'capital'. This problem is not unique to the UK. Governments throughout the world have to tackle this problem. In general, people are reluctant to vote for parties which will raise taxes, which makes it increasingly difficult to finance care in this way. One of the alternatives is that of insurance-based funding, either to totally or partially meet the costs of care. However, this is generally expensive and, unlike life insurance, 'may not be collected'; only a minority of people will ever need any form of institutionalized care.

Financial support for private residential or nursing-home care in the UK is available via local authority funding. As mentioned above, it is means-tested. It is also subject to an assessment by the local social work department, on behalf of the local authority. Budgetary constraints on local authorities have a part to play in this and in many areas the number of local authority-funded placements is rationed, making fiscal considerations more important than the need for care. Private care is more easily and more rapidly accessible to the relatively rich.

The purpose of Attendance Allowance and Disabled Living Allowance, and their independent living benefits, is to buy appropriate care. They can help to a greater or lesser extent in maintaining individual patients in their own homes. But very large amounts of money will be needed to make proper community care a realistic possibility for the majority of sufferers and so lessen the burden both on relatives and on institutional care. Again, *case management in the community* is intended to direct money which was previously used for funding residential and nursing-home care into helping people remain at home. It is unlikely to bring enough money with it to achieve this in most cases, and may even achieve the opposite effect.

In fact, some contradictory things are happening in Britain. The fight for better community care is going on in parallel with a growing tendency for elderly people and their relatives to accept the idea of going into residential or nursing home care. And there are political and financial pressures and 'market forces' which may encourage the latter trend, despite all the enthusiasm for community care.

Availability of services

Money can only buy what is available. A patient's desire to go into care, or the desire of her relatives to give up caring at home, can only lead to admission if a place in a home or hospital is available. It is easy to see that, if one form of care is not available in a particular area, there will be pressure on other services. They will be asked to do a job which they do not consider is theirs to do. They will be asked to take patients who are too fit or too unfit for their service as they see it. The full implications of this are seen in the 'balance of care' model (Table 3.5).

In the table we can see that not only is there a range of types of care (support at home, day support and residential care), but a range of providers of this care (health services, social services, voluntary bodies and private organizations.) Whenever help is needed from one of these services then whether or not the service

Table 3.5 The balance of care

Type of care	Providers of care (examples)		
	Health service	Social services	Voluntary and private
Home care	Nursing	Home helps Meals on wheels	Sitters and helps Nursing
Day care	Day hospital	Day centres	Day centres
Respite care	Hospital	Residential homes	Residential homes Nursing homes
Residential care	Long-term hospital	EMI homes Residential homes	Residential homes Nursing homes

is given depends largely on whether it is available. If the service is not available then a load falls on the services on either side or up or down the same column of the table.

If there is no day-hospital service for dementia sufferers in a particular area, then other day-care services will be taking some of these patients. These other services may justifiably protest that they were set up to do a quite different job – either to be a social club for older people or, in the case of medical day hospitals, to be a centre of nursing, physiotherapy and occupational therapy for people with specific medical problems (p. 375). Other patients and their supporters will have to struggle on at home with too little support, or may put a load on home-care services that they should not have to carry. Some families, with the backing of their general practitioner, solicitor or other advisors, will feel they cannot cope and so the patient will be prematurely admitted to care of one sort or another.

To give another example, the widespread absence of EMI homes means that many dementing patients who require supervision and simple basic care are having to be looked after in local authority residential homes which are not staffed or organized to give the necessary supervision and care, in private homes which may or may not have the necessary staffing, or in hospitals where the levels of staffing and training may actually be more than is needed, so that money is wasted.

At its simplest, the balance of care model shows that we need to have both adequate community services and adequate residential-care services if the problem of dementia is not going to be one merely of desperate 'gate-keeping', buck-passing and crisis decision-making. It also suggests that, in the meantime, the different services in a particular area should know as much as possible about each other in order to coordinate their planning and use of resources, so that the burden of care for patients who need a service that is not yet available is shared equitably.

The situation is made still more complicated by the fact that, to a greater or lesser extent, entry into or discharge from each 'box' in the balance table is determined by the policies of the 'gate-keepers' and these policies are all too often devised in a professional vacuum (Table 3.6). The British Geriatric Society and the Royal College of Psychiatrists have drawn up guidelines to help distinguish between a typical 'geriatric' dementing patient and a 'psychogeriatric' dementing patient, but most other

Table 3.6   Admission policies to care

Organization	Service	Contract	Compulsory powers	Who pays
NHS	Hospital long-stay care	'Treatment contract' not often explicit	Mental Health Act powers rarely used	Free at point of use Pension reduced
Social service departments	Residential care	Signed application	Guardianship rarely used	Client with SS support
Voluntary organizations	Residential care	Signed application	Guardianship rarely used	Client but SS support available
Private organizations	Residential or nursing care	Application may be made by relative or lawyer	Guardianship rarely used	Client but SS support available

admission policies are drawn up by organizations in isolation, and even the BGS/RCPsych guidelines can easily lead to dispute in a particular case.

What makes some of these admission policies unhelpful is that, while they determine admission or non-admission to some extent, other factors already mentioned are equally or even more important. Thus, a local authority may set up its residential home system with a policy of only accepting residents who have given informed consent to admission. If they stick rigidly to this then the care of dementing people who cannot or will not give this consent falls on the community, on the private sector or on hospitals – the balance of admission policies determines where a patient ends up. However, if there is a shortage of community supporters or of hospital services in the area, pressure for admission will outweigh the local rules about admission. Admission policies would be more effective if they were discussed and agreed between the different services (p. 383).

Transfer of responsibility for care

A further twist to this complicated tale is brought about by the growing enthusiasm for hospital closure and the transfer of hospital patients to private nursing homes. This may bring better, more accessible care in some cases. In others it may simply bring a change of institution and in a few cases may lead to worse care. It will certainly bring a change in the 'balance of care' and mean that to our list of forces pushing people into one form of care rather than another must be added government and managerial decisions and even managerial financial convenience.

There is some obvious unfairness in the present system. One person with dementia may be receiving the same type of care in a nursing home as a similar person is receiving in hospital. The first pays, the second doesn't. A person whose care needs are such that care in her own home is very expensive, but wants to stay at home, may be forced into even more expensive and unwanted nursing care, because it is more easily subsidized. It is for governments to find fair solutions to these problems.

CONCLUSION

We will return to these issues later when discussing the proper organization of help for dementia sufferers in Chapter 11. The importance of looking at these factors now has been to highlight the constraints within which we are all working in trying to care for a dementia sufferer.

The next six chapters will deal with the actual management of a case of dementia. We will concentrate on how the problems of dementia sufferers and their families arise. We will see that assessing problems and their causes can lead to clear ideas of the best management. But, at the back of our minds, we should be asking whether our plans to help are practically possible. Are the facilities available to manage our patients properly? Will our management materially alter the circumstances of the patient? Or will factors beyond our control determine what happens to her? This may seem a rather pessimistic stance. However, only by being aware of the constraints on our optimism can we see how to improve the outlook for the dementia sufferers of the future.

4

The losses of dementia

In this chapter we will look at the most obvious cause of problems in dementia – progressive damage to the brain causing gradual failure in its function. As we have just seen, the *problems* that bring dementing people to medical or other attention are varied and are not all to do with this central process of decline. Some problems arise from the symptoms of disinhibition and reactions to the illness (described in Chapters 5 and 7), while others are more to do with family interactions, social factors or the sufferer's previous personality. In assessment (Chapter 10), we will see that it is helpful to pin down and list these problems and then to look at what is causing them. So each of the next chapters is about a different *type of cause* of problems in dementia. We will see that one problem, say restlessness (see Table 5.2, p.

172) or depression (see Table 7.3, p. 221), can have a number of causes and will therefore appear in a number of chapters. First, though, we will look at how loss of brain function leads to problems for dementing patients.

Localization of function in the brain

As widespread areas of the brain are progressively damaged in dementia, the functions of those areas decline. We might expect that we could deduce the total effect of a dementia by adding together all these losses of function.

Localization of special functions

As Figure 1.2 (p. 4) shows, there are some parts of the cerebral cortex, such as the visual, auditory, sensory and motor areas, that do very specific things. Here, electrical activity in the neurones in very clearly defined tiny areas of the brain can be linked to very specific sensations or actions, for example, light shining on a specific point on the retina, sound of a precise frequency, touch on one area of skin or the tiny movement of a particular muscle. Damage by injury, operation or disease to one of these areas, or to the pathways to and from it, can lead to the loss of its specific action or sensation. An epileptic discharge in which the electrical charge is localized to a tiny bit of one of these areas (called a *focal* fit) would lead to its specific sensation or action occurring out of the blue. These three types of evidence, from measuring electrical activity, from 'lesions' (foci of local damage) and from the effects of focal fits, together with anatomical evidence of *connections* with other areas, have led to a better understanding of what these parts of the brain do. In fact, the diffuse damage of DAT and most other types of dementia tends to spare those areas which have very specific functions, at least until very late in the illness. In VaD, however, a localized stroke may damage such areas, or their connections, resulting in a paralysis or a gap in the field of vision, for example.

Wider areas

In other parts of the cortex quite specific functions are carried out by wider areas. Examples include those areas of the temporal and frontal lobes which are concerned respectively with the reception and expression of speech, the secondary sensory areas of the parietal lobe, where we appreciate shape, space and the other aspects of perception that translate sensations into patterns which can be recognized as objects, and the hippocampal region in the temporal lobe which is involved in recent memory. These wider areas are usually all affected in dementia, and loss of their functions is one of the most obvious aspects of the syndrome. So important is loss of the controlling function carried out by wide areas of the frontal lobes that it is the subject of most of Chapter 5.

In the last few years the PET and SPECT scanners (see p. 339) have been able to show that patients who have lost one or other of the functions have reduced blood flow and metabolism in just the parts of the brain that we might expect. This confirms that the damage in dementia can be quite clearly localized in the brain and that it can directly explain the impaired abilities of the patient.

General functions

But there are yet more subtle types of brain function. Functions like thinking, imagining, storing distant memories, intelligence, emotional responses, personality attributes and social habits are all carried out by making connections all over the brain. So it is impossible to localize any particular area which is specifically involved. It is to these functions the the 'law of mass action' applies (p. 11); the more damage, the more loss of function, no matter whether that damage is patchy or is worse in one area than another.

In reviewing the losses of dementia, we will see that these very general losses are much more insidious in their development, that they have very general effects on the life of the patient but that there is very little that can be done to help them. In the case of damage to more specific functional areas, assessment of the loss of function is simpler, and it is easier to work out how to help.

Complications in assessing losses

Simply adding up losses does not, unfortunately, describe the whole situation. There are complications.

Patients start their dementia from differing levels of function

A baseline is most important in assessing how much has been lost, but it is difficult to work out in retrospect what someone was like before dementia began. Even relatives can find it hard to be clear about how she functioned previously, and very careful questioning is required. Putting a specific date on memories of her past can be particularly helpful. 'She used to be able to count her grocery bill quicker than the check-out girl'. 'How long ago was that?'

Losses gradually increase

Dementing patients are rarely static at a particular level of function for long; they will usually be getting worse. Assessment of losses should therefore be a continuous process, not once-and-for-all. And each particular treatment or way of helping will have to be repeatedly reviewed.

Losses appear to vary

As well as this slow decline and the 'stepwise' variations in course which may occur in VaD (p. 29) there are other reasons why a patient's performance may be different at different times.

Time of day. Many relatives and staff describe a change, somewhere around 4 p.m. or later, after which the patient becomes more disorientated, muddled and restless (sometimes called *sundowning*). In some cases the pattern is reversed and the patient is worse in the morning, though this can also be a hint of a hidden depression. There are a number of possible explanations for this *diurnal variation* including fatigue, a natural search in the evening for familiar surroundings, diurnal variations in hormones and changes in light. Assessment should take both the morning and evening levels of performance into account.

Fatigue. We can see the effects of mental fatigue on a patient if we ask her to keep doing something such as reading or mental arithmetic for a period. Quite a small 'load' of mental effort fatigues her, she loses concentration and begins to make mistakes. This limits how much assessing and how much activity she can take part in at one session. It also indicates how much 'mental work' she can cope with in her day-to-day life.

Attention. Wandering attention is part of fatigue. As we shall see (p. 117), this is a major problem in dementia. How well the patient performs depends on whether she can attend to the task in hand or whether there are distractions which take her attention away. A noisy or busy environment will make her perform worse.

Emotional state. When the patient is angry, suspicious, anxious, depressed or uncooperative she is less likely to perform well than when she is in a good mood, confident and inclined to cooperate.

Who is present. Some people have an approach that helps patients to perform. They are probably calmly encouraging and know how to help the patient use her abilities to the fullest. They sense when her attention is wandering and know to give her a break. Others seem not to be able to do this. The result is that there can be two quite different assessments of the same patient. Sometimes this leads to argument, but in fact both types of information are important. One tells how good the patient can be in the right circumstances and suggests what we should be aiming for. The other points out how bad she can be and emphasizes problems that can arise. Instead of arguing, the people who are assessing should realize that together they have a fuller picture of the patient's ability.

Losses mean different things at different stages

As a particular deficit increases, two things may occur which alter its importance. First, its relation to other losses may change, so that the pattern of loss changes. For example, a patient's understanding may change faster than her ability to cope with money. At first her insight will match her deficits and she will realize that she is not managing perfectly. But later the loss of insight is greater than the loss of coping. Although she is now less able to cope with money she thinks that she has little or no problem.

Secondly, different degrees of loss may have different *practical significance*. Thus memory impairment in early dementia may lead to some silly mistakes but no major risk; later on the greater impairment leads to major risks, of fire, gassing, flooding; later still, if she goes into care, the practical importance of her severe memory loss becomes less again, because there will be people around to help fill in the gaps in her memory for her. As well as reassessing the degree of loss and the pattern of loss it is therefore also important to reassess the practical consequences of losses for the person's present life.

Losses interact

Because of the multitude of different types of loss of function that occur in dementia it is not surprising that losses affect each other in complicated ways. We will see that many different functions must interact to allow a patient to say what time of day it is (p. 118). And if one of these functions, say sense of the passage of time, is lost, all the other interacting functions, such as the ability to name, the ability to remember, etc., are rendered useless.

One loss can also make another *appear* worse. Thus if speech difficulties are present, either in comprehension or expression, the patient may seem more disorientated than she actually is, because she cannot understand the question or because she cannot express her answer. Another example of this interaction between losses is the apathetic lady, who has lost her motivation to look after herself as a direct result of brain damage (p. 136). We might show that her other deficits do not prevent her cooking for herself – she has all the necessary skills – but when we try to get her to cook she does not have the *will* to manage. The two deficits add together and she performs less well than she 'should'.

Disconnection

Very often a particular function seems not to be too badly damaged, but the *connections* between it and other important functions are lost. Thus a patient may be able to understand the word 'sit down' perfectly; she may be able to sit down perfectly; but if she cannot make the connection between the words and the action she will be unable to carry out this simple command, and so will appear extremely confused (or obstinate). Disconnection is extremely common in dementia. It interferes with many abilities and it is very difficult to overcome. We will see several other examples later in this chapter.

Other losses

By the time someone has developed dementia, many other losses may have occurred which are not directly a result of the pathological process itself. Older people have often lost many of their roles in life, sometimes due to death. Thus they have lost being a parent, a spouse or a sibling. Often they have lost independence, and may have lost being a householder. Health and general fitness levels have often deteriorated with age. The decline associated with dementia will make it much more difficult to come to terms with these losses.

From assessment to management

As we now examine some of the losses of dementia in detail we will see some general principles of assessment and management emerging.

Management often depends on looking at a loss in two different ways. The first is 'What can the patient not do?'. But perhaps more important is the second question, 'What can she still do?'. Assessment needs to be able to answer both questions. And the answers to the two questions will suggest different approaches to treatment. We can try to *fill the gap* of what is missing by external aids. Or we can try to ensure that she is using what she has left to the full – we can *stimulate* and encourage functioning. In a few cases *retraining* can actually extend the amount she can do and reduce the gap. We will see how these different approaches suit the various losses to a greater or lesser extent.

First, we will consider impairment of the ability of the brain to take in information, for everything that we do depends on our understanding of the world about us. Then we will look at failures in the ways that the brain stores information. Next we will examine general losses in the processing abilities of the brain, and finally in expression and action. This is the best sequence to follow, for each of these types of loss interferes with the next, and there is less interaction back along the list. A difficulty in understanding speech affects the patient's ability to express speech (p. 115). But a difficulty in expressing speech will not affect her ability to understand others.

RECEIVING INFORMATION

PERCEPTION

Agnosia

Many difficulties in perception can be caused by the progressive damage to the parietal lobes which is common in DAT, but occurs also in other dementias. For example, the functions of feeling or seeing the shape of something, appreciating the position of an object in space, distinguishing right from left and recognizing faces all involve parietal areas. These are part of the process of perceiving what objects are.

The practical effects of such losses, which mostly go under the name of *agnosia* (Greek for 'not knowing'), can be enormous. If common objects are not perceived properly they may be used for the wrong purpose or become useless. Agnosia goes some way to explaining why a dementing lady puts the milk in the sugar bowl or does more risky things like putting her underclothes under the grill, although poor attention, dyspraxia (see p. 140), perseveration (p. 153) and poor connections in her thinking may also be involved. Impaired ability to see where things are in space may explain why she misses her chair, although poor mobility may also play a part. Poor localization of bodily sensation or failure to recognize parts of one's own body (called *autotop-agnosia* – 'not knowing one's own place') create difficulties in complaining about or diagnosing physical illnesses. Agnosia puts a great barrier between a patient and the outside world. It can lead to dangers in the home and limit her ability to use everyday objects, or indeed to do anything to care for herself.

Recognition

An added problem is that the sense of *familiarity* of an object, place or person may be lost. In focal epilepsy of the temporal lobe a patient may have the experience of *déjà vu* (the feeling that an unfamiliar object has in fact been seen before) or *jamais vu* (that a familiar object has never been seen before). We can therefore guess that this type of recognition is a function of the temporal lobes. In dementia this function is gradually lost. The result is that even though the patient perceives her room as *a* room, and can understand what the objects in it are, yet she does not recognize them as *her* room and *her* objects. The consequences of this jamais vu or strangeness can be that she wants to 'go home' from her own house, or that she thinks people are bringing in strange furniture or objects, or that she wishes to put the 'strange man', who is actually her husband, out of the house.

This particular problem of not recognizing faces has been called *prosop-agnosia* and of course can be distressing to relatives.

In another version of it – *autoprosop-agnosia* – the patient does not recognize her own face in the mirror and may complain of intruders in the house – the so-called *mirror sign*. (This term has also been used to describe the tendency that some people with dementia have to simply stand and stare at themselves in the mirror for long periods of time.) A third version is the *picture sign*, in which the patient does not recognize that photographs or characters on the television are not real and may talk to them or complain of their presence.

The forms of agnosia may largely explain some of the delusions which people with dementia may suffer from.

Perception of speech

The recognition of words out of the millions of sensations of sound that go to the auditory cortex is a function mainly of the temporal lobes. Damage here leads to a lack of understanding of what is heard, called *receptive dysphasia*. Dysphasia means 'difficulty with speech'. Reading ability resides in the parietal lobe and damage here can lead to *dyslexia*. In earlier stages of dementia patients seem still to be able to read and pronounce even quite complicated words, though not necessarily to understand their meaning or use them in speaking. This retained ability can be used to indicate how intelligent the person was before their dementia began. At later stages receptive dysphasia and dyslexia become more obvious.

These difficulties in recognizing words in speech or writing apply not only to what we say or write to the patient. They also affect *her own* words. She does not know whether what she has said or written makes sense or not, and so may produce rubbish words without realizing it. Any attempt to communicate with her or by her becomes extremely difficult. She may become annoyed that people do not understand her and may think they are being deliberately difficult or are playing games with her.

Understanding

At a 'higher', more general level, the dementing person's capacity to grasp her situation and understand what is going on, to get meaning out of it, declines. Consequently, she may misinterpret her situation or be bewildered by it. Again, she will have difficulty in realizing the problem and so may appear unconcerned or get annoyed. She understands little, but acts as if she appreciates the situation fully.

These problems of general grasp usually involve loss of the connections between perception and logical reasoning. A patient may, for example, see that it is dark outside and be able to say so, and yet not connect that accurate perception logically, so she says that it is the middle of a lovely day. She may see and understand the meaning of the word 'Toilet' on a notice, but walk past it because she does not connect it to the feeling that she needs the toilet now. Her good perception has been useless.

Assessment of perceptual losses

There are a number of 'parietal lobe tests' which identify agnosias. For example, deficits in this area can be shown by difficulties in recognizing by touch alone objects placed in the hand, and by difficulties in copying shapes accurately without missing bits out or distorting them. Receptive dysphasia is most easily tested by checking if the patient can follow instructions of an increasingly complicated nature, starting with, say, 'Stick out your tongue', going on to 'Touch your right ear with your left little finger'. It is important also to test reading ability.

Management of receptive losses

Most of the ways we try to help disabled people require that they understand what is happening – instructions, physical aids, activities. It is very difficult, therefore, to help someone who has a problem in perception of understanding. If she is not aware that there is a problem, as is so often the case, things are even worse, for she will not see why we are trying to help her.

Simplifying

The first principle is to lighten the load of information. We should give very simple instructions, use simple aids and activities, and avoid confusing matters by long explanations which may merely be misinterpreted. The patient also needs to be encouraged to simplify her speech and actions. We should intervene and try to pin her down to simple answers, or to doing one action at a time. For she will tend to ramble on, not realizing that her speech and actions are not making sense.

Getting round the problem

A second approach is to avoid the problem and try to get information across by another route. Thus, if reading is difficult, picture messages or 'charades' may help, though unfortunately much of our thinking, even about pictures, is done in words. If recognizing objects or places is a problem then a label or notice (TOILET) can sometimes help. The speech therapist may have particular ways of getting round problems of reception of speech. But there will be great difficulty in giving any form of help when it is the more general aspects of understanding that are impaired. We are likely to end up having to do things for the patient rather than help overcome the problem.

ATTENTION AND CONCENTRATION

Attention is the ability to *focus* one's mind and consciousness on a particular object, task or thought (see p. 149). Concentration is the ability to *sustain* attention over a period of time. Even if we can gain the patient's attention, and even if she can perceive what we say, she may not be able to keep concentrating long enough to take in all the information we give. Poor concentration is very common in dementia and it causes enormous problems, not only in understanding the world, but in doing things as well. Relatives frequently complain that they could cope much better if only the patient could sustain some activity. She sits down with the paper and attends at first, but quickly loses concentration and wants to do something else. She starts to cook a meal and drifts off in the middle, leaving a saucepan to burn dry.

This inability to settle at anything inevitably leads on to the problem of restlessness. But most of all it interferes with our attempts to help. Any retraining or activity programme may founder because the patient's concentration cannot be maintained. She simply gets up and walks off. This can make group activities in particular rather disorganized affairs. In severe dementia the ability to attend is lost completely so that engagement in any activity is impossible and little in the outside world 'gets through' to the patient.

A repeated and active effort by family or staff to gain the patient's attention can overcome the problem to some extent, but she may then become easily fatigued or, feeling the pressure on her, collapse in emotion (p. 161). Games and other activities in which she can feel involved can improve concentration, sometimes quite dramatically. It might even be possible to devise simple variants of the video games which engross younger people and so extend concentration in time, but it remains to be seen how much of this improvement would generalize to other activities.

ORIENTATION

Orientation is not a simple process. There is no 'orientation centre' in the brain. Our knowledge of where we are in time, place and person depends on the combination of a number of functions, all interconnected.

In order to know what time of day it is, we need an inner sense of the passage of time and continuity; we need a recent memory of what has already happened today or when we last looked at the time; we need a longer-term memory of what usually happens at this time of day; we need to have evidence from our senses, about the light, about what other people are doing; we need to be able to connect all this logically to a particular time. Alternatively, we need to be able to read a watch or clock and understand the significance of what we have read. Or we must be able to recall what time we were told it was by someone else. To know the day, week, month or year requires even more memory function, and all require the ability to grasp the question being asked, process it properly and express the answer in words either to ourselves in thought or to others in speech. Similar skills, together with a sense of space and the ability to recognize objects, places and faces, are required for orientation in place and person.

Verbal and behavioural orientation. We can describe two general types of orientation, *verbal* orientation and *behavioural* orientation, depending on whether the ability to speak is involved. Many patients cannot *say* where they are, or cannot use words to *think* where they are, but are nevertheless orientated to the geography of where they are living. Many cannot tell the time, but will still do roughly the right things at the right time of day. This is behavioural orientation based on using the senses, both outer and inner, as opposed to verbal orientation. Other patients can say what the time is, or where they are, but act as if they were disorientated because they cannot connect their verbal knowledge to practical action.

Testing orientation. The questions which test orientation are: 'Can you say what time it is, what day is it, what month, what year?'; 'Where are you, what is this place?'; and 'Who are these people around you?' (not 'Who are you?' which is a question of *identity*). As with all tests of mental function, orientation tests need careful interpretation to work out which actual functions are impaired. And remember that another single serious defect, for example, in sight or speech, can make someone appear much more disorientated than they actually are.

Importance of orientation. Orientation questions, properly interpreted, can clearly be useful as part of a very general test for brain damage. It is important, though, to assess also the *practical importance* of orientation for the patient. A person at home needs a general sense of time of day, and at the very least a sense of day and night. They usually need to know what day it is, for example, that the home help comes, or which is pension day. Months and years are less important. In a residential home, knowing meal times is useful but other orientation in time is not essential, for the staff will fill the gap. Orientation in space is vital in one's own home, and not knowing where one is when outside can be disastrous. In a residential home knowing the name of the home is not important, but knowing the way to the toilet and to the bedroom are. Orientation in person can prevent a patient at home being exploited by bogus workmen. In care it is merely reassuring to know who people are.

Helping orientation depends on helping each of the skills involved in this complex process. But there are some general ways of helping, including reality orientation programmes and orientation aids.

Reality orientation (RO)

This technique was first used in the USA in the 1950s, in the back wards of big mental hospitals, where elderly long-stay residents (many not suffering from dementia at all) tended to have withdrawn and got out of touch with everyday life. The results later encouraged the use of RO for dementia sufferers.

Suitable patients

Basically, the technique consists of presenting the facts of orientation repeatedly to patients, either in a group or individually, with positive reinforcement and encouragement. We could not expect such a technique to reverse the process of dementia, and in patients who have some specific deficit in speech or spatial sense, etc., it is unlikely to be helpful. Furthermore, it is particularly unlikely that patients who are severely demented would be in touch enough to be helped. On the other hand, RO is likely to help patients with milder dementia who are withdrawn, and are therefore not using their remaining faculties to the full, and also those who are lacking in confidence.

Group RO technique

A group of dementia sufferers, no more than six if possible, sits in a group. Communication is difficult for bigger numbers and distractibility becomes a major problem. Special help should be available for those who are partially deaf, so that they can hear the rest of the group, and for the partially sighted. It is important to focus the attention of the group, by repeated reminders of the subject and by the use of a reality orientation board, which has the questions of orientation on it. The questions on the board should be answered during the session. The patients are thus actively involved in putting on the board the day, date, etc., the place, the weather, items of news or events happening in their lives or in the world at large.

The group leader adopts an encouraging attitude, not showing up a patient's disorientation but helping her work out the facts, encouraging questions and praising her when she is even moderately successful. The group members should also be encouraged to help each other in working out the answers. The leader does not criticize or blame patients for failure. What is said in later sections (p. 327) about the need for a slow pace, calm, simplicity, repetition, cueing and forced choice to help recall memories are all vital if RO is to be effective.

Effects

The question whether RO like this is effective remains open. There is some evidence that it is partly effective over short periods for some people. What is certain is that the technique has a generally stimulating effect on patients and can improve morale and interest among staff. So it should not be dismissed.

24-hour orientation

Possibly more important than the specific technique of RO groups is the idea that has grown from it, of carrying on RO techniques as part of individual care plans throughout the day. It is, after all, unlikely that patients will remember the facts of orientation learnt in a 'classroom'. In fact, the techniques used in '24-hour orientation' are really designed to help a number of the different deficits that add up to disorientation, and so will be discussed in other sections as well.

Family and staff are asked to remind the patient repeatedly of orientation and to correct disorientation. This should not be done in a disapproving way and not by simply telling her the right answers. She can be asked to use her senses to work out where the place is, reminding her of familiar objects or people – 'Who are those people there?', 'Nurses.' 'So where are we now?', 'A hospital.' She can be asked to use her memory and logic to work out the time – 'Have you had your lunch yet?', 'Yes.', 'So what time of day will it be now?', 'Afternoon.' As with RO, a positively encouraging approach works best. This enables her to use her abilities to the full and it may even be that with training she will improve her ability to work out where she is or what time it is. The *verbal* element (knowing the name of the place, for example) is always less important than the *behavioural* (finding her way around), and gaining her active *participation* (helping her find her way to the toilet by herself) teaches better than simply *giving* information ('The toilet is the third door on the right').

Orientation aids

External aids to orientation are also important. Clear, simple labelling of rooms or objects can help, but once again the active participation of the patient in learning to use aids is vital. It is not helpful just to put up a 'Toilet' sign. The patient should be directed to it, asked to read it and then reminded of the association between going to the sign, reading it and finding the toilet. The placing of signs is important. They should be at eye level, and they should stand out clearly from the background so that there are no distractions.

The orientating attitude

Encouraging orientation depends most of all on the attitudes of family or staff. If they take the attitude that a dementing person is bound to be disorientated and therefore cannot be expected to tell the time or find her way around, they will tend to take over and allow her to give up working out where she is. The result is that she will withdraw from day-to-day reality. If they assume that 'dwelling in the past' is normal in dementia, they will let her talk of long-dead people as still alive, or talk of going to work, without helping her correct her mistakes. If they take a critical view they may argue with her over orientation.

The 'orientating' attitude is one which gently reminds her of the present reality and gently corrects mistaken ideas. If she loses her way, we help *her* to find it again. If she thinks she should be at work, we help *her* remember how long it is since she retired. She is *actively involved* in working these things out and so should not feel criticized. This attitude involves hard work, time, repetition and patience. It will not succeed in completely orientating the very disorientated, or correcting all mistaken beliefs. But if it works at all it can help the patient's confidence in using her own senses. It can make her feel less detached and improve the relationship between family and patient or staff and patient.

This is not true in all cases. A few sufferers are upset or irritated by attempts to help them orientate and it is most important that these techniques should be used sensitively and with respect, not as a blunderbuss 'therapy' for anybody and everybody who has dementia.

STORING INFORMATION

MEMORY

There are several stages involved in memory. If we come across a new word, say 'Alzheimer', we must first be able to hold it in *attention* and *perceive* it properly. Then we *register* it in a store, *coded* in a way that will help its recall. Thus to register it better we must make links with *dementia* – it must have some *meaning*. If there is some *emotional* connection with the word (a relative suffers from DAT) or it is otherwise important (for an exam, for example) that will encourage registration. And we can further improve our chances of recalling the word if we note that it begins with 'A', sounds German and is part of 'DAT', using mnemonics. When stored there may be a *time* or *place* coding as well as coding by meaning ('I first heard the word *then* and *there*'). So we can place memories in sequence. The store will gradually decay (we *forget* the memory) and we need reinforcement or *rehearsal* of the memory from time to time if it is to persist. Finally, we need to be able to *recall* it, using its code or codes to look up the correct files, as it were. So, when we think of types of dementia, or other associated ideas or feelings, the word Alzheimer is 'waiting' ready for use and can be easily retrieved.

Short- and long-term memory

The very short-term retention which consists of keeping some bits of information in mind for a few seconds is called *short-term*, *immediate* or *primary memory*. There is a limit to the number of items that we can normally keep in this memory store; this can be checked easily by testing the number of digits that we can keep in mind long enough to repeat back immediately (the 'digit span' test). Most people can manage no more than the seven figures of a telephone number (unless they can 'code' a number into chunks, as in 10661939452468). Retention for any longer than seconds involves a more elaborate mechanism called *recent memory*; and retention from months or years ago is called *remote memory*. Many psychologists make no distinction between recent and remote memory calling it all *long-term memory* or *secondary memory*. So long-term memory may involve anything from remembering what we had for breakfast (recent) to events from our school days (remote). Most items of memory enter the secondary stores from the primary store. If we do not have a special reason for storing the word 'Alzheimer' and so do not encode or rehearse it, it will disappear from memory after a few seconds of first reading it. Seeing it or hearing it several times and realizing its importance helps get it stored in the recent or remote memory. To confuse matters, many doctors and others call recent memory 'short-term'. It is therefore best to avoid the use of the words 'short-term' and 'long-term' altogether; this will prevent confusion.

Types of memory

There are many different things which we have to remember. Most is known about memory for words and numbers, and memory for events (*episodic memory*). But there is also memory for other information from the senses, including visual memory for shapes, objects and people, memory for non-verbal sounds such as music, memory for smells, tastes and bodily sensations, *geographical memory*, which is the ability to remember one's way around by having a mental map of an area; there is a sort of muscular memory or memory for actions or gestures that we use (*procedural memory*) and there is even *future memory*, the ability to remember what you were going to do (the ability to follow the instruction 'Come and see me in 5 minutes' for example).

Although these different types of memory probably share some pathways and mechanisms in the brain, they are also likely each to involve specific areas or connections. So damage to one area of the brain may impair one type of memory more than another. A good example of this is that damage to the left temporal lobe often causes impairment of verbal memories but leaves musical memories intact.

Memory in dementia

Since the ability to register, store and recall memories involves attention, perception, thinking and imagining (to work out coding), sense of time and place, the capacity to store enormous quantities of information and the ability to recover it when needed, and since all the various different types of memory just mentioned are needed for daily survival, we can guess that a good memory requires that many areas of the brain and their interconnections are working well. There are problems in all aspects of memory function in dementing patients. Many psychologists have found particular problems in coding of memories and in retrieval from the memory store in DAT, and have suggested that in the 'subcortical' dementias retrieval only may be impaired. There are still some arguments among the experts about which aspects are more or less affected in different groups of sufferers, but these only apply to the milder stages. In the most severely demented people we must assume that there is little or no registration, storage or recall of any type of memory.

The temporal lobes are particularly important in recent memory, and they are damaged in most, if not all, dementing people. Indeed, in DAT there is quite selective damage to the hippocampus and surrounding structures. This is the area which is also damaged in Korsakoff's syndrome (p. 69), in which recent memory becomes very severely impaired. But the more widespread damage in dementia means a more general destruction of memory functions.

Immediate or short-term memory

Unlike patients with Korsakoff's syndrome, many dementia sufferers show an impairment of immediate memory. This is connected with their difficulty with attention (p. 117). The result is that, except in the mildest stages, a dementing person will be able to hold fewer items in the short-term store than a normal person. So she may be unable to keep a telephone number in mind while she dials it, unable to keep the shopkeeper's total bill in mind while looking in her wallet, or keep the amounts of money she is counting in mind as she counts it. She may not be able to keep anything more than a simple instruction in mind while carrying it out (such as 'Go through that door and turn left'), and this applies to her own instructions to herself ('To work the cooker I have to turn that knob and then that one'). The widespread and disastrous effects on every aspect of life that follow this loss can be easily imagined.

We cannot trust the short-term store of a dementing person. We should expect her to be able to cope with only one or two bits of information at a time. We should split information into small components, or else try to use other types of memory if more complex information has to be remembered.

Long-term memory (recent and remote)

But longer-term memory, both recent and remote, is impaired as well. Recent memory is most affected in the earliest stages of Alzheimer's dementia. Most of the recent memory loss is due to hippocampal damage, but part of it follows from the short-term memory problem. For if a patient cannot hold a memory, for example a telephone number, in the short-term store for a few seconds she will not be able to register it in the recent memory store to remember it a few minutes later. And if, because of damage to the hippocampus, she cannot keep the number in her recent memory in order to rehearse it, or realize that it is important, it will not get into long-term storage. Remote memories from before the dementia began are in the store already, and so do not suffer because of the short-term and recent memory problems. So, for a time, some important old telephone numbers will be remembered. But these stored remote memories decline too and are forgotten. So a well-known telephone number, such as her own, will gradually be forgotten. Gradually in fact the patient remembers less and less of her earlier life, leaving only islands of very firmly fixed memories, and eventually nothing at all.

In the early stages of DAT the greatest memory defects are in coding and retrieval of recent memories. The patient has difficulty in putting a *meaning* on the memory by associating it with other things, so as to store it in a particular mental compartment or file. She has difficulty associating the word Alzheimer with the compartment labelled 'dementia' and linking it with other ways of remembering, such as 'begins with A', 'German name', 'DAT', to retrieve the memory. And recognition must be impaired – she cannot recognize the word as one she has seen before, even though it has been properly stored (p. 114).

Testing memory

There are very many different tests of memory, covering all the different stages and varieties of memory. In normal practice psychologists and doctors test immediate memory by asking the patient to repeat something back, say a list of numbers. They ask her to keep a name and address, if she can register it, in her recent memory store for a few minutes. And they ask questions from his history, or historical dates that she should know, to test whether she has a good remote memory store. If the patient is dysphasic, visual tests may be used, for example remembering pictures. These tests help in diagnosing dementia, and in working out how severe it is, but may not tell us much about the practical effects of memory problem (see Table 3.4, p. 98 for examples).

Management

Self-help

How can we help these problems? Retraining memory to improve it might seem attractive, but there is no evidence that this works. However, the patient may be able to find ways of making more effective use of her existing memory. The difficulty of registering memory may be helped if she rehearses the memory over and over again, and by mnemonics (coding by initials, rhymes or other associations). The problem of storing can be overcome if she writes things down, so that the memories do not have to be stored mentally to the same extent. She will be able to learn these techniques up to a point. However, we should always assess how far she can go. The patient who ends up rehearsing a name but cannot remember its significance, or who remembers a mnemonic but cannot remember what it is for ('I had to remember something beginning with N'), or has a pile of scraps of paper with reminders which she cannot understand, will simply be anxious or frustrated.

Outside help

We may be able to encourage better use of the patient's memory by outside help. Registration of a word or fact may be helped by offering links and mnemonics to help remind her of its meaning. Storage may be helped if the information is repeated from time to time. Recall may be helped by two useful methods. One method uses *cues* and involves giving a hint of the answer or part of the answer, or reminding the patient of a mnemonic. Some mildly demented people can use cues very well ('What you had to remember was about your money'). The other method is *forced choice*. A list of possible answers is given and the patient is asked to pick out the correct one. If her recognition of memories is retained better than 'free' recall, then this method can be particularly helpful. We should not say, 'Who visited you?' but 'Was it the nurse, or the doctor, or your sister who visited?'.

A particular problem is the time coding of memories. Almost all dementia sufferers mix up the timing of their memories, thinking that some old event happened recently or that things happened in a different order than they actually did. It is this problem which makes the question, 'How long has your memory been bad?' so nonsensical. We may have to try to put in the correct time sequence for her ('That happened a long time ago, didn't it?', 'That was before you retired?'). In general it has to be said that if a patient has lost the ability to code memories into the memory store in the first place, then no amount of help will recall them.

Using the different types of memory

Another way to help memory is to use the different types of memory more extensively. If verbal memory is most affected, then visual presentation may be more effective: not, 'I'm leaving your money in the drawer,' but 'Look, here's your money, I'm leaving it in that drawer there'. Better still may be memory through action – procedural memory: 'Come, we'll put the money in the drawer,' 'Do you remember where you put the money? Show me where it is'. Best of all is to use as many types of memory as possible for the same thing. In reminiscence work, where the idea is to stimulate old memories, talking over old times is not enough. Pictures, music, dancing, actions (using an old-style iron, visiting an old school, going over actions used at work) and even tastes or smells can often bring a much richer recall that is both satisfying to the patient and informative to others.

Lightening the load

Where these techniques do not work, or have limited effect, we may have to lighten the load on the patient's memory. The most obvious way to do this is to *simplify* the information that the patient needs to remember, and advise her against trying to remember too much ('There are only two things you need to remember today').

The other way is to provide an *'external store'*. I have already described how she may learn to do this for herself by making notes or 'memoranda'. More often the store has to be provided by others. Thus, if she has to remember that Tuesday is pension day, the memory can be stored on a notice board, or in a relative's memory. She then finds out by looking at the board (assuming that she has a way of knowing which day is Tuesday and can find the board!) or the relative can ring up to remind her. She will need a lot of encouragement to use the aids that we provide ('Always look at the board'). Many mildly demented people admit that they have given up using their own memory and instead use their spouse or children as a memory store.

The future

Few people over the age of 40 have learnt to use computers early in life when very fixed memories can be formed. New learning

(p. 131) is extremely difficult for dementia sufferers. This means that it will be some decades before significant numbers of elderly sufferers will be familiar enough with computer techniques to make much use of their artificial memories. If electronic aids to memory are to be devised they will have to be in a form that the patient can cope with. Even a digital watch or a pocket calculator are likely to be, and remain, mysteries to the majority of sufferers who did not learn their use as children or young adults. And messages that appear on a TV screen are more likely to bewilder and frighten a dementing person than to help.

However, simple memory aids can be developed. The most useful is a clock or watch which can give a spoken or printed reminder of something the patient has to do at a particular time. This can help pill taking, getting up in the morning, eating a meal that has been left. But the patient has to be able to understand the messages and will need considerable training in using such aids.

Reminiscence

Reminiscence is a normal part of old age. It is normal for an older person to look back over life, review its ups and downs, perhaps dwelling especially on the good things, and try to put it all in perspective. This 'life review' is healthy and can be very enjoyable. For many the sharing of memories is stimulating. From this has arisen a variety of activities ranging from local history groups to 'reminiscence theatre', from old-time song and dance sessions to slide shows of old scenes.

Reminiscence like this is recreational. But it may also be therapeutic. For older people may have unfinished business from the past – regret, bitterness, sadness, anger, guilt and disappointment – which still affects their lives. There may be a relative who has never been forgiven, some distressing event that has never been talked about in the family, wishes and hopes that have never been fulfilled. Discussing these things can help the process of putting the past in perspective.

In both recreational and therapeutic reminiscence, sensitivity is needed. For one person's past joy is another's disappointment, and we can be surprised at the distress caused by old memories. Some people are actually stuck with their memories and do not wish to change. They have bad memories but have no wish to forgive or forget them. They do not use reminiscence positively but dwell on these bad memories. Others avoid any bad memory and look at the past through rose-tinted spectacles.

Reminiscence in dementia

For dementing people this review of remote memories can be useful, particularly as a stimulating recreation. In the absence of new recent memories being laid down, the dementing person has only her remote memory to fall back on. And with the uncertainties and confusion of her present life, those old memories can be an important solid support. They are almost the only real evidence she has of her identity as a person.

So her confidence can be improved by reminiscing. And the amount of material that comes from her store of memories can be surprising. Using the different types of memory – old tunes, pictures, going to old haunts, using scrapbooks, handling old household implements, going to a local museum, even cooking – can help her get access to that store in a way that her day-to-day life does not. The delight of recognition and the even greater delight of being able to explain something to a younger person is a great help. There too, emotional reactions may vary, however, for some old memories can be upsetting.

It is best if reminiscence is combined with a reality orientation approach (p. 119). We should not expect dementing people to do much therapeutic work on the past; they are unlikely to be able to change their attitudes to people or events of the past, to come to terms, to reconcile or otherwise put the past in emotional perspective. But we can try to use memories to help the patient understand the passage of time – that those things happened years ago, that things are different now, that those relatives are now dead and that another generation has come along, that it is 20 years since retirement, etc. Once again, sensitivity is needed. This reality can be very shocking. Finding out, as if for the first time, that one's spouse is dead, or that one is no longer at work, is distressing. If we do introduce reality, we must be prepared to cope with these reactions. We must learn to remind gently and not force the truth on to the patient.

Reminiscence work for people with dementia is, however, generally very rewarding. The stimulation of memory, the release of positive emotions and the confidence gained from remembering at all seem to increase the patient's interest and alertness, at least temporarily. Even more than with reality orientation, reminiscence helps family or staff to see the real person, her background, achievements and personality, in a way that improves their interest and respect. It is engaging for both. But like RO it should not be seen as a 'therapy for all'. It should be used sensitively with those individuals who can benefit from it.

NEW LEARNING

During the long decline of dementia, patients have to cope with many new situations both due to the ordinary changes of life and as a consequence of the illness. They have to cope with new home situations, new people, new places and new routines. Unfortunately, they have great difficulty with new learning. Learning is another very general function of the brain and requires the making of multiple complicated connections. It overlaps, of course, with memory function but requires other abilities as well.

For example, if a patient needs to learn to use a new cooker, she must remember that it is new and not try to work it like the old one, remember the instructions on how to use it, think out how it works and then learn to manipulate the controls semi-automatically. As well as having specific deficits in these areas, she will show a general loss of ability to learn new actions. We should not expect her to do well.

It is a wise general rule, therefore, to keep new learning to a minimum. If it is vital for her to learn something new then the task should be simplified, the instructions should be repeated often and she should be actively involved (using *procedural memory* rather than verbal instruction). Like all other deficits, it is not the case that the ability to learn is lost absolutely; it is slowed down and more difficult. Repeated reinforcement, reminders, praise and rehearsal will be necessary to ensure any significant amount of new learning. It is no wonder that dementing people avoid new experiences and fall back on what they learned years ago. Indeed, before thinking of teaching her something new, we should ask ourselves whether her old way of doing things could not still be useful. Thus, if she was not safe with the gas, could the gas cooker not be made safer for her, rather than her having to learn new skills with a supposedly safer electric cooker or microwave oven?

OLD LEARNING

Much of what we do is done by routine. We learn slowly over many years how to go to the toilet, to feed, to shop, to cook, to follow social customs, to communicate with others, to relate to others, to have sexual relationships, to do our job, to pursue interests and activities. Thereafter, all these activities have an element of routine about them. Our brains have a vast store of this learned behaviour ready for our day-to-day needs. Again, we have no special cerebral learning area; to store and retain all this learning we use billions of connections made all over the brain. So it is no wonder that the store of learned behaviour is gradually lost in dementia and that what is left can be difficult to retrieve when necessary. The result is that all these habits decline and the person is less and less able to perform them according to her routine.

Take social habits as an example. Normally we respond to others in routine ways. If someone comes up and smiles, we look at them and smile back, we exchange pleasantries, we do things by gesture and facial expression which encourage them to speak. All these actions were learned years ago. If, however, we were to lose the ability to behave in these ways we would seem unresponsive and would not encourage other people to respond to us. They would not be inclined to go on with the conversation and might even think that we were being rude.

Similar problems can affect all our routine and not-so-routine activities. Indeed, it is the less routine that will disappear first. A lady may seem to be able to cook, preparing the same one or two dishes every day. It is when she tries to cook a dish that she has only occasionally done in the past that the loss of learned habits becomes obvious. Loss of old learning can thus hide behind routines. In general, Ribot's law (p. 9) applies – things learned earliest in life disappear last. So social habits tend to decline before personal care, cooking skills before eating skills. And it is also probably true that very old sufferers rely on their routines even more than younger sufferers. But this is only a very general rule.

Can patients be retrained? The answer is probably that retraining the patient in abilities that have *recently* declined is more likely to work than trying to train her in completely new activities. It is generally easier, for example, for a dementing person to relearn old routines in her own house than to learn a few simple new routines in a new house. For the old learned patterns are not lost altogether at first. They are merely less accessible, though eventually they will disappear. Unfortunately, some professional staff seem more willing to be involved with assessing deficits than to spend their time and patience helping dementia sufferers relearn some of their old habits. Time spent in practising simple but important skills such as cooking, dressing, or using money can be invaluable.

PROCESSING INFORMATION

GENERAL LOSSES

Speed

All older people may be slower mentally than they were in their younger days (p. 49), but dementing people slow even more. This slowing affects every aspect of mental activity – reception, storage, central processing and expression – and it progressively worsens.

Anyone who has to deal with a dementing patient must also slow down, for there is no way of remedying the loss of speed. That means talking slowly, moving slowly, allowing her time to think. It means that, given enough time, she may slowly dress and wash herself, slowly learn her way around a new house, slowly change from subject to subject when talking (p. 153), slowly remember that her husband has died.

Intelligence and problem-solving

Intelligence is a mixture of many abilities. It is mostly concerned with the ability to solve problems but may best be defined as 'what is measured by intelligence tests'. As we age, our scores in intelligence tests may fall, but some of this is due to the normal slowing and cautiousness of old age (p. 50). In dementia, there is a definite progressive decline in intelligence, particularly where the tests involve solving new types of problems rather than going over well-learned material. This explains a great deal about the behaviour of dementing patients. They do not handle new problems well and try to avoid them, while they cling repetitively to their remaining old knowledge in a way which can be exceedingly boring and frustrating for their carers.

Thinking and imagining

Most thinking involves words, and therefore declines as speech deteriorates in dementia. Much of our thinking is also to do with problem solving – 'using' our intelligence. But there is a more abstract form of thought which involves letting ideas float freely through our minds, and which includes imagination and imagery, fantasy and day-dreaming, and multitudes of unconscious thoughts. Although this is not directly to do with solving problems it forms the background of much of what we do. What we think of people, our attitudes to various courses of action, our wishes and desires, are all dealt with by this sort of thinking. Both thinking and imagining involve abstraction, the ability to move away from the particular object or situation to general concepts and ideas. And there is often an emotional content in our thinking.

Like all general functions of the brain thinking of either sort requires multiple and widespread connections; there is no specific 'problem solving' or 'imagining' centre in the brain. And having new thoughts must involve the ability to make new connections.

All these abilities decline in dementia. So dementing people imagine less, cannot think abstractly as well as they used to and do not make new connections, or make mistaken ones (p. 228). In the absence of new thinking the patient has to fall back on the remnants of old thoughts. So her mind will be relatively empty apart from repetitive stereotyped thoughts and platitudes which she cannot develop.

EMOTIONS

Experiencing and expressing emotion are complex processes. A person's emotional state changes depending on what he sees or hears, what he is thinking or imagining, what relationship he has with the people or things around about him. And there is a steady state of emotion, the 'mood' that we are in. The *expression* of emotion (see also below, p. 160) involves coordination of many of the body's mechanisms, for smiling, laughing, crying, blushing, angry gestures, frightened or anxious reactions, sexual expression. Both the content and the tone of what we say are involved. The *experience* of emotion is partly the experience of going through these expressive actions, and partly a more internal, abstract experience. Widespread areas of the brain, especially in the temporal lobes and deep in the centre of the brain (the *limbic system*), are involved in emotion, so it is no wonder that all aspects of emotion may be damaged or disconnected in dementia.

Emotions in dementia

Poverty. The principal result is a gradual decline in emotions, called *poverty of emotion*, or *apathy*. The patient simply does not feel or express so much emotionally as she used to. The expected ups and downs in mood do not happen. The eventual result is a patient who seems to show no emotion at all and is totally bland. Since emotional reactions are an essential part of one's personality this decline contributes to the *loss of personality* often described in dementia. It tends to make the patient less interesting to others; she is less colourful. And it affects her motivation, so that she is less moved to action by her emotions. But it also allows her not to feel the full horror of her situation.

Disconnections. Disconnection between emotions and their causes, and from their expression, are also common. For example, someone may talk about a distressing personal subject without apparent emotion. Another may say that she feels distressed but does not express the feeling in her face and gestures. Another may do the opposite and be in tears about something distressing but then say that she is not feeling distressed. These phenomena of lack of emotion and loss of emotional connections contrast with the loss of control of emotion described in Chapter 5.

Management. There is no way of putting back the lost emotions. We simply have to learn to live with a patient who does not respond emotionally. However, there are also many dementia sufferers who *appear* to have become dull and emotionless when in fact they have simply become withdrawn (p. 229). These patients can 'come out of their shell' with the right stimulation. It is also important to distinguish poverty of emotion from depression, either as a reaction to dementia (see Table 7.3, p. 221), or as part of a depressive illness; to distinguish it from the poverty of *expression* which occurs in parkinsonism; and from the dulling effects of other illnesses and of certain drugs. All these other conditions are potentially treatable.

Motivation

To a large extent motivation, the drive and energy to do things, depends on imagination, reasoning and emotions. But some people with dementia are much more inactive and apathetic than we expect them to be. They seem to have a specific loss of motivation. Attempts to get them to 'get up and go' are frustrated and lesser goals have to be set. This can be one of the most disappointing aspects of dementia for optimistic energetic helpers. Family or staff have to fill the gaps in motivation by using their own energy, but it can be a soul-destroying task. Lack of motivation may explain some cases of self-neglect. It is often due to damage of the frontal lobe of the brain. It must be distinguished from *depression*, where the patient's low spirits make her disinclined to be active. And sometimes antidepressants (in the USA even amphetamine-like drugs) have been used in an attempt to improve motivation, usually with little success. It is, however, important not to miss depression, and often a trial of antidepressants may be of value.

PERSONALITY

Personality (p. 202) is really a mixture of many of the functions mentioned in this chapter – learned social skills, attitudes and other characteristic ways of thinking, learned habits of behaviour, typical emotional reactions and habitual reactions to various stresses. It goes without saying, therefore, that we almost always see a gradual decline in all aspects of personality in dementia. This 'death of the personality' is most distressing for relatives (p. 237). It is important that staff who have never met the sufferer before get to know what she was like *before* the illness began, and do not assume that the rather dulled, blank person they meet is her original self. Life-story books (p. 309) or other reminders of the person's previous self should include plenty of evidence of her previous personality, attitudes and personal style. Again it is important to distinguish *apparent* decline due to depression, social withdrawal, physical illness or drugs from the real decline of dementia. *Change* in personality, where dementia causes new personality traits to emerge, is dealt with in the next chapter.

EXPRESSION AND ACTION

SPEECH PROBLEMS

We have already (p. 115) seen the difficulties which dementing people have in *receiving* speech, whether it be spoken or written. Often the processes of understanding meaning are more affected than the simple perception of words and grammar. We find something similar when we look at the *expression* of speech.

Even if a person has understood a question such as, 'What did you have for breakfast?' and has enough memory to know the answer, there is still a very complex process to go through in order to produce an answer which will be fully understood. Some sense of the meaning to be got across is necessary; the right sounds and syllables must be used to construct the correct words, which need to be assembled grammatically; this must then be translated into muscular action and actual expression.

Speech and language in dementia

Dysarthria

Eventually in dementia most of these expressive aspects of speech will decline. The severely demented patient may be mute, or give out only scattered inarticulate, meaningless fragments of speech. But, until near the end, the physical mechanism of the muscles of the larynx, the *articulation* of speech, is usually quite normal. In VaD, a particular stroke may affect the controlling centres of articulation, causing what is called *dysarthria*. Other neurological conditions, such as parkinsonism, can also lead to disorders of articulation. But most people with uncomplicated dementia articulate speech quite normally.

Language

The difficulties for dementing people lie more in *language* than in speech. Indeed, the individual sounds, the syllables and words that result, and even some simple aspects of grammar, are relatively normal in earlier stages. It is the more complex processes of getting meaning across that decline first.

We find sufferers gradually using a smaller vocabulary and simpler, shorter sentences when they are talking, and find them becoming quite muddled when trying to get across more complex messages. Many also show a particular difficulty in naming objects they are shown (called *nominal dysphasia*), which can be easily tested, and in making up lists of, for example, flowers, pieces of furniture or colours, again easily tested. These problems, which are akin to the problems of coding memories into 'boxes' have considerable effect on the patient's *fluency*. She will be frustrated in her attempts to get her meaning across and may try roundabout ways of describing things, called *paraphasia*. Her family find her speech both less interesting and more frustrating. It is little wonder that communication between the patient and her family declines. Nor is it surprising that patients come to rely on stock phrases, old stories and platitudes in their attempts to get some meaning across.

All these difficulties in expression will be made worse if the patient also suffers from *perseveration* (p. 153), or from a difficulty in excluding irrelevancies (p. 168), so that the clarity of her message gets lost because of repetitive or meaningless intrusions.

Dysphasias

Neurologists have defined specific dysphasias or difficulties with speech, either receptive or expressive, which are due to damage to quite specific areas of the brain (in the temporal lobe and the parietal lobe respectively and usually on the left side of the brain in right-handed people and the right side in left-handed people). Some patients with VaD will show one of these specific dysphasias. However, the speech problems of most dementing people are far too general and complicated to be defined so clearly. In one patient there will be some receptive dysphasia, much difficulty in comprehension and the formulation of meaning, some more specific expressive dysphasia, and some loss of control, all mixed together. It is no wonder that speech therapists have tended to be pessimistic about helping dementing people, that patients themselves tend to communicate less and less, and that relatives and friends are tempted to give up communicating with them. Only if one type of dysphasia predominates will specific help be possible.

Dysgraphia

A further problem which can arise is deterioration of writing, called *dysgraphia*, which can, for example, interfere with the patient's ability to remind himself of things by notes. It can be just as frustrating a problem as dysphasia.

Assessment

Speech and language problems are best assessed simply by listening to the patient speaking, either spontaneously or in answer to questions. Can she produce the right words, with the right grammar, does she get her meaning across, does she articulate properly? Or we may ask her to repeat some words back, to recite something she knows well or to read. These tests show up expressive dysphasia. Can she name things or give lists of things when asked? These tests show nominal dysphasia. It is again important to judge how practically important her speech difficulties are. Do they mean that she cannot state her needs or are they merely frustrating?

Management

If someone has expressive problems but few receptive problems, she will likely be *frustrated* by her inability to say clearly what she wants. We can lessen the frustration by guessing what she wishes to say. Relatives of dysphasic patients become good at this guesswork, knowing that, for example, when she says something about going for a walk she wants the toilet. The relief for the patient in knowing that she is understood is enormous. Alternatively we can ask questions to find what she is trying to say. The forced choice technique is useful. 'Do you want the toilet?', or 'Are you hungry?'. In this way she gets across her meaning simply by a 'Yes' or 'No', or by a nod. A further method uses printed or written words. If she can point out the word that she needs she does not need to be able to say it properly.

On a more general level, we should keep our sentences and questions to the patient simple. If we invite a complex answer it is unlikely to come clearly. Remember that poor short-term memory does not allow lots of material to be in her mind at once. And there is little value in letting the patient ramble on in an attempt to make sense, when she is losing sight of the subject and getting frustrated. It can be more helpful to interrupt and bring her back to the subject. If there are more severe speech problems it may be useful to try to find other methods of communication. Touch and guidance by hand, pictures and photographs, and 'charades' which she can copy can all be helpful.

Unfortunately, as we have seen, many of the speech difficulties of dementing people are not of one sort or another, but are mixed. If she has difficulties in reception of speech, then our attempts to help her get over an expressive problem will be limited because she will not understand fully what we are saying. In VaD there may be quite specific, single, speech difficulties and in such a case a speech therapist should be asked to give advice.

It is only when we see the effects of dysphasia that we see how important speech is in every aspect of everyday life. We should remember that not only does communication with others depend on speech but most of our internal thoughts are spoken. So speech difficulties interfere fundamentally with the patient's ability to understand her situation, to solve problems and to think logically.

COORDINATING ACTION

The primary motor cortex (see Fig. 1.2, p. 9) is not affected in early DAT, although in VaD a stroke may affect this area or its connections. However, the motor cortex only controls the individual movements of muscles. The everyday actions that we carry out require interconnections with other regions of the brain, for they are complicated, involving different groups of muscles working together and depending on sensory input and learned habit. Actions such as dressing, going to the toilet, feeding and cooking all require very complex coordination. Impairment of this coordination is called *dyspraxia* and is mainly due to damage in the *parietal lobe*. Dyspraxia, agnosias and disorientation are together all common features of DAT, and are also often found in VaD. They are less common in subcortical types of dementia (p.

43). Dyspraxia may cause the patient to *dress* in the wrong order, put his bottom clothes over her head, get right and left mixed up or be unable to manipulate buttons. She may have no problem of muscular weakness, stiffness or tremor but still be unable to carry out the essential actions of dressing. Dyspraxia can affect any of our activities which require to be coordinated, such as cooking, eating, work activities, driving, even sitting down, standing up and walking. For someone who is still at work, trying to carry out complex tasks becomes impossible. For the patient at home, we can see how even at mild stages it can lead to the need for outside help to prevent risks and neglect. The *practical importance* of dyspraxia depends entirely on the individual patient's situation.

Dyspraxia can be assessed by getting the patient to try to arrange play blocks in a particular pattern – showing what is called *constructional dyspraxia*. Trying to draw the face of a clock can also reveal dyspraxia, even at early stages of dementia (p. 318). More practically, she can be asked to carry out various tasks of daily living (p. 333). We need to be on the look-out for any other specific deficit, such as an agnosia or right–left disorientation, which is adding to the problem. Our aim is to fill in the specific gaps in the patient's ability as best we can. This means assessing not only what she cannot do, but what she can do. It may be, for example, that simply leaving out her clothes in the correct order solves the problem of a dressing dyspraxia; it may be that we have to get each item the right way round for her to be able to put it on, or it may be that she only needs help with buttons. Simpler garments with 'Velcro' fastening get round the problem at later stages, but in early stages the patient may feel better if she has been able to get 'proper' clothes on with only a little outside help. Almost all patients eventually need to be dressed and undressed completely. Similar remarks apply to all the other actions which may be impaired by dyspraxia.

MOBILITY
Alzheimer-type dementia

Much of the need for physical help with dressing, washing, etc., in DAT comes from the decline in learned habits and from dyspraxia. The great majority of DAT sufferers remain otherwise remarkably physically fit until the late stages of the illness. Major paralyses like strokes are not usually found, as they are in VaD (though they can occur, making diagnosis difficult). However, as the disease progresses, patchy damage in various parts of the *motor* system of the brain, those complicated pathways involved in the voluntary and involuntary control of muscles all over the body, gradually has more and more obvious effects. The result may be some *weakness* of various muscles, some increase in muscle *tone*, leading to reduced mobility and stiffness, or *tremor* and other abnormal *involuntary movements*. Eventually almost all patients show some of these changes. Because they are patchy and rather vague, it is difficult to decide on methods of treatment. The danger is that the patient's ability to walk independently can be lost. She is in danger of falling, loses her confidence and causes alarm in her carers. She may become chair- or bed-bound. These problems of mobility can also affect her use of her hands, eating and swallowing and all muscular movements.

Assessment

Other causes should always be considered before concluding that dementia is the cause of poor mobility or other disorders of movement. Parkinsonism, stroke and the side-effects of drugs are all common causes. In particular, the *phenothiazine* drugs such as thioridazine and other similar drugs can cause parkinsonian symptoms of muscular rigidity, tremor and poverty of movement. A shuffling gait with a tendency to take progressively smaller steps, difficulty in initiating movements, a blank, mask-like face, a regular tremor of the hands of 'pill-rolling' type and excessive saliva should suggest parkinsonism due to Parkinson's disease or to these drugs. In older people the typical tremor is often missing, and it is easy to fail to realise that poverty of movement may be due to prescribed drugs. Other drugs can cause mobility problems because of their sedative effects, because they lower blood pressure, or by causing tremor.

Management

In dealing with mobility problems, preventative action is best. Because of the tendency to withdraw socially the dementing patient may be inclined to sit in a corner 'not bothering anybody'.

But this stores up physical problems for the future. Inactivity in any older person very quickly leads to loss of power in the muscles. Regular exercise can prevent loss of muscle power and delay the decline in mobility. Relatives should be encouraged to take the patient out for walks every day for, besides its benefit as 'physiotherapy', this is stimulating for her and may reduce restlessness at other times, particularly at night. In group situations such as day care, residential home or hospital, the daily exercise group is of vital importance. It can be led by a physiotherapist, remedial gymnast or any member of staff.

If there is a more specific problem, such as localized weakness, rigidity or a tendency to fall, then referral to a physiotherapist is advisable before the patient becomes too immobile. There are, of course, problems for dementing patients in physiotherapy. They may not understand the exercises they are asked to do; they may have dyspraxia or agnosia and use aids in the wrong way; they will be unlikely to be able to practise on their own. However, once a patient is chair-bound, the situation can become irreversible. Muscles develop contractures through misuse and she will be unable to use her limbs properly again. There is also a danger of pressure sores. Passive exercises to prevent contractures and encourage freedom of movement are essential. However, not many patients will have access to enough physiotherapy time to carry out these treatments effectively. The physiotherapist should be prepared to instruct and advise nurses, care staff and families in the principles of active physical rehabilitation and passive exercising. If immobility or contractures are developing, then specialist physiotherapy should always be sought.

Walking aids – the stick, tripod and walking frame – are important aids but, like all gap-fillers, should only be used if, after assessment, it is clear that the patient cannot cope at a higher degree of independence.

Falls

These can cause a great deal of anxiety to families and staff. They can of course be dangerous, and a significant number of dementing people suffer fractures of the femur and other bones. These are much more likely to happen if the patient is on sedative or other similar drugs. Mobility problems and carelessness due to poor judgement also contribute. Patients with dementia of Lewy body type (p. 33) are at particular risk of falls, and are also at particular risk of side-effects from phenothiazine drugs. The persistent 'wanderer' is at risk if she has some degree of muscle weakness or other mobility problems. She is also at risk if she tires herself out. At the beginning of the day she may appear entirely fit, but by late afternoon she is 'falling on her feet'. The temptation is to confine her to a chair for her own safety, for no one likes to feel responsible if there is a risk and it has been ignored. But once confining to a chair becomes habit, the patient's mobility declines more rapidly. It is far better if staff or family can spare the time to walk with her under supervision, or even try to get her to walk more rather than less. A ward or home which does not have the staff to do this has too few staff (or the wrong sort of resident). A family who cannot do this needs outside help.

Vascular dementia

In addition to the problems just mentioned, which are likely to affect all dementia sufferers, patients with VaD may have more specific mobility problems. The strokes that they suffer can cause varying degrees of paralysis in one or other parts of the body, ranging from minor weakness of one or two muscle groups, to hemiplegia (paralysis of one side of the body). The vast majority of strokes in VaD, however, will not have any of these neurological manifestations, but will simply add to the general decline. Specific medical, nursing and physiotherapy attention will be required for any significant paralysis.

VaD sufferers may also be more prone to other physical problems including 'funny turns', 'drop attacks', faints, dizziness, all of which lead to falls. Such episodes should not, however, be assumed to be simply part of the dementia but deserve medical investigation.

WEIGHT LOSS

Weight loss is very common in dementia. This is particularly well-documented in DAT, where patients may lose considerable amounts of weight. It is not confined to the later stages of illness. Weight loss demands medical investigation, for it might be due to any number of other physical causes; however, in most cases no cause other than the dementia is found.

Forgetting to eat may be a contributory factor, as may dyspraxia with eating utensils. People with dementia are often very slow in their activities of daily living, and it is important in the various long-term care settings, and at home, that they are given sufficient time to complete their meals, with assistance where necessary. Agitation and restlessness may mean that someone may not sit long enough at the table to finish their food; additional between-meals eating is then necessary to maintain weight. Likewise, low mood and apathy can contribute to poor dietary intake.

Poor coordination of swallowing is common in the later stages of dementia, and may contribute to eating difficulties. It may make patients reluctant to eat for fear of choking, and may make carers reluctant to encourage eating. In many patients, however, there are no such causes; they eat well but still lose weight. There are control mechanisms for appetite and weight maintenance in the hypothalamus in the centre of the brain, and this area is often damaged in many types of dementia. Indeed this may be part of that general, but vague, physical decline which leads eventually to the death of the sufferer.

Eating difficulties, including swallowing problems, are most common in later stage dementia. Patients become susceptible to aspiration of food, both solid and liquid, into the lungs, and this can lead to life-threatening pneumonias. Many ethical issues surround this. Feeding and hydration can be maintained in various ways such as by giving nutrition intravenously, via a naso-gastric tube or via a gastrostomy tube (a tube inserted directly into the stomach via the abdominal wall). Patients with dementia will often not understand the reasons for such interventions, and will find them uncomfortable. They may therefore try to remove intravenous or naso-gastric tubes. The decision to use (or indeed, not to use) such means of feeding needs to be made on an individual basis, and this involves discussion between relatives, carers and all the professionals involved. Where possible the sufferer's wishes should be taken into account. She may have expressed opinions about life-support prior to the development of dementia, and the existence and knowledge of such previous opinions can make a decision easier to come to for those caring for the patient (see Chapter 9).

The final decision will rest with the doctor who must weigh up the risks and benefits of the situation, including in his assessment a judgement on the patient's quality of life with or without artificial feeding, and any associated suffering. One crucial consideration is whether the feeding is likely to be temporary or 'endless'. The doctor must consider how much he needs to interfere with the inevitable last stages of a terminal illness.

CONCLUSION

Most dementing patients suffer most of the above losses to a greater or lesser degree. In VaD the losses are often patchy, so that some of the more general functions – personality, emotional reactions, social skills or even memory – are maintained until quite late in the dementia. In DAT, as well as the general losses, there is concentration of damage in some temporal, parietal and frontal areas. But most patients eventually have most losses – dementia is truly a devastating condition.

We can summarize the stages in the management of deficits and impairments of dementia as follows:

1. Establish a baseline – what were the person's past abilities?
2. Assess the losses – what can she not do now compared to the past?
3. Assess what is left – how much can she still do?
4. Assess the practical importance of the losses – how much do they matter?
5. Exclude causes other than dementia – particularly other illnesses and drug treatments.
6. Attempt retraining where possible.
7. Help the patient use her remaining abilities to the full.
8. Simplify the tasks she has to carry out.
9. Provide external help to fill the gaps.
10. Do not take over completely until necessary.

This last point requires special emphasis. No loss can be considered complete until the very last stage of the dementia. The patient is *losing* her abilities. Our chief aim should be to ensure that she uses what she still has as much as is reasonably possible, no more and no less.

5

Behaviour and dementia

So far we have considered dementia as a decline, as a failure of brain function. And that of couse is essentially what it is. But how can we explain the fact that dementing people sometimes behave in ways they never did before, and sometimes even seem like a different personality? A mild-mannered man, for example, may become irritable and aggressive, a quiet lady become noisy and demanding. This is one of the most distressing facets of dementia for relatives, especially if they have been in a close relationship for many years. It is difficult enough to cope with a relative who is chronically ill with an incurable disease, and more difficult still when this illness involves the gradual loss of her whole being as a person, to a state of complete dependence on others. But it is extremely difficult if at the same time the family has to get used to totally new behaviour, or a new type of relationship with a person they hardly recognize.

The problems of declining memory and declining ability to carry out daily living activities such as washing, toileting, dressing and feeding, undoubtedly put a substantial burden on carers. In general these problems develop gradually, and carers develop methods of overcoming the difficulties in various ways. However, the stress associated with behaviour problems can be much greater than that associated with cognitive decline in itself, and these problems are probably the commonest reason for admission to care. Indeed, they are the commonest reasons for any particular care arrangement breaking down. There is a common tendency to see *positive* behaviour such as aggression, uncooperativeness, wandering and restlessness as posing the most difficult problem, particularly since these actions have a more direct effect on others. However, we must not ignore the management of *negative* behaviour, such as lethargy, withdrawal and apathy, which affects only the sufferer herself.

Why do behavioural problems occur? Many of these *new* experiences of dementia can be explained as variations on a general theme – the failure of one of the most important functions of the brain, to compare with standards, control or inhibit.

Inhibition in the brain

The messages which pass from one nerve cell to another by chemical transmitter (see Fig. 1.4, p. 19) are of two main types: messages which *increase* the likelihood of the second cell reaching the point where it fires electrically to send a message to yet another cell (called *excitatory* messages), and messages which *reduce* that likelihood (*inhibitory* messages). Much of the workings of the central nervous system depends on the complicated interplay between billions of these 'yes' and 'no' messages passing between billions of cells.

On a larger scale, we can define certain areas of the brain which seem to have a generally controlling effect on what other areas do. They monitor how these other areas are working compared with how they ought to be working, and if necessary prevent them from overworking by inhibiting their actions. Much of the activity of the frontal lobes and their connections with other parts of the brain (see Fig. 1.2, p. 9) seems to be of this supervisory or 'executive' type. Such control can affect the amount of information coming into the brain (sensory *input*), particularly how much of this information we focus on and are consciously aware of. It can also affect the *output* from the brain, for example, expression in speech and in emotion, as well as our social and other behaviour. It helps us to say and do what we want to and only that.

We also need to have control over the interconnections of the brain and the processing of information, for example in thinking and solving problems. *Planning* what we want to do, the *standards* which we aim for and our *judgement* and *conscience* about whether we are right or wrong, in our thinking as well as in our actions, are all part of this controlling function. And there are more physical, *neurological* aspects of this comparison and control, for example when we want to carry out an action and need to monitor how well we are doing it.

Because the brain is damaged so widely in dementia, and particularly since the frontal lobe is damaged in DAT, it is not surprising that there is some loss of this ability to compare with a standard and have self control. So, on top of the decline in abilities described in Chapter 4, the sufferer may be taking in irrelevant information – may be saying or doing things that she would normally not say or do – may appear to have a changed personality. And these changes may be minor failures of judgement or major disinhibition.

LOSS OF CONTROL OVER THE INPUT TO THE BRAIN

ATTENTION

Only a tiny fraction of the information from our senses can be allowed to reach our consciousness. If we were consciously aware or perceived every bit of what was in our field of vision as equally important, if we consciously heard every sound around us all the time (people who wear hearing aids complain of something like this experience), if all the sensations in our body claimed our attention, we would be bombarded with a jumble of information which we could not disentangle. We have to *filter out* all the extraneous and unwanted information and *focus* on what is immediately relevant.

This filtering process involves inhibition, the playing down of those unwanted messages, and is called *attention*. It is a function of those parts of the brain which are involved in consciousness, including the reticular activating system (p. 62) and the frontal lobes. It is closely linked to *consciousness* since consciousness means being aware of the world about us. We wake when someone calls our name, we become alert and attend to or focus on the voice. When we are less conscious it is more difficult to attend, whether the lowered consciousness is due to sleep, coma or the clouding of delirium (p. 62). The level of consciousness and its daily changes are not actually altered in dementia until late in the illness; patients are fully awake by day and sleep fairly normally at night. But the ability to focus attention is often impaired. The dementing patient is thus easily distracted by irrelevant things in her surroundings; the filter is not working.

Dementing people may also be able to hold fewer bits of information in attention at one time. This can easily be tested by *digit span*, the ability to attend to and repeat back a series of 3, 4, 5 or 6 numbers (many psychologists call this ability *short-term memory*, and the two functions are indeed almost identical).

'Stuck' attention. Once attention is gained, a dementing person may 'get stuck' on that object. It can be very puzzling to see someone absolutely engrossed in some sound or sight which has little relevance at the moment. In severe dementia the patient has little ability to focus attention at all. It may be impossible to get her to attend to a voice out of the jumble of sounds in a ward, as she may be visually distracted by all sorts of things around her, and by nothing in particular, or she may spend hours engrossed in 'stuck' attention.

Management

In practical terms, we must make a greater than usual effort to gain the attention of a dementing patient. We should *simplify* information, giving only one or two simple items rather than complicated messages, avoiding the need for codes (p. 123). We should make whatever we want the patient to attend to stand out clearly from its background and we should *lessen distractions* as much as possible.

HALLUCINATIONS

Visual hallucinations, and to a lesser extent other types of hallucination, are characteristic of delirium (p. 64). Whenever visual hallucinations occur, particularly if they begin quite suddenly, this diagnosis should be our first guess. However, hallucinations can occur in dementia sufferers, especially those with Lewy body dementia who seem particularly likely to experience bizarre visual hallucinations.

The usual story is of a lady who is alone at home. She mentions visitors, but describes them as rather strange. They do not speak, they seem to appear from nowhere and disappear into thin air, or through the wall. She does not feel paranoid as they do not appear threatening. But she is bewildered and amazed, especially if she has made tea for them! She may realize that the experience is ridiculous and have some insight, but their very real appearance is likely eventually to convince her that she is not imagining them. This sort of experience usually occurs in early dementia, and the patients involved are likely also to have *eye problems* such as cataract or glaucoma. It is possible that loneliness and the wish for companionship at a time of failing faculties may encourage imagination. However, it is likely that much of this phenomenon is due to a failure in the filtering out of irrelevant visual information by the brain. A similar sort of experience occurs when we walk along a very dark lane and shapes on the edge of our visual field seem like figures, or seem to move, and when we imagine we hear sounds in a silent house at night.

In more severe dementia, when there is a more severe breakdown of the attention process, when reality and imagination are less clearly differentiated, disorganized hallucinations occur. Patients may be observed talking to long-dead relatives or to people who never existed. When asked, they can only vaguely describe whether they are seeing or hearing these people.

Hallucinations in dementia often have a very bizarre quality. Examples of this include seeing very small people all around, seeing disembodied heads, or seeing people who appear and disappear at will.

There are other causes of hallucinations in older people, not associated with dementia. These must be kept in mind. Older people with visual impairment and no mental disorder may develop visual hallucinations, the so called *Charles Bonnet syndrome*. A similar process is sometimes found in those with auditory impairment, who begin to hear music or singing – *musical hallucinosis*.

Though small doses of neuroleptic drugs may sometimes be helpful in managing these particular problems, the results are often disappointing. The hallucinations themselves are not usually distressing, but the fact that they may be constantly present can be irritating to the person.

Detection

The detection of hallucinations is quite difficult, particularly in later stages of dementia. Only if the patient can actually tell us of her experiences can we be sure. Often the only evidence is that she seems to be seeing things that are not real. It is easy to misunderstand hallucinations and describe what is happening as 'disorientation' or 'memory impairment' because the patient is preoccupied with her experiences and does not see them as abnormal, but acts oddly and appears out of touch with reality. The result is that she may appear to be more impaired than she actually is. So it is doubly important carefully to check orientation, memory, etc., in any patient who is having hallucinations.

Management

First, the other signs and causes of delirium (see Table 2.3, p. 61) should be looked for and that diagnosis ruled out. Drugs which might be causing the hallucinations should be stopped. Secondly, we should ensure that the patient's eyesight and hearing are checked and aided as much as possible. Thirdly, we should make the real environment stimulating, though simple, engaging her attention in ways that she can understand, with as few distractions as possible. Hallucinations are often worse at night when it is more difficult to make sense of what we see or hear. A night light is therefore advisable.

These measures may reduce the likelihood of hallucinations but, once the hallucinations are established and firmly believed in, are unlikely to take them away completely. Drug treatment may therefore be necessary, but only after the other measures have been tried. One of the antipsychotic drugs such as haloperidol, pimozide or sulpiride may help. Unfortunately, drugs are not likely to be completely effective. It is unlikely that a large dose will do anything more than a small dose and may merely oversedate the patient. It is also important to remember the paradox that bizarre distressing hallucinations are often a feature of Lewy body dementia, and that these patients are particularly sensitive to neuroleptic drugs.

PRINCIPLES OF MANAGEMENT

Summarizing the management of a dementia sufferer who has a disorder of attention or hallucinations we can begin to see some general principles which will apply to other disinhibitory phenonema:

- Look for causes other than dementia
- Look at the circumstances in which the abnormalities occur. Can these be changed to lessen the problem?
- Can we encourage more normal experience and behaviour?
- Drug treatment is a last resort and should be used in smaller doses only.

LOSS OF CONTROL OVER THE OUTPUT FROM THE BRAIN

DISINHIBITION IN SPEECH

In Chapter 4 we looked at the deterioration which occurs in the various aspects of speech in dementia. In addition, any problem in attention that the patient has will mean that she cannot focus properly on the spoken and the written word; she cannot filter out the irrelevant from the relevant. This will worsen problems of *comprehension*. But failure of comparison and control may also explain three other abnormalities that occur in the *expression* of speech, namely perseveration, 'stuck' speech and disinhibited content of speech.

Perseveration

This can be defined as difficulty in shifting from one subject to another, of changing what is called 'mental set'. We have already seen something similar in relation to attention. Normally, when we answer a question, when we call someone's name, when we express something, we realize that we have said what is necessary and can prevent ourselves saying it again. We then

move on to the next subject. This is, in fact, another monitoring
and inhibiting mechanism in the brain. We are not talking so
much about that conscious social inhibition, which prevents us
from 'going on' about something when we see that others have
got our message or are bored. That is to do with our personality
and our social awareness (p. 168). Perseveration is a much more
basic problem which can make a person *unable* to shift from
subject to subject. As with other inhibitory mechanisms the
controlling mechanism which is damaged in perseveration seems
largely to be a function of the frontal lobes.

Perseveration in diagnosis

At the early stages of dementia, perseveration can be a very
important diagnostic sign. It is most easily detected when we ask
a series of questions of the patient – the time, the day, the date,
the year, the patient's age. She may answer a question with the
previous answer, even to the extent of getting stuck on the first
answer and giving it for every question. Or parts of an answer
may carry over to later answers, so that if the time is '11', the year
becomes '1911'. The patient may or may not be aware of making
these mistakes. People who do not suffer from any form of brain
damage very seldom show evidence of perseveration. So it is a
useful sign of organic brain disease, even when orientation,
memory and other brain functions are not greatly impaired.

Management

We should be aware of perseveration in talking with dementing
patients. We may have to move from subject to subject very
slowly, or give a lot of extra clues to ensure that the patient has
moved her whole attention on to the new subject. ('How old are
you? We're talking about your age and how many years old you
are. You understand?')

'Stuck' speech

At later stages, and occasionally early in dementia, more extreme
forms of perseveration can occur. A word, a phrase or a story
may get repeated over and over again as if a record was stuck –
the *gramophone sign*. If this happens in early dementia the patient

may be aware of what they are doing but seem powerless to stop it. Later on they are less likely to be aware. The classical examples are patients in a ward who shout for a relative continually, or cry 'Nurse, nurse, nurse', despite having no obvious physical or psychological distress. They continue this even when the relative or nurse is present and they cannot explain why they wanted them.

Management

Following the four principles mentioned above, we can work out how to try to treat this sort of repetitiveness.

Other causes may be contributing. Real physical distress or unhappiness of any kind will naturally make the patient more likely to call for help, to the person who seems most likely to respond. If she forgets that the person has already responded then she is likely to repeat the call for help. A thorough search for any causes of distress or discomfort (Table 5.1) is therefore most important, before we start treating disturbed behaviour as due to a loss of self control (see Chapter 7).

Circumstances and environment. Even if a patient is repeating words or phrases during large parts of the day, it is unlikely that she is doing it all the time, or at the same intensity all the time. This variation in behaviour gives us an opportunity to modify it by altering the circumstances.

The first step is to *define the problem* carefully and agree the definition of the behaviour among all concerned. If this is not done, people are recording and discussing slightly different problems. What type of speech is to be considered as repetitive? Is it particular words? How many times does it have to be repeated to be considered repetitive? Is only shouted speech to be considered?

These and other clarifying questions prepare for the second step which is to *record when it happens*. This is best done using a behaviour chart (Fig. 5.1). The first type involves observing when her behaviour is most obvious and recording the circumstances in which it is happening. This is most appropriate for recording things which a patient does relatively seldom, such as being incontinent, so it is less useful in a case of repetitiveness than the second type. This involves *time sampling*. No one is going to be able to record every instance of very repetitive behaviour. Either a record can be kept of what the patient is doing, say, every hour

Table 5.1 Some causes of noisiness

Cause	Management
Deafness	Speak clearly or use communicator or writing Hearing aid
Noisy surroundings	Remove the cause (e.g. noisy radio or TV)
Internal noise	Treat if possible (e.g. tinnitus or hallucinations)
Overcoming dysphasia	Speech therapy
Physical discomfort	Treat the cause of discomfort
Emotional distress – anxiety or depression	Reassure, discuss cause, counsel and treat with drugs if necessary
Anger or frustration	Discuss cause and ease it Drugs should not be necessary
Self stimulation from loneliness	Arrange more company and activities
Looking for 'lost' relatives	Reality orientation Give other comfort and reassurance Arrange company and activities
Loss of control	Encourage normal activities External control (rarely effective) Behaviour modification Drug treatment

Note that each cause has a different treatment
Note also that in one patient several of these factors may be important at once, and each needs attention

on the hour; or she can be observed more closely for, say, quarter-hour periods at various times of the day. The circumstances to be recorded include, 'What time of day is it?', 'What else is the patient doing?', 'Is she engaged in activity or not?', 'Where are other people in relation to her?', 'What relatives or staff are around?', 'How do other people react to her behaviour?'.

From the chart, a pattern will probably emerge. Perhaps it is seen that she behaves in the undesirable way with staff but not with relatives. The behaviour chart can then be modified to look more closely at the types of interaction that occur and particularly at how the two groups of people react to her shouting. Then, by altering the circumstances, the behaviour may be modified and lessened. And this is true even though the damage to the control systems in the brain is an organic change which cannot be reversed.

Type 1 (This patient has only occasional episodes)

Time of noisy episode	Circumstances	Reactions of Staff	Outcome
9·15 a.m.	After breakfast, alone by bedside	Asked to join others in day room	A bit quieter
1·05 p.m.	After lunch, sitting by bedside	Ignored	Later seen joining others
4·00 p.m.	Relatives have just left	Told that relatives would return	Remained noisy for 1 hour then stopped

This patient was only disturbed when 'left alone'.

Type 2 (This patient has very frequent episodes)

Time sampled	Number of noisy episodes	Where was patient?	Who was around?
9 - 9·15 a.m.	1	Bedroom	Alone, nurse nearby with another patient
11 - 11·15 a.m.	3	Day room	In exercise group
1 - 1·15 p.m.	2	Dining room	With 5 patients at table
3 - 3·15 p.m.	0	Day room	With relatives

This patient was more disturbed when with other patients.

Fig. 5.1 Two types of behaviour chart.

Behaviour modification is most effective if we can identify something which has been rewarding or encouraging the patient's behaviour. If when she shouts she always gets attention, that attention may actively encourage her to shout more. Attention may consist of a kind word, physical contact, something that is thought to be pleasing such as a sweet, or something to read to divert her attention from the shouting. Even a 'telling off' is a form of attention. Attention can come from family, staff and other residents and is usually given with very good motives. So withdrawing these rewards can sometimes seem cruel. However, it is often effective. If a lady is calling for help it is easy to feel obliged to go, even if we are almost certain that she is 'crying wolf'. But it may be important to stop going in order to lessen very distressing behaviour. Equally important, she must get extra attention at times when she is not behaving in the undesirable way (see below).

Consistency is important in carrying out such a 'behaviour modification' programme. If some relatives or staff are prepared to carry through a programme which means lessening their response to calls for help, while others are not, the programme is unlikely to be very successful. Continuing the charts during the 'treatment' is an important check on consistency. But more important is to get everybody's agreement beforehand that they are prepared to be consistent in their approach. Unfortunately, such behaviour modification programmes are often sabotaged by relatives, by well-meaning domestic staff or, most often of all, by other residents, dementing or not, who cannot stop themselves reacting in a instinctive 'helpful' way when a patient seems to be distressed. A lot of explanation and support is needed throughout a behaviour modification programme if it is to succeed. Much depends on the persistence and enthusiasm of the person in charge of the programme.

Furthermore, taken to extremes, such programmes can be cruel, if they involve completely ignoring patients or if they involve 'time out' and other techniques that are near to punishment. The dementing patient will be unable to understand what is going on and may be put under considerable unwarranted stress. The need to involve all relatives and staff and the need to keep a programme under review should prevent such excesses and make sensible behaviour modification more effective.

Occasionally, much of this effort is not needed. The extra general attention to the patient and the fact that staff have to record their own responses are sufficient in themselves to bring an improvement in the problem. The difficulty then becomes one of maintaining the improvement.

Encouraging normal behaviour. The behaviour chart will show times when the patient is quiet, perhaps during meal times, perhaps when visitors come, perhaps in the morning, perhaps when others in a day room are quiet. The other side of reducing interaction with her when she is noisy is to increase interaction when she is not, so encouraging her to be quiet for longer periods. Once again, an examination of the behaviour chart may show which factors encourage quietness. These can then be increased. Most commonly, attention and physical contact given at quiet times and engagement in engrossing activites will be helpful. Increasing attention at these other times will also help family or staff feel less unhappy about reducing attention at the noisy times.

The sort of attention or 'reward' that is given should be chosen for the individual patient. It should be rewarding specifically for her. Not everybody likes physical contact, or the chance to go out and about, or sweets, and some people are rewarded by quite 'odd' things like being alone, being allowed to go to bed or listening to music or television programmes which others do not like.

The timing of reward and attention is also important. Especially for dementing people, rewards cannot be delayed, for the patient will forget and the link between what she is doing and the encouragement gets lost. There is no point in promising a reward later, it has to be given at the time. Indeed the best reward is in the activity itself. Put at its simplest, if a patient is engaged in something normal and enjoyable, she will have neither the time nor the inclination to be engaged in abnormal behaviour such as shouting.

The clinical psychologist is the expert in behavioural techniques and will help in devising charts, planning treatment programmes, continuing supervision and discussing any difficulties which arise.

Drug treatment. This is the last resort. As we have already said, it is unlikely that a big dose will bring more effect than a small dose and oversedation and poor mobility are the likely consequences of overdosing. The choice of drug has to be by trial and error. The drug which works is the best one. It may be an antipsychotic drug or neuroleptic such as haloperidol, risperidone or sulpiride. It could be a tranquillizer such as chlormethiazole or a benzodiazepine drug such as oxazepam. The benzodiazepine drugs can occasionally actually cause disinhibition so they must be used with caution. And phenothiazines can cause restlessness (called *akathisia*) which can be mistaken for a worsening of the behaviour problem. Other drugs being used include carbamazepine, originally an antiepileptic, and antidepressant drugs which help the action of the transmitter 5-HT in the brain, such as trazodone and fluoxetine, which seem to have an effect on repetitive behaviour.

All this being said, it is also important to remember that the abnormalities in behaviour that we are describing are due to organic damage, if other causes have been ruled out, and so the chances of total success are by no means great. Nevertheless, an improvement in repetitive shouting which makes a dementing lady more tolerable to live with and avoids having to send her to long-stay hospital care is worth considerable effort. And working out a treatment programme, rather than assuming that nothing can be done, transforms our attitude to the dementing patient.

Disinhibited content of speech

Since this is akin to other problems of social behaviour we will discuss it under that heading (p. 168).

EMOTIONAL DISINHIBITION

The ability to control emotions varies from person to person and is an important aspect of personality. Some people are throughout their lives impulsive, some are irritable, some easily moved to tears, some placid, some over-controlled in their emotions. But we are all capable of a wide range of emotional reactions. Even the coolest person is aware that they could, if they 'let go', be much more openly emotional, and even the most emotional person does not express everything that he or she feels. The mechanism of emotional control is again a function mainly of the frontal lobes and their connections, and so is likely to be impaired in all forms of dementia, but particularly if there is a lot of damage in the frontal area.

Two main types of problem can occur: emotional lability and 'stuck' emotions.

Emotional lability

Labile means 'prone to change easily'. Emotional lability is changeability of one or more than one emotion. What happens is that something causes an emotional response which would usually be fairly minor, for example, the mention of the patient's long-dead father. Instead of her normal slight sadness on thinking of him, an emotion which is under control, she loses control and bursts into floods of tears. Likewise, a tiny argument with her husband can lead the patient to an outburst of anger, out of all proportion to the cause, and even end in physical aggression. And other emotions – fear or laughter for example – can be involved. In some cases there does not even have to be a cause at all and the emotional outburst comes completely without warning. This is called *emotional incontinence*. In either case the swing of emotion usually starts very suddenly, within a few seconds, and there is just as sudden a recovery. What is more, the patient may have complete insight. In other words, she realizes that her reaction has been excessive, cannot explain why it has happened and is very embarrassed by her behaviour.

An extreme form of emotional lability has been called the *catastrophic reaction*. Here the patient has been subjected to a series of questions in rapid succession, has been posed a complicated problem or has been otherwise 'overloaded' mentally. Having lost the skill to ask for more time to give herself space to think she begins to be upset. Lability of emotion then brings a very sudden burst of severe emotion, whether tears, fear or anger, which brings the interview to an end.

Management of lability

Using our principles of management of disinhibition we can often help emotional lability to some extent.

Other causes. We must first ensure that the emotions expressed are not due to some other cause; that they are not real emotional reactions to a difficult situation (Chapter 7) or the outcome of disturbed relationships with family or staff (Chapter 8), and that the lability is not due to delirium or to the effects of drugs such as benzodiazepines or antiparkinsonian drugs.

Circumstances. Using a behaviour chart the pattern and circumstances of the lability can be recorded after clearly defining the problem. The type of chart on which each episode of disturbed behaviour is recorded (Fig. 5.1) is more often useful here, since episodes of lability are often quite widely scattered over time. The factors which are causing the lability to occur may well include circumstances which 'raise the emotional temperature'. Even quite severely demented patients can be sensitive to the emotional atmosphere long after their ability to express feelings in words is lost. People who meet a dementing patient will vary greatly in the degree of calmness or emotional expression with which they react to her. Those who are anxious about the patient, upset by her, frustrated by her or confrontational will induce an emotional reaction which, in the absence of proper control, can lead to a labile response. Other exacerbating factors may include situations which bewilder or frustrate the patient – confusing surroundings, too many questions, too much choice or situations which will show up her disabilities.

Having identified the exacerbating factors we can look into ways of modifying them. We may need to teach each other how to be calm with the patient, or we may need to simplify her surroundings and activities, to avoid frustrations where possible.

A most distressing vicious circle can develop if a relative or staff member assumes that the patient's emotional response is intentional. If, for example, a dementing wife becomes angry in a disinhibited way with her husband he may feel that she is getting at him and react just as strongly back. Or a relative may try to shout down the patient who is getting emotionally upset, instead of lowering the emotional temperature. These reactions disturb the patient even more and the whole situation can get out of hand, even ending in violence. It does not take a chart to see what is happening. But if the relative's excessive reaction to the patient has been a lifelong habit it will be very difficult to get him to change. Often the only thing which helps is for the relative to leave the room for a while until both settle down.

This sort of over-reaction by relatives shows up very clearly if the patient attends day care or goes into respite care. A problem of emotional lability at home turns out to be no problem in the other setting. Partly this is because people are on their 'best behaviour' when they go among strangers. But partly it is because of a different emotional 'level'. Unfortunately the ordinary, warm emotional bond between husband and wife can be enough to increase the likelihood of lability, without anything being wrong in their relationship. This is one of the reasons why caring husbands or wives need a regular break. But it is also worthwhile spending effort in trying to teach a relative how to distance himself emotionally from the patient – learning how to 'cool it'.

Normal behaviour. The 'normal' times when the patient is not labile give clues as to what helps her feel at ease. This is likely to be a calm, simple, non-frustrating, non-bewildering environment. There is little more that can be done to encourage these settled times. The treatment of lability consists mainly of reducing the labile episodes.

Drugs. Once again the choice of drugs is wide and trial and error must be used. Sometimes an antidepressant drug may be helpful if the patient is generally in low mood as well as suffering episodes of labile tearfulness or other distress, and drugs like fluoxetine may be particularly helpful. Sometimes a small dose of a phenothiazine or similar drug helps best.

'Stuck' emotions

Here the ups and downs of emotion are lost and the patient seems unable to move away from a particular emotion. Thus she may be constantly anxious for no apparent reason, or persistently irritable, or spend long parts of the day in tears. The curious dissociation between emotional expression and actual subjective feeling which occurs in lability may also apply here. So, in contrast to someone suffering from depression, the tearful lady may say that she does not know what is upsetting her, or even that she feels perfectly happy. In other patients a search for meaning makes them identify some cause for their emotion. Needless to say this cause may be quite imaginary. If the emotion is sadness, she may complain that a parent has gone away, or that she is going to die. If it is anger, she may make a paranoid interpretation, that someone is getting at her. If it is anxiety, she invents a danger of fire, harm to relatives, etc.

More common than these distressing emotions, though, is 'stuck' happiness, a state of vacuous *euphoria* which is the permanent emotion of many dementia sufferers especially in late phases of the illness. To some extent this is due to the gradual loss of all other emotions (p. 135), but at the end of this decline patients often seem positively happy, and certainly happier than they might be expected to be, suffering such a dreadful illness as dementia.

Management

Management of these disorders of mood is quite difficult. Euphoria is usually seen as a blessing rather than a disorder, and few would wish to 'cure' it by presenting the awful truth of their condition to the happy sufferers. And it is difficult to estimate how subjectively distressed patients with other 'stuck' emotions are. Do they actually feel the emotions or not? Even if they do not feel distressed, or forget that they have been like this for months, it must be a bewildering condition to be in and, of course, it is extremely distressing for relatives and others to see the patient apparently in severe and constant distress.

The behavioural approach is worth trying, but often does not identify clear causes. Distracting the patient into other engaging activities can be very helpful but even in the new activities the emotions may return, upsetting other people around her. Often drug treatment must be used, trying to match the drug to the emotional state – an anti-anxiety drug for anxiety, an antidepressant for depression, a phenothiazine or similar drug for anger, especially if associated with paranoid thinking. Once again the choice is made by trial and error, but larger doses of drugs may be required than in lability. However, as before, success cannot be guaranteed and a few patients have to survive in this apparently distressed state for long periods.

The period of disturbance eventually comes to an end in most cases. This is because the decline of the dementia eventually affects the ability to feel or express any emotion at all. So the emotional disturbance dies away. Both lability and 'stuck' emotions are more often (though not always) problems of early and moderate dementia. Indeed this is a general rule of disinhibition in dementia, that *the problem is likely to be worse in earlier stages and to lessen as the dementia becomes more severe.*

DIFFICULT BEHAVIOUR

A lot of the experience and activity that we have been discussing in relation to attention, speech and emotion has been learned.

Much of our self control and many of the inhibitory mechanisms in the brain are also learned. When we turn to social behaviour (how we interact with other people and how we behave in relation to the 'rules' of society), a great deal of learning over many years must be involved in order to develop a sense of what is 'right' in a particular situation and what is 'wrong'. By Ribot's law, we would expect loss of social controls to be quite an early problem in dementia. Indeed it can be the first sign.

What is difficult behaviour? Difficult behaviour is behaviour which is found to be difficult to manage by those looking after the person with dementia. The description *difficult* is often as much a function of the person describing it as it is of the behaviour itself.

Causes of difficult behaviour

These will be considered in turn.

Factors directly associated with dementia. These relate to the particular type of dementia, and to the areas of the brain affected. It has been reported, for example, that vascular dementia is more likely to be associated with aggression. This may at least partly be related to the fact that these patients tend to retain insight into their disabilities more than those with Alzheimer's disease. This, naturally, leads to frustration and anxieties, which in turn may lead to verbal outbursts.

Many different parts of the brain may be involved in dementia, and, as with other features of dementia, this influences the behaviour of the patient. The frontal lobes are involved in the comparisons of standards which help us control our behaviour. Functions such as conscious social awareness, self control, moral ideas and judgement seem to be largely carried on in this part of the brain and through its connections. Damage here leads to a decline in this learned control, leading to disinhibited behaviour, and since much of our description of personality depends on how a person behaves socially, it is these changes which are usually meant when families talk about a dementia sufferer having a change of personality. At its mildest this change affects many minor judgements the sufferer has to make from day to day – standards of cleanliness, choice of clothing, what is a sensible price for something, table manners, road sense. Relatives may report a general but vague decline in standards, and say that the patient does not seem to care about these things in the way she used to. She is careless and does not seem to realise it. More serious lack of judgement and self control can cause considerable distress and embarrassment or put the patient and others at great risk. Sexual disinhibition is one group of behaviour problems that can be very difficult to manage in any care setting. Likewise, these patients may be more prone to aggression, which may be verbal or physical. Dysphasia (p. 137) is common in the later stages of Alzheimer's disease. There is a clear association between this and aggresive behaviour, presumably because of the communication problems which these patients have.

Parietal lobe damage can lead to degrees of dyspraxia, that is, difficulties with visio-spatial orientation. Thus, the patient may have problems dressing, or of finding the way to her bed or to the toilet; this may lead her to go to the wrong bed, or to do the toilet in inappropriate places. These problems are often very distressing for relatives (and indeed for professional carers), and can seriously compromise the dignity of the patient.

A lack of comprehension as to what is going on round about can cause many difficulties for the patient with dementia. Thus, when approached for help with bathing or dressing, the patient may well be unable to recognize what is happening and may see the approach in terms of an assault and may quite understandably then try to 'defend' herself.

Environmental factors. People with dementia are often cared for in far from ideal conditions, whether this be in their own homes, a hospital ward or residential or nursing homes. Features such as large group living, lack of activities, locked doors and communal meal times are often unfamiliar to the person, and her reactions may well lead to problems. Her behaviour might well be behaviour-seeking as a result of boredom or to what she sees as lack of attention. It is impossible to be dogmatic on what is the ideal environment for those with dementia; however, as much as possible we should adapt the environment of any care setting to the residents, rather than expecting the residents to adapt to the environment.

Loneliness is perfectly possible in a crowded situation. We can all feel alone in a room or in a street full of strangers; in dementia, sufferers may lose the ability to recognize those around them and so feel constantly alone. Loneliness can be a source of discomfort or even distress to any of us.

Inappropriate noises which may be repetitive, unusual or simply unidentifiable are a potential source of agitation. The nursing home or hospital ward with constant shouting, door alarms and fire alarms going off, and competing noise from the television and radio, is setting itself up for agitation in its residents.

Previous personality of the person with dementia. By the time someone with dementia has been admitted to a long-term setting, many losses have been experienced. As well as the loss of cognitive abilities, there has been a loss of lifetime roles (as a spouse, parent, householder, etc.), a loss of independence, perhaps loss of a loved one, loss of choice and loss of individuality. How anyone copes with losses depends very much on their previous life experiences as well as with his or her general 'psychological' make-up. These losses may often cause a loss of purpose, resulting in perhaps aimless wandering or frustration.

A man who has worked in a steel works and has enjoyed male company in pubs as his main form of entertainment may well swear and act aggressively when confronted, but this might well be a reflection of his personality rather than due to his dementia – should it be managed medically? Likewise someone may be overfamiliar, interfering, rude, withdrawn, constantly on the move – is this necessarily due to dementia? We all know people like these!

Thus, there are many factors in the genesis of difficult behaviour in dementia. We must keep them in mind when dealing with it, as it is more appropriate to alter the circumstances leading to a problem than to tackle it from the effect it may have on ourselves or on others.

Let us look at examples of poorly controlled disinhibited behaviour before examining ways of managing such problem behaviour.

Perseveration of action

The sort of difficulty of moving from one subject to another, mentioned above under speech, can occur also in relation to actions. The patient who tries to change from one action (say pouring the tea) to another (say adding sugar) finds herself unable to do so, and ends up pouring tea into the sugar bowl. She may or may not be aware of the problem.

Old habits

An interesting phenonemon which is due to disinhibition is the reappearance of old habitual actions, often an action which was used at work. Such actions have been learned and repeated many, many times over years, but may have last been performed 20 years or more previously. Loss of inhibition allows their return. This usually causes no problem, but may be a great puzzle until an old workmate or a relative recalls its original meaning. Repetitive dusting actions may even be put to some present use!

Rituals

New repetitive actions may also emerge. Failure of control allows a repetitive habit to continue and become established. Such rituals as turning on and off taps (sometimes with disastrous consequences), folding pieces of paper or touching certain objects are quite common. They may have started as early reactions of the patient to her dementia (Chapter 7), perhaps as attempts to keep a crumbling world in order with reminders or routine, but they can become fixed and meaningless.

Conversation

Unnecessary or meaningless words can get into speech by loss of the normal inhibitory mechanisms. However, the content of our speech is also controlled by our understanding of what is proper, what is acceptable to the person we are talking to. Loss of this control may lead a polite lady to start using swear words, or a careful lady to say just what she thinks about someone else. Sometimes the amount of speech is affected and someone who was very quiet speaks endlessly.

Table manners

A coarsening of table manners is often seen in dementia, ranging from being sloppy to eating everything in sight (even including the soap and the house plants).

Dressing and undressing

Normally how we dress depends on the standards of those of our own sex, age and social group. Some dementing people, quite apart from their declining ability to dress properly (p. 141) or remembering to change their clothes, seem to choose to wear eccentric clothes. They seem to have lost the concern for their own appearance which is part of our social relationships. In other cases the problem is one of undressing in public, the patient losing her usual concern about privacy and propriety. She may go out half-dressed or undressed in the street, or undress in front of other residents.

Undressing can be an extreme problem, the patient dressing and undressing repeatedly for no apparent reason. There may be some physical or mental distress that makes the patient feel uncomfortable. She may be too hot. She may be uncomfortable because of incontinence, a desire to urinate, or constipation. She may feel unwell or be made restless by drugs. She may be anxious, depressed or frustrated. She may, of course, be particularly frustrated by a dressing dyspraxia. She may have a curious condition which is sometimes found in dementia, *hyperaesthesia*, an extreme sensitivity of the skin which makes normal touch seem like pain. But often there is no clear cause and the problem seems to be purely due to disinhibition.

Excreting

Children learn quite early in life that it is considered correct to urinate or defaecate in a toilet. If this learned social control is lost, then anywhere will do. We need, however, to distinguish this type of *inappropriate excretion*: first from disorientation or ignorance of where the toilet is, which may force the sufferer to go somewhere else and will be highly embarrassing to her; secondly from urgency, a need to rush to the toilet but perhaps not get there in time, caused by bladder problems; and thirdly from true incontinence where *physical* control of urination or defaecation has been lost (an example of neurological disinhibition, see p. 180). Of course many dementing patients lose their conscience about these other causes of 'accidents' as well and so do not feel as embarrassed by them as a normal person would.

Another associated problem is that of faecal smearing (*scatolia*) which usually arises from the patient touching her own faeces (usually, but not invariably, when defaecating), and then trying to clean her hands on anything available, combined with a lack of awareness of the consequences. Like sexual disinhibition, this can be 'the last straw' for carers.

Common causes of faecal smearing and faecal incontinence are:

1. *Constipation* – when there is a blockage in the rectum or higher up in the intestine, the movement of food becoming faecal waste continues and may overflow past the blockage. The result is foul-smelling, poorly formed, incontinent faeces. Relief of the constipation will cure the problem, but if the constipation has been a problem for some time, retraining of the bowel will not be immediately effective. Often it is necessary for the doctor not only to examine the patient rectally, but also to take an X-ray of the abdomen to check whether there is high-up constipation, and later to check that the blockage has completely cleared. Scatolia is not uncommon among dementia sufferers, and is very distressing to their carers. They usually assume that it is due to poor personal standards, or carelessness. However, scatolia is in fact almost always a sign of constipation. Presumably the patient is trying to cope with the vague discomfort of constipation, or attempting themselves to clear their blocked bowel by hand. A laxative or enema will often solve the problem.

2. *Laxatives* – on the other hand, overuse of laxatives can produce incontinence. Some patients are dependent on laxatives, and may even take them secretly, but usually this cause is easily found and corrected.

3. *Bowel diseases* – food poisoning and other infections which cause diarrhoea, diverticular disease and less common illnesses, including ulcerative colitis and cancer of the bowel, may all lead to incontinence of faeces. If constipation and laxative overuse have been ruled out as causes of the incontinence, then these causes should be considered.

4. Having ruled out these medical causes, the problems of *self-neglect*, *loss of 'conscience'* and *inability to find or reach the toilet* should be considered.

5. Incontinence due to *loss of control* occurs late in the illness – there is no medical treatment which is likely to reverse this type of incontinence. Much depends on avoiding constipation, good diet and regular toileting. Although it occurs relatively late in the disease, faecal incontinence can still be very distressing to the patient. Prompt cleaning and changing are the best service that

can be given. Under no circumstances should the patient be blamed for being incontinent.

Incontinence of either urine or faeces is a medical problem. It always deserves careful investigation before assuming that nothing can be done.

Physical contact

Social taboos prevent people from picking their noses or touching their own genitals in public. They limit the amount that people touch each other both sexually and non-sexually. Older people in general do accept ordinary touching much more readily than younger people, perhaps because some of the sexual meaning of touch has been lessened. But in dementia the taboos may be lost.

The good side of this is that touch can be used to help dementing people, to reassure and support them, to calm or to help engage them in activity. The not-so-good side is that patients may look for sexual contact in a disinhibited way. The patient's spouse may find it very distasteful or embarrassing if their wife or husband starts being sexually interested after years of lack of interest, especially if that interest is shown in an uncontrolled or demanding way which is out of character. The worst situation of all arises when the object of sexual desire is apparently a completely new one, for example a happily married man who begins to show a disinhibited sexual interest in children.

Respect for others' possessions

When this social standard is lost (partly due to a loss of the ability to recognize what is one's own), the patient may lift other people's belongings without concern. Patients then tend to believe that these items are their own, and trying to return them to their rightful owners can lead to a great deal of aggravation. Mildly dementing people at home may become shoplifters. In a residential home or hospital a hoard of other people's possessions or items belonging to the establishment may be found in a resident's locker. Even exchanging false teeth is not unknown.

Asking for attention

In the section on speech (p. 154) we discussed repeated calls for help that are meaningless and due simply to a 'stuck' word. A more general change can occur, whereby the patient loses the patience to wait for help and becomes insistent, demanding of attention, even histrionic in her demands. Linked with some disinhibition of emotion, this can change a polite, patient, uncomplaining lady into a rather unattractive, cantankerous one who demands immediate attention for real or imaginary complaints and who loses her temper or acts out physical or mental distress if her demands are not met.

Restlessness

There are a number of different causes of restlessness in dementia which must always be considered (Table 5.2). Disinhibition is only one and often, indeed, more than one type of cause applies. The other types of cause are physical discomfort, physical illness, delirium, drug side-effects and emotional distress (including searching for familiar territory, anxiety, depression and frustration). Only when all of these have been ruled out should disinhibition as a sole cause of restlessness be considered.

Our activity is usually set at a particular general level, though where this controlling function is located in the brain is not

Table 5.2 Restlessness

Cause	Management
Physical discomfort e.g. pain, constipation, heat	Find cause and treat it
Delirium	Find cause (Table 2.2) and treat
Drug side-effect (akathisia)	Reduce dose
Need of customary exercise	Exercise
Searching for familiar people or territory (which may or may not still exist)	Reality orientation (RO) Find alternative activities

Distress
  anxiety
  depression
  frustration
	Reassurance, RO, drugs
	Support, counselling, drugs
	Assess losses, fill gaps

Disinhibition	Behaviour management, drugs

Again each cause has a quite different treatment, and several causes may co-exist.

known. There are of course variations, some people feeling active and energetic in the mornings, others in the afternoon, some feeling less inclined to be active as it comes to night-time in preparation for sleep. We have mentioned before the decline in activity and apathy which affects the majority of dementia sufferers (p. 133). For a minority, however, the opposite occurs. They lose the normal control mechanism and have an increase in their energy and activity. As with ritual behaviour, some of this may arise from early distress and agitation but then the disturbed behaviour gets 'stuck'. In its extreme forms this overactivity, like mania or akathisia (general restlessness of the muscles) due to phenothiazine and related drugs, can appear unstoppable. The patient is unable to concentrate on anything or to relax for any length of time and seems to need to be in constant motion. Sleep may be lost and sitting long enough to have a meal becomes a problem.

More common than this constant overactivity is the change in the usual diurnal variation in activity mentioned on p. 63. For reasons which are obscure, the patient is settled throughout the morning, but beginning in late afternoon there is a build-up of restlessness until sleep comes. Relatives frequently report the disruption that this 'sundowning' can bring to family life. Or they complain that day care is provided at the most settled part of the day. And staff who only work in the morning and early afternoon wonder why evening and night staff are complaining.

MANAGEMENT OF BEHAVIOUR DISINHIBITION

Most of the steps in management have already been covered in the four principles on p. 153, though some additional principles apply particularly to social disinhibition.

Identify the problem. Be absolutely clear that all are agreed what behaviour is being discussed. Once that is done we can begin to look for causes.

Is it normal for this person? If she cannot tell this herself it will be important to ask her family or someone who has known her well for years. Only behaviour which is a change from normal should be considered.

Other causes. Delirium, and particularly certain drug reactions, should be ruled out before deciding that disturbed behaviour is due to disinhibition. Among drugs, we should consider antiparkinsonian drugs such as L-dopa and bromocriptine which can be potent causes of restlessness, sexual disinhibition and other behaviour disorders, as well as causing delirium. Depression (p. 221) can cause restlessness and agitation. Mania (p. 75) can lead to disinhibited behaviour of all sorts and needs to be differentiated very carefully from dementia. The sort of lists shown in Tables 5.1 and 5.2 could be made up for all the different behaviour problems.

Assess the significance of the problem. Questions to be asked are, 'Is this behaviour posing a real problem?', 'Does it upset the patient or does it upset others?', 'If it is other people who are upset, is that because they have an intolerant attitude which might be changed?'. Only if the problem is really *significant* should we be trying to 'treat' it.

While difficult behaviour may lead to problems providing care to a patient, it is important to remember whom we are in fact treating. Some behaviour patterns cause great stress or even distress to carers or to other patients; but the patient herself is totally oblivious to this and not at all worried. *How far is it right to treat* someone in this situation?

Attitudes to disinhibition. It is important to look further at our attitudes towards the behaviour that is released by social disinhibition. We all know of things that we would like to do if only we were less inhibited. But it is not fair to dementia sufferers to assume that the disinhibited things they do are 'naughty' things that they have wanted to do for years and are now released from inhibition. All of us are capable of behaving in all sorts of ways that we have never even thought of. It may be tempting to see a lady's disturbing behaviour as a protest at past over-control. But this is only our fantasy unless we have real evidence that she actually wanted to act in a more disinhibited way. We should be tolerant of disinhibited behaviour in dementia, for it is due to organic brain disease and the patient cannot help what she is doing, but we should not encourage it because it is colourful or seems rebellious.

External controls

Disinhibited social behaviour can be seen as due to a loss of conscience. Can we fill this gap by an external conscience? We behave 'properly' not only because of our internal conscience but also because others show disapproval if we behave 'improperly'. In dementia the ability to understand and respond to external disapproval or advice is gradually being lost so it may have little effect, especially in later stages of the illness. But it is worth consideration.

What we are suggesting is simply that if the patient has lost the ability to say 'No, don't do it' to herself, then someone else should say it to her. There is a danger, however, that we may become too punitive. The decision to use external control should, therefore, be based on very careful assessment. Will she understand what is being said? Does this external control make her embarrassed, guilty or frightened, by making her realize that what she is doing is 'wrong'? Does it make her angry or resentful without affecting her behaviour much? Or does it have to be done so often or so strongly that it causes 'overload' and a catastrophic emotional reaction? Do other patients and visitors understand what is being done and do they approve? Most important of all, does the attempt at external control actually encourage the behaviour it is supposed to stop, by constantly bringing up the subject?

All this being said, there is a definite place for external control. It is used by relatives, but they often feel quite guilty about what seems like scolding their spouse or mother. It is used by staff in hospitals and homes to control eating habits, or undressing in public, inappropriate urination or sexual misbehaviour. It should never be done in bad temper. And it should not be used willy-nilly on all patients. It is better decided upon after full discussion among everybody who is working with the particular patient.

Circumstances

Charting the circumstances of the patient's abnormal behaviour and others' reactions to it can again be very useful in identifying what makes it happen more often. For antisocial interactions, the most important factors are likely to concern *to whom* the patient behaves towards in a disinhibited way and *what response* she gets from them. Further, the response which reinforces her behaviour may not be the obvious one. We might expect that anger or disgust would stop undesirable behaviour. Paradoxically, such reactions can actually encourage it, probably because they represent some sort of attention and interaction and so fulfil a basic human need. This is particularly a problem when nobody is interacting much at all with the patient except to shout the occasional 'Stop that!'. Thus attempts at external control of the behaviour may actually have to be discouraged. Often, though, it is more general attention which has been reinforcing. People only notice her when she is doing something odd or startling and automatically pay more attention during these times. Withdrawing attention, rather than changing from being nice to being nasty, will be most helpful. But, of course, there may be protests, both from the patient and from relatives, other patients or staff who see the withdrawal of attention as dereliction of duty, especially if the patient is being antisocial, so any thought of withdrawing attention should be carefully discussed with all concerned, and the arguments and decisions recorded carefully.

Normal behaviour

In some cases it is possible to retrain patients to a limited extent. Sloppy habits in eating or dressing are likely to be most easily helped this way. In general, encouragement, praise and reinforcement that is appropriate to the individual should be tried. It should be given immediately after the patient has properly performed what at other times she does in a disinhibited way. Again, success is likely to be limited. But a combination of reducing reinforcement of abnormal behaviour and positive reinforcement of more normal behaviour, together with judicious use of external controls, can bring enough improvement, helping an undesirable, unpopular patient to change and become a more acceptable and likeable person who has a better quality of life.

Some of this change will have been brought about by changing circumstances. But some assumes an ability to learn, for behaviour therapy is largely based on theories of learning. The improvement achieved by any of these techniques must be limited by the declining ability of the patient to learn (p. 131). Indeed, at later stages of dementia, learning ability is so slowed as to be effectively absent. Furthermore, the patient's ability to make or receive any meaningful contact with the outside world is declining, so behaviour modification is likely to be less effective later on. On the other hand, behaviour and experience are often simpler at the later stages, so simple modifications of circumstances can occasionally bring surprisingly good results. The most obvious examples of this occur when a demented lady moves from one environment to another, or when she becomes physically ill. Behaviour which has been disinhibited and troublesome in one set of circumstances can disappear overnight. The lesson is that behaviour modification should always be given a chance.

Alternative activities

Once again it needs to be said that the dementing person who is involved and enjoying some interesting activity is not going to have any time or enthusiasm for disturbed behaviour. 'Changing the subject' may be the most effective therapy. Even a change of scenery can seem to help in itself. The restless patient is not causing a problem if she is going for an enjoyable walk with someone. The sexually disinhibited man is not offending anyone if his need for interaction with women is being met by a sing-song or a quiz.

Maintaining improvement

If behaviour has improved, there is always a tendency to relax and fall back into old ways of responding. Whoever is in charge of a behaviour programme should ensure that its principles are continued and should remind family or staff from time to time of what it was that helped. If the behaviour returns, a repeat programme may be justified.

Drugs

The same principles apply as before. As a last resort small doses of tranquillizers or the other drugs mentioned on p. 160 may help to control disinhibited behaviour. An apparent improvement that is merely caused by oversedation is undesirable. The oversedated patient is likely to be more muddled, less physically able, and less able to cooperate – a combination which will add to rather than lessen the difficulties of her behaviour.

There is often a tendency to use drugs as the first line of management. We must avoid this, and try all other management techniques first. If a drug is to be used, it should be in as small a dose as possible, and it should be stopped as soon as possible. Before we resort to drug treatment we must think 'Have other management strategies been tried?', 'Who are we treating?', 'Is the difficult behaviour really intolerable?', 'Can the patient consent to treatment?'. Once it is prescribed we must continually review the need for its ongoing use, and monitor for any possible side-effects (Chapter 6). The common practice of prescribing these drugs as 'repeat prescriptions' should be resisted, and each time a new prescription is to be issued, the doctor should stop and think whether it is really necessary.

Disinhibition of thinking

We have earlier described the usual poverty of thinking of dementia sufferers (p. 134). But often we come across odd or quite bizarre ways of thinking among patients. Some of these are caused by attempts to make sense of what is happening (p. 163) in the absence of proper information from senses or memory. But the fact that the patient seems to accept these peculiar ideas as normal requires some further explanation.

Within our minds thoughts are judged by a standard of acceptability that we learn. We treat whatever is not accepted in a variety of ways – as dreaming, as imagination, as contradictory, as something that it is not polite to think. If this controlling mechanism is not present, then previously unacceptable thoughts become acceptable and unacceptable thoughts are not dismissed.

Often a patient will hold ideas that contradict each other, or contradict reality. An example is the person who says that her parents are alive and yet also knows that she herself is 85. This 'double orientation' is partly due to memory loss, but there must be an absence of something inside her, saying 'That must be nonsense'. If such contradictory thoughts become fixed she can be said to suffer from a *delusion*, which cannot be shifted by reason. She is absolutely convinced that her parents are alive. This type of loss of judgement contributes to the paranoid delusions which some dementing people develop to explain their memory lapses (p. 228).

In most patients, however, the odd ideas do not become fixed, and they may be held for very brief times. Some *illusions*, in which the patient misinterprets what she sees or hears (see also

p. 64) are due to faulty judgement, as well as showing poor perception.

Perseveration of thinking and 'stuck' thoughts can occur. The extreme of this is obsessional thinking, in which the patient is forced, against her will, to think the same thought again and again. More often there is a simple difficulty in moving from one thought to another, so that clear thinking becomes very difficult.

Planning

Another aspect of this sort of controlling mechanism of thoughts is planning, which is used to build up complicated courses of action and to prevent us from rushing into things. We have already seen one example of lack of planning in relation to people who behave in a demanding way (p. 172), wanting immediate responses, rather than seeing that a more planned and organized request for help might be more effective. One of the very first subtle signs of dementia is often that the patient stops making plans for the future, and so comes to dwell on the present and then more and more in the past.

It takes only a little thought to see how vital to all that we do is this ability to foresee and plan ahead. It actually affects every single action that we carry out.

Management

Problems of planning and judgement affect the patient's ability to understand her current circumstances and make rational decisions (Chapter 9). There is little that can be done to recover the power of judgement once it is lost. Presenting facts in a simple way and reinforcing reality by repetition can help, but drug treatment may be needed if the patient is deluded, and decision-making may have to be taken away from the patient if her thinking becomes out of touch with reality.

NEUROLOGICAL DISINHIBITION

The theory of how disinhibition can cause symptoms is largely due to Hughlings Jackson, a neurologist of the last century. He saw the brain as divided into less advanced 'lower' parts and more advanced 'higher' centres. The latter had a largely controlling function over the former so that, when higher centres were damaged, one result would be loss of this control and the emergence of more primitive functions. Looking at disinhibited social behaviour as an example, we can see that this theory fits quite well. We learn with our 'higher' frontal bits of the brain (parts that are much smaller in 'lower' animals) to control our social behaviour. Failure of frontal lobe function means that 'lower', less advanced types of functioning re-emerge.

Jackson's experience, however, was neurological. For example, damage to the frontal lobes can lead to the emergence of primitive reflexes such as the sucking reflex and the grasp reflex which usually are only present for a short time after birth and then disappear. They have been inhibited during all those intervening years, but the possibility of them recurring has remained and is released by the loss of inhibition.

INCONTINENCE

The commonest type of neurological disinhibition in dementia, however, is incontinence. From the base of the frontal lobes, an inhibitory mechanism passes down the spinal cord to the bladder, preventing it from opening. Normally this inhibition can only be overcome by the voluntary decision to urinate, and of course we are reminded of the need to do this by messages coming up from the bladder which indicate that it is full. If the inhibition from the brain is lost, then the bladder may empty without voluntary control. A somewhat similar, though less sophisticated, mechanism controls defaecation.

In dementia sufferers there are a number of ways in which inappropriate urination and defaecation occur, not all of which are true incontinence. The true loss-of-control incontinence of dementia should occur relatively late in the progress of the disorder and urinary incontinence should occur before faecal incontinence, according to Ribot's law (p. 9). So incontinence occurring earlier in dementia is more likely to be due to other causes. There are some exceptions to this rule. In normal pressure hydrocephalus (p. 36), and occasionally VaD, loss-of-control incontinence occurs early in the course of the illness.

Urinary incontinence

The common types of urinary incontinence met with in dementing patients are (see Table 5.3):

1. Incontinence due to a *urinary tract infection* – when incontinence starts, especially if it occurs suddenly and if there are symptoms of an infection – frequency, discomfort during urination, pain in the lower abdomen or loin, raised temperature – a midstream specimen of urine must be taken and checked for infection. Urinary infections are usually treatable, though recurrence is a problem, especially in women. If continence has been lost because of an infection it usually returns after treatment, but a little retraining may be necessary. It is not clear to what extent urinary infections without symptoms cause incontinence.

2. Incontinence of urine due to *constipation* – the mass of faeces in the rectum disrupts the mechanics of urination and can lead to incontinence of urine. This will improve after the constipation is relieved.

3. *Diuretic treatment* can lead to or exacerbate incontinence – in particular, a diuretic drug (a water tablet) given later in the day

Table 5.3   Common causes of urinary incontinence in dementia

Cause	Management
Urinary tract infection	Antibiotic
Constipation	Treat and prevent constipation Good diet with plenty of roughage and fluid
Diuretics	Reduce dose or change drug
Self-neglect	Social stimulation
Loss of conscience	Behaviour management
Inability to get to the toilet in time	Help mobility Signposting and easy access Training how to get there
Stress incontinence	Gynaecological advice
Bladder dysfunction	Specialist incontinence clinic
Loss of control	Regular toileting Learn warning signs Incontinence aids

can give rise to night incontinence, and the night-time cup of tea can make things worse still. Diuretics should be given in the morning, in the mildest form and the lowest dose that are absolutely necessary. Unfortunately, these are very widely used drugs and patients tend to continue taking them for years with little review.

4. *Self-neglect* incontinence – the patient who has withdrawn and become depressed or apathetic may not bother about her self-care and gradually become incontinent. Social stimulation and improved morale can reverse this.

5. Incontinence due to the *loss of 'conscience'* – the patient with frontal lobe type of damage loses social concern and judgement and may urinate in inappropriate places. This is a form of disinhibited behaviour needing behavioural management (p. 169) by general stimulation, encouragement of normal behaviour, retraining and avoidance of attention.

6. *Inability to get to the toilet* – memory impairment and disorientation leave the patient unable to find the toilet and, especially if she suffers urgency or frequency of micturition, incontinence is the result. Poor mobility leads to the same problem. Anxiety and embarrassment result and can make urgency worse and so, by a vicious circle, increase the incontinence. Good signposting and a regular toileting programme to suit the particular patient can often solve this problem. Patients with poor memory may need to be taken along the route to the toilet repeatedly before they begin to learn the way. The poorly mobile patient, or the patient who suffers urgency, will feel much more relaxed if she can sit within sight of a toilet. At night the provision of a commode or a bottle or bedpan can avoid considerable problems (though the patient has to remember that these aids are there!). It is important to learn just how the patient feels, complains or behaves when she needs to urinate, especially if she is unable to say directly and needs help to get to the toilet.

7. In women, symptoms of *stress incontinence* and the related problems of vaginal prolapse can range from the passage of small amounts of urine when the patient coughs to severe loss of control – symptoms are likely to have been present long before the onset of the dementia, but may be exacerbated by one or other factors above. Gynaecological help is required to treat this.

8. In men, incontinence may be related to *prostate enlargement* – the most common problem is frequency of micturition by day and night, the patient passing small quantities of urine with difficulty, but very often. If there is a problem of finding the toilet, this can easily lead to incontinence. Alternatively, urine may be retained in the bladder and then overflow past the blockage caused by the prostate. The patient has no control over this 'overflow' incontinence. A failed prostatectomy operation can also lead to incontinence. Specialist surgical advice will be needed in such cases.

9. *Bladder dysfunction* – it is now known that the bladder mechanism may go wrong in a number of ways, and these can be investigated by special X-rays and pressure measurements in the bladder. For example, some incontinent patients have a large bladder which has poor muscle tone and empties spontaneously when the volume of urine reaches a certain amount. Others have a small but 'irritable' bladder which empties small quantities of urine with no warning. These and other related forms of incontinence are not uncommon, but they are not directly due to dementia. They may require special investigation at an incontinence clinic.

10. *The incontinence of dementia* – in the true neurological incontinence of dementia the patient has a normal bladder but the inhibitory messages from the brain are not being dispatched from the frontal lobes (in disease or injury of the spinal cord these messages are interrupted on their way to the bladder and incontinence also results). The patient's bladder opens when it reaches a certain size and pressure. The messages to the brain telling of the bladder pressure and of urination may also be appreciated less and the patient is completely unaware of the problem. At early stages, however, some awareness is present and the patient may react with embarrassment, or by attempts to hide wet clothes.

Management

As with all the other forms of disinhibition, we should search first for the remediable causes or exacerbating factors listed above. In many patients there is more than one cause for the incontinence.

Retraining can be very useful if the incontinence of dementia is of recent onset, giving regular reminders to the patient that she may need the toilet and praise for success. Criticism of failure is more likely to cause incontinence than cure it. Regular toileting at 2-hourly or hourly intervals can help reinstitute continence, calm and praise once again being used to reinforce success. Like external controls in social disinhibition (p. 174) this technique provides a message from outside ('It is time to urinate') that previously came from inside.

On the other hand we must not fall into the situation of 'the toileting round' where all patients in a ward or home are toileted on a rota system. Not only is this degrading for the patient, it leads to loss of choice and of individuality. It certainly does nothing for job satisfaction of care staff.

Eventually, most dementia sufferers lose urinary continence for good and require incontinence aids.

Drugs such as oxybutynin (Ditropan) are often used to treat incontinence in older people. However, their use should be reviewed. They often do not work, and they have strongly anticholinergic effects which may lead to increased memory impairment and delirium, often with vivid hallucinations.

Incontinence aids of many types are available. Special absorbent pads or pants can be useful for both urinary and faecal incontinence. Learning how to use them, and indeed accepting a need for them, is often difficult for people with dementia. Protective bedding can reduce the discomfort, smell and damage of incontinence. Incontinence laundry services provide regular fresh sheets. For men a sheath and bag arrangement may help, especially at night, but if the patient feels uncomfortable or is restless, he may not tolerate it. Occasionally an indwelling catheter may be necessary and is tolerated by the patient. In severe dementia it is likely to be impossible to explain to the patient what is being done, so it is quite common for the catheter to be pulled out.

FITS

Fits are common in both DAT and VaD. They may be caused by scarring after damage to the brain; this is certainly the case in VaD. The scarring acts as a focus of irritation and the electrical disturbances so caused lead on to a fit. There is an element of loss of control, though fits are not true disinhibitory phenomena. The fits of dementia may be of various types – focal, petit mal or grand mal.

A *focal fit* is a discharge of activity in a particular area of the cortex leading to an experience or behaviour that relates to that area (p. 108). In a fit in the motor area, specific muscles may twitch. In a temporal lobe fit, the patient may hear sounds or experience other unusual experiences (called an *aura*). Such a fit may become more generalized and turn into a grand mal fit. But *grand mal* fits can also occur without warning. These are 'major' fits, and are caused by electrical disturbances in the central parts of the brain. Because the centres which control consciousness are in these central regions (p. 62), the patient becomes unconscious during the fit, while there is at the same time a generalized discharge in all areas of the brain. This leads to a contraction of all muscles (the 'tonic' phase) followed by irregular shaking of the muscles (the 'clonic' phase). After this the patient goes into a coma, a deep sleep, a delirium, or any combination of these. A *petit mal* fit is not a lesser version of a grand mal fit; it is different. There is a characteristic pattern of electrical discharge in the brain, again due to central disturbance, but the only outside evidence of the fit is a sudden and usually brief loss of consciousness, or *absence*.

Complex partial seizures can be difficult to diagnose and treat. These are seizures which go on for long periods of time, often hours or even days, leading to episodes of bizarre behaviour or memory loss, or of other changes in thinking. Patients with this condition show dramatic differences in mental state from time to time, of an intermittent nature. Like other seizures, episodes like this are often followed by periods of drowsiness. It is important to diagnose, as this is a treatable cause of intermittent confusion.

If fits occur early in dementia, or repeatedly, they need investigation by a neurologist and EEG examination to rule out other, possibly remediable, causes such as tumours. If the fits are part of the dementia, and are happening repeatedly, then an anti-epileptic drug will be required.

However, the problem in dementing patients is that, although classical fits do occur, many 'turns' are not so classical and it can be difficult to be clear about what is an epileptic fit, what is a dizzy turn and what is a transient ischaemic attack (TIA) (p. 30).

Many severely demented patients have repetitive twitching movements in one or a few muscles. These are called *myoclonic jerks*. They may respond to anti-epileptic treatment although they are not true fits.

CONCLUSION

Table 5.4 summarizes the principles that we have seen to be useful in dealing with various types of loss of control in dementia. These are all problems which cause great distress to families and staff, and sometimes to the patient herself. They are what make a dementing patient 'psychiatric'. If they can be relieved, then the course of dementia can be smoother and less stressful.

Table 5.4 Disinhibition and its management

Steps in assessment	Management
Define the problem behaviour carefully	
Look for causes of the problem other than dementia	Treat cause
Examine attitudes to 'problem'	Discuss among staff and family
Look at external controls	Are these being under- or overused?
Identify circumstances of behaviour	Modify if necessary
Identify reactions of others to behaviour	Modify if necessary
Look at circumstances of 'normal' behaviour and reactions to it	Encourage this behaviour
Check that improvements are maintained	Reinforce improvement
Assess whether these techniques have worked or whether behaviour is too disturbed	Drug treatment if necessary

6

Drugs and dementia

DRUGS AND OLDER PEOPLE

Prescribing drugs for older people involves a different set of considerations than it does for a younger population. The presence of dementia increases any potential difficulties.

Drug distribution in the body, the breakdown, and the excretion of a drug are significantly different in an older person. The most important factor in this is renal excretion; most drugs are removed from the body through the kidneys. Mild or even more severe impairment of kidney function is regularly found in older people. Liver enzymes, involved in the breakdown of many drugs, often function at a lower level, and thus keep the dose in the body higher for longer. As a result of these changes the concentration of a drug in the tissues may be greatly increased, as may the half-life of the drug (a measure of the time it remains active in the body). It is important to consider these factors, and change the prescribed dosage of a drug appropriately, in order to ensure that a patient receives the minimum necessary dose and therefore avoids side-effects where possible.

As we age, our bodies are likely to suffer from increasing numbers of diseases, and thus more and more drugs may be prescribed. This can lead to polypharmacy, that is, being prescribed several different drugs at the same time. As a result, there are side-effects because of interactions between the drugs. Polypharmacy also increases the likelihood of mistakes in compliance with treatment.

Older patients may have difficulties in taking tablets. These can vary from difficulties in using child-proof containers and blister packs for those with arthritis or sight problems, to difficulties in swallowing.

The British National Formulary gives the following guidelines for prescribing in older people:

- Is a drug necessary?
- Use a limited range of familiar drugs
- Start with a low dose
- Review repeat prescriptions regularly
- Simplify regimes
- Explain clearly, and label containers properly with instructions (avoid 'as directed')
- Instruct patients what to do when drugs run out.

ANTI-DEMENTIA DRUGS

ALZHEIMER'S DISEASE

This is an exciting time for all of us working in the field of dementia. For the first time, drugs are becoming available to treat the condition (Table 6.1). In the UK, donepezil, rivastigmine and tacrine have been licensed for the treatment of Alzheimer's disease. It is too early to say what effects these drugs will have in the care of dementia patients, but there is no doubt that some patients show significant improvement in cognitive function.

Ideally, a drug for dementia should be able to prevent or reverse the disease process. However, the treatments available to date do not do this. They act by enabling one of the neurotransmitters (acetylcholine) to be active for longer. This substance, as we have seen (p. 20), is depleted in the brain of those with DAT. The drugs slow down its breakdown, making the remaining acetylcholine more effective. Unfortunately, they do not affect the underlying progress of the disease. They are said to put cognitive functioning

Table 6.1 Drugs for Alzheimer's disease

Anticholinesterase inhibitors	tacrine (Cognex)
	donepezil (Aricept)
	rivastigmine (Exelon)
	metrifonate
	galanthamine
Neuroprotective drugs	propentifyline
	selegiline (?)
	oestrogen (?)
	anti-arthritis drugs (?)

(mainly memory) back to what it was 6 months previously, but only in some patients. Many health authorities remain unconvinced of the benefit, and at the time of writing prescribing remains restricted. Potential benefits in improving those skills needed to look after oneself (activities of daily living, or ADL) have still to be clarified.

Acetylcholine is by no means the only neurotransmitter implicated in Alzheimer's disease. Dopamine, noradrenaline, glutamate, serotonin and others are also involved. Future *cognitive enhancers* may well have to affect these other transmitters to be more effective.

Some work is going on into the effects of other drugs which work on various different systems in the brain. These include oestrogen, anti inflammatory drugs such as ibuprofen, enzyme inhibitors such as selegiline and psycho-stimulants such as methylphenidate. However, as yet, there is no strong evidence for useful benefits from any of these. Some studies have suggested benefits from the use of vitamins E and C.

Animal studies have shown that a substance called nerve growth factor (NGF) can maintain neurones, and help to effect their repair. At present, however, NGF can only reach the brain by direct infusion into it. Work continues on this substance and there may be other related drugs which emerge from further research.

Vascular dementia

There is a place for drugs in the management of risk factors for VaD, in particular for treatment of hypertension, but also in managing high lipid levels. Low-dose aspirin is effective in lowering the risk of other vascular problems (such as strokes) and may have a role in slowing the progression of VaD, especially if it is of the multi-infarct variety. However, there is no clear evidence that these measures influence the progress of established dementia.

Cerebral vasodilators such as naftidrofuryl oxalate and co-dergocrine mesylate have been used in attempts to increase the brain blood flow. It has been claimed that they improve mental function, but there is actually very little evidence to support this. They probably do not help dementia. There were hopes that calcium channel blockers such as nimodipine might be of value in treatment, but again this has not proved useful in practice.

Research continues into drugs which may protect neurones from the toxins implicated in vascular damage, but at present we are unable to be certain of whether there will be any clinical benefit from such drugs.

PSYCHOTROPIC DRUGS AND DEMENTIA

Patients with dementia are often prescribed one or other of a variety of psychotropic drugs, often for symptoms such as depression, anxiety, insomnia or behaviour problems (see Chapters 5 and 7). Doctors tend towards over-prescribing, particularly the 'neuroleptic' (or 'antipsychotic') drugs. We will now consider the various groups of psychotropic drugs.

HYPNOTIC ANXIOLYTICS

This group of drugs includes the benzodiazepines (such as diazepam, nitrazepam, chlordiazepoxide, temazepam and lorazepam). They are commonly used to sedate, or induce sleep. Older people are at particular risk of side-effects, which include prolonged sedation, unsteadiness leading to falls, slurring of speech, and confusion. In general, longer-acting sleeping tablets such as nitrazepam should be avoided. Dependence is a common problem, and can occur after only a few weeks on these drugs. Long-term prescribing, especially using automatic repeat cards, is considered to be bad practice medically, but these drugs can be invaluable in the short-term in tiding over a crisis.

ANTIDEPRESSANTS

As we have seen, depression is common in those with dementia, though it is often missed. Treatment with antidepressant drugs can lead to great improvements in the quality of life of a person with dementia and depression. There are many different groups of antidepressants, with different modes of action.

Tricyclic antidepressants (e.g. amitriptyline, clomipramine, lofepramine) were, until a few years ago, the first choice drugs. However, they have many side-effects including heart rhythm irregularities, low blood pressure, constipation and confusion, and many doctors feel that they should be avoided in older people. They also tend to be more toxic in overdose, always a risk in people with depression.

Specific serotonin reuptake inhibitors (SSRIs) such as fluoxetine, paroxetine, citalopram and sertraline are, in general, safer. They are usually given as a single daily dose, making for ease of compliance. However, they themselves are not without side-effects, such as nausea and increased agitation with some, and drowsiness with others.

Monoamine oxidase inhibitors (MAOIs) are an older group of drugs which are often tried in patients who have not responded to other antidepressants. Potential interactions with cheese, one or two other food stuffs, and other drugs mean that careful monitoring is essential. There are, however, some newer MAOIs available with a lower risk of problems (e.g. moclobemide).

Other new antidepressants are now available; at present they are not usually used as first-line treatments. These include drugs such as venlafaxine.

NEUROLEPTICS (ANTIPSYCHOTIC DRUGS)

These are drugs (Table 6.2) which were originally developed to manage schizophrenia. Their development revolutionized the management of this condition. They are used specifically in the management of two aspects of dementia – for psychotic symptoms (that is, hallucinations and delusions) and in the management of behaviour disturbance. The rationale for the former use is much more clear than for the latter.

Older people are more susceptible to the side-effects of neuroleptics. The side-effects can be divided into various groups.

Table 6.2 Neuroleptic drugs and suggested starting doses

Chlorpromazine	10 mg twice daily
Haloperidol	0.5 mg twice daily
Thioridazine	10 mg twice daily
Risperidone	0.5 mg twice daily
Sulpiride	100 mg once daily

These include oversedation, *anticholinergic* side-effects and *extrapyramidal effects.*

Anticholinergic side-effects include constipation, urinary obstruction and confusion, sometimes in fact leading to hallucinations. Drugs such as chlorpromazine and thioridazine are particularly prone to cause these effects. Extrapyramidal side-effects are commoner with drugs such as haloperidol. The word extrapyramidal refers to the part of the nervous system which is involved with the control of muscle tone and movement but is not under voluntary control (the voluntary muscle system uses a pathway through the brain stem called the pyramidal tract).

Side-effects include:

- *A Parkinson's disease-like state* of rigidity, slowness and difficulty initiating movement which is often wrongly attributed to underlying dementia and depression rather than to the drug. The typical tremor of Parkinson's disease is less commonly seen.
- *Akathisia or motor restlessness,* an inability to sit still or stay in the same place; it is often mistaken for increased agitation. If a doctor assumes that the restlessness is due to agitation, there is a danger that he will prescribe even more treatment and get into a vicious circle, making the side-effects even worse.
- *Tardive dyskinesia,* repeated or abnormal movements of the muscles of the mouth, limbs or trunk. It is called *tardive* because it often takes weeks or months to develop after starting the drug treatment. It is commoner in older people, who may also develop it in a much shorter period of time and at lower drug doses than younger people.

Akathisia and tardive dyskinesia, once established, do not always recover on stopping the offending drug. They are difficult to treat. Treatment with neuroleptic drugs should not, therefore, be undertaken lightly. The lowest possible doses should be used, and we should continually review the need for treatment, keeping in mind the ratio between the risk and benefit. *Start low, go slow* should be the policy when deciding on dosage.

There is sometimes place for depot injections of a neuroleptic drug, i.e. the drug is given in an oily base, usually into a muscle, so that it has a prolonged action which may last up to 4 or even 6 weeks. For example, this can be used when there is a problem with compliance with oral medication in a patient who needs ongoing treatment to treat paranoia. These depot drugs are particularly likely to cause extrapyramidal side-effects, so, with their long course of action, very particular care needs to be taken to watch out for any side-effects developing.

DELIRIUM

Many drugs can be implicated in the development of delirium and of course polypharmacy increases the risks – delirium has been discussed in Chapter 2 (p. 56).

COMPLIANCE AND DEMENTIA

It is difficult at the best of times for those of us on regular medication to remember to take it. Memory and other cognitive impairments add greatly to this difficulty. The patient may not remember to take a tablet, or how many to take. She may not even accept that she has any illness, and therefore believe she does not need medication.

For those in nursing-home or hospital care, or with readily available carers, there are fewer difficulties since staff or carers can remember for the patient. There may still be problems if the patient refuses to take medication which is prescribed. Strictly speaking, when a doctor prescribes a drug the patient should be given the necessary information to understand why it is being given, the risks involved in taking it and in not taking it, and on that basis she should come to an informed decision about whether or not to accept the drug. In other words she should give her full and informed consent. Where this cannot be given, we can only justify giving medicine if it is necessary to prevent death, serious deterioration in the patient's condition, or serious suffering or distress.

Things are straightforward enough when someone readily takes a tablet, but problems arise when the patient actively refuses to take it or gives no indication of consent or refusal. The problems apply not only to psychotropic drugs, but also to drugs for such conditions as heart disease or chest infections. There is no easy way to deal with this (the issue of consent is discussed further in Chapter 9).

Sometimes it is possible to change how medication is given (e.g. always having the same person giving out the drug, changing from a tablet to a liquid form of the drug, or using a different tablet which may be smaller). A pharmacist can be of great help in discussing these possibilities. There is a widespread practice of trying to conceal medicine, perhaps by adding it to food or drink. This practice is ethically dubious, and we would not recommend it. If it is felt that there is no option but to do this, this should be discussed with all involved, including the patient if possible, an outside second opinion should be sought, and the discussion and decision should be well documented in the patient's records.

The discussion on how far to go in insisting on giving medicine to a patient, without her consent, or in the face of resistance, should take into account her previous attitude to illness and treatments, as well as any advance directive (p. 286). The views of relatives, though they are not in any way legally binding, must also be considered. Account must be taken of the quality of the person's life if the condition is not treated (including distress and any risk) and of the risks and benefits of the treatment, including any possible side-effects.

Whether to treat or not is the doctor's decision, but he should know about any difficulties there may be in administering any treatment and consider these very carefully before making his decision. Nursing or other care staff, or relatives who are involved in helping the patient to take medication, should make clear to the doctor any problems in administration. It is potentially a form of assault to give medication without consent. All concerned, therefore, need to be extremely thoughtful and follow the best possible practice if they wish to help those they are caring for, but not be open to complaint or criticism. Many of those with dementia live alone and here the strategies to improve compliance are different. Helping the person keep her own control of medication is part of maintaining her independence and dignity, and as long as it appears safe to do so, we should continue this.

In order to do this, it is useful to keep the number of times a day a medication is given to a minimum – once- or at most twice-daily medication should be used. At the same time, however, we must remember the risks of building up the blood level with long-acting preparations. We should also avoid 'polypharmacy'. Where there are people such as relatives, home helps or other carers going into the house regularly, times of medication should be coordinated with the times of their visits if possible.

Good compliance not only means taking medicine when it is meant to be taken, it also means not overusing medication. Frequently a person with dementia might forget they have taken a tablet, and then take more at a later time in the day leading to potential problems with overdosage.

COMPLIANCE AIDS

Aids are available for people who are able to manage their medication, but who are simply unable to remember which tablets to take, or when to take them. Compliance aids are devices which enable the medication to be put into separate compartments labelled with when they should be taken. They are available for various periods of time, from daily to weekly. With the help of a community pharmacist, a prescription can be dispensed in these containers. Alternatively, a carer can put the tablets into the appropriate boxes. In dispensing drugs for those with dementia, the container for the medication should be easy to access. We should avoid using child-proof containers and complicated blister packs.

As well as reminding the person to take her tablets, these devices enable those providing care to check whether medication has in fact been taken. In order to use them, the user must be able to understand their use, must be able to see any labels, and must have some degree of manual dexterity. Many different devices are available, and can usually be obtained through the community pharmacy. Some of those available are Medidose, Dosett, Redidose and Dispensatab. The community pharmacist will discuss with carers which device might be most appropriate in any given situation.

The experience of dementia

We can now understand the main changes that happen during the course of dementia, the losses and the new behaviour. They are directly caused by damage to the organic structure of the brain. The function of the damaged parts gradually fails and the person changes. But these changes are happening to a person who lives through the experience of dementia and reacts to it, though, since experience and reaction are also functions of the brain, these too will be modified and failing. In this chapter we will see the various ways in which patients react to the experience of dementia and how these reactions sometimes pose problems for the patient or for others. We will also look at how to manage the more distressing aspects of these reactions.

Severe dementia

What is it like to suffer from dementia? How do patients feel about the experience? To some extent these are unanswerable questions. If we take a severely demented lady, who is apparently unable to understand, who shows no evidence of any thoughts or feelings and who is unable to speak, we can have little idea of what she is experiencing. Anything which she does experience will be quickly forgotten and she will be unable to give a coherent account of it even to herself.

We must remember that dementia is not only loss of memory and other cognitive functions. There is also loss of personality, of judgement and of insight. These are concepts we cannot properly understand – we have not 'been there'. We do not know, and we cannot know, how we would feel if we had severe dementia.

A fragmentary world

It is most unlikely that such a patient with severe dementia is 'locked in' with lots of thoughts and feelings that she cannot express, as can happen to people who suffer severe speech disorders or severe parkinsonism. It is much more likely that there is very little mental activity at all and that she is living in a world of fragmented experience, a world of meaningless sights, sounds, smells, tastes and bodily sensations, partly experienced consciously and unconnected to her equally fragmented emotions and actions.

We can have little concept of what these fragmentary sensations or thoughts are like, or what a fragmentary emotion is. We may be able to recognize in ourselves the experience of half-remembered ideas, or half-understood perceptions, of fleeting emotions or vague motivations, but we experience these from a normal base. When fully conscious, our minds also contain other, more coherent ideas, our sense of self and of the world around is clear and we see these fragments as on the verge of our experience. What, however, if these were the only things in our minds and if that sense of 'I' was incomplete too? Would it be like the bits and pieces of experience that go through our dreams? Or is it like recalling what we can of a delirium? The answer is 'neither', because there would never be a time when we would 'wake up' to recall what we had experienced.

Objective and subjective experience

What we can be sure of is that the experience for the onlooker is different from the experience for the sufferer. The onlooker sees the decline, the emptiness of the patient's mind, her inability to do anything for herself, her disintegrating personality, and so may feel a sense of loss, of pessimism, of emptiness, of degradation.

The patient herself, on the other hand, is unlikely to be aware of or feel any of these changes in a coherent fashion. She will not recall all the things that she used to be able to do and so she will be unable to recognize the change in herself. She will not be able to feel the humiliation of her dependent position. She will not sense the passage of time. Or she may experience the wrong feelings, or jumbled bits and pieces of feelings, some appropriate, some not. It is important to remind ourselves of this, when we think of the plight of the severely demented. Our feelings about what is good or humane for a very severely demented patient cannot come from an understanding of what she feels as an individual, or of what she 'wants'. These concepts are meaningless and so any real understanding is impossible. At the final stages the patient may be assumed to have no real subjective awareness, no sense of self at all, and to be in this sense mentally 'dead'.

Respect for the severely demented

We could conclude that it does not therefore matter what we do to a severe dementia sufferer, for she will not understand or react. This is tempting, but it is not humane and denies the right of the individual to reasonable care and attention when she is ill. It is hardly what we would like to happen to ourselves. We should instead realize that her position of helplessness demands that we pay *special* attention to her needs and treatment. It requires of us a dignified, humane approach to the dementing person which can be difficult to sustain. We forget this approach when we treat all dementia sufferers in the same way. We remember to do it when we recall with respect who that patient was before the illness began and ask ourselves how she would have wished to be treated. This special attention is not so vital for the non-demented, for they can usually answer back, can feel offended or grateful, can remember who is treating them well and who is treating them badly and complain if necessary. People who are mentally impaired are unlikely to be able to complain if they are abused or neglected.

The 'second childhood'?

It is also very tempting to think that the life of a very demented lady is just like that of an infant. It is true that an infant is likely to experience both the world around and its own mental content in an incomplete way. But even at early stages there is some structure and pattern to the way an infant begins to understand, feel and express itself. Despite Ribot's law, the breakdown of the mind in dementia does not exactly reverse that sequence of development. So, trying to make sense of the utterances or expressions of the victim of severe dementia is unlikely to be successful. These are the random, often inappropriate, expressions of a disintegrating mind, not the half-formed products of a developing mind which will later become more organized.

We remember not to infantilize sufferers when they remind us that they are not children or when we recall that they are actually adults with a wealth of experience behind them, usually far more than we have had in our shorter lives.

Milder dementia

Although it is impossible to understand the experience of severe dementia, we must not assume that we cannot understand the earlier stages, even when the person's mental abilities are very obviously impaired. It is true that the further the process of dementia continues and the more distant from her normal experience the person becomes, the less we can comprehend of what she feels. But we can try to understand her experience. Some of our understanding comes from patients with other illness, such as strokes. These may damage only one or two brain functions, leaving unchanged the patient's intellect and her ability to react emotionally. In addition, although the dementia victim may not be able to explain clearly *all* her experiences, many early sufferers have quite good insight into what is happening and can describe their feelings very well. From this evidence we can try to piece together a picture of what it feels like to be dementing.

The value of understanding reactions

What value will this picture serve? It is, of course, humane to try to empathize with people who are ill, to know and understand what they are feeling. If we do not empathize, we distance ourselves from them and are in danger of seeing them as things and not as people. But there are more practical reasons for wanting to understand the experience of dementia. We would, after all, expect sufferers to be horrified, to feel depressed and anxious, even hopeless about the future. They need understanding and practical help to cope with these feelings. But they sometimes appear to have no reaction at all or react only partially. Furthermore, some react in ways which we would not expect, such as by hoarding money for security, by blaming neighbours for mistakes they have made themselves, by becoming aggressive when frustrated or put under pressure, by pretending that they are perfectly well.

These reactions may puzzle us. We do not know how to respond. If we could understand *why* they were happening, we might respond more appropriately and devise treatments which could help the patient. Life might then be more tolerable both for the patient herself and for her supporters.

FACTORS AFFECTING REACTIONS TO DEMENTIA

To move from *guessing* what we would expect the patient to feel, to *understanding what she does feel*, we need to consider several factors (Table 7.1):

1. her personality before the illness developed
2. her expectations of dementia
3. her insight into what is happening
4. the changes in her personality and reactions brought about by the dementia.

Table 7.1 Factors affecting reactions to dementia

'Normal' reactions	Effects of dementia
Personality and attitudes	Degree of insight modified by denial
———————————→ 'Expected' reaction ———————————→ Actual reaction	
Expectation of dementia	Personality and emotional reactions blunted or modified

PERSONALITY

In Chapter 4 we saw that individual patients retain many of their personal characteristics a long way into dementia, even if these are eventually lost. If we can describe the patient's *lifelong* personality we will understand many of her reactions to the illness, especially in the earlier stages.

'Personality' and 'personality disorder'

There is no exact science of personality. Psychologists argue about whether we can define it at all or whether it is just a ragbag of habitual ways of behaving which could easily be modified by changes in circumstances. And attempts to define particular personalities have varied from the description of broad types (e.g. extroverts and introverts) to a more individual description of personality 'traits'. In psychiatry, categories of 'personality disorder' are described. But it is quite difficult to say what is a 'normal' personality and what is abnormal or disordered.

To avoid some of these criticism it is best to take a position that is not too dogmatic. There *are* some characteristic patterns in the way people behave, in how people deal with crises, in their ways of relating to others, and in their attitudes and interests. These can be roughly described and categorized as different personality *types*, but such descriptions are not very reliable. Sometimes a person may wish that her own personality type were different, or other people may complain about it. She can be said to have a personality *problem* or *disorder*. Let us look at how people of different personality types are likely to react to dementia.

Types of personality and their reactions to dementia

Extroverts and introverts

People who are extroverted and sociable often cope quite well with dementia. If they keep their personality they are popular patients and they accept help cheerfully. On the other hand, people who are introverted or schizoid (detached and emotionally cold), while they may not mind the isolation of old age, being usually quite self-sufficient, often dislike the communal aspects of care such as going to day care or living in a home with a group of other people. It is unfortunate for such people that so many services are organized along group lines.

Dependent personality

Some people look at the world as if they could not achieve much by themselves, they feel the need for someone or something as a crutch, they may actually be quite capable of coping but feel that they cannot. We might expect such people to adjust well to dementia, because they will accept the need for outside help readily. They tend to ask for services, sometimes even ending up with too much help. On the other hand they may be reluctant to show initiative or to keep active and independent by using their remaining abilities. We may have to spend time encouraging these 'dependent' people to feel that they can cope alone or do more for themselves.

Independent personality

Others are of more independent types and dislike relying on others. They will resist the increasing dependence of dementia, even when they actually do not have the capacity to cope. Thus they may often be 'bad' patients, since they may refuse the help that family and others offer. They may even end up requiring compulsory measures to ensure that they get help (Chapter 9). They are 'good' patients, however, if independence is needed. So they may do well in retraining programmes, though they will be impatient with their helpers and sometimes unrealistically optimistic about their ability to cope.

Basically, such people need to feel that they are in charge of their own destiny and that they will 'die with their boots on'. So an 'infantilizing' or patronizing approach will not work with them. Family and staff should contrive to let the patient feel that she is making the decisions, even though that is something of a white lie. She is likely to protest strongly when help is introduced without her full agreement or when she has to move into care. But in fact it is remarkable how often that protest is short-lived, for secretly she can appreciate the more dependent position.

Paranoid personality

The paranoid person tends to be suspicious or critical of the outside world, especially when anything goes wrong. Such a person is also likely to be extremely independent-minded. When dementia occurs, she may blame others when *she* makes mistakes and may be suspicious of the motives behind offers of help. This type of reaction is discussed further on p. 228.

Obsessional personality

The person who is orderly, punctual or rather rigid by nature, or the person who is prone to recurrent self-doubts and who needs to check repeatedly that everything around her is exactly right, will find the experience of dementia distressing, for she is faced with a disintegration of order, forgetfulness of time, loss of control and lowering of standards. And the changes brought about in her personality due to the dementia are likely to be very obvious to her family. For both these reasons obsessional people tend to be referred for help very early in dementia.

Hysterical personality

A person who tends to live on the surface of things, dramatizing little problems, needing the attention of others to feel good herself, perhaps playing people off against each other, but forming few deep relationships, is said to have a hysterical personality type. Faced with the multiple problems of dementia she may in fact cope surprisingly well. But sometimes such a patient will behave in a more typical demanding way, acting 'iller' than she actually is. There is always the danger that real illness or distress is overlooked, that she 'cries wolf' too often. Such a patient requires the same attention as others, no more and no less, but working out her actual needs can be difficult.

Psychopathic personality

The psychopath is concerned only with her own immediate needs. She is impulsive and demanding, uses people without concern for their needs and may be aggressive or even criminal without conscience. Many psychopaths seem to 'cool down' or 'mellow' in old age, so psychopathy is not a major problem among dementia sufferers, but one or two can add to the management problems of a ward or a home.

Normal personality

There is no such thing as a normal reaction to dementia, for there is really no such thing as a normal personality type. Most individuals have little bits of one or more of the above personality traits within them, though some are classic examples of a particular type. Each person deserves to be understood as an individual.

EXPECTATIONS OF DEMENTIA

If asked how common 'confusion' is among elderly people, both young and old people regularly overestimate, some guessing at a figure as high as 50% rather than the true figure of less than 10%. Those who work in the health or social services are particularly likely to overestimate because, as mentioned in Chapter 3, they see a concentration of dementing people in their care. But the tendency is probably part of that general set of negative attitudes to old age which has been called 'ageism'. The corollary of this sort of belief is that people who are not demented in old age are treated as remarkable, particularly if they remain active, socially involved and able to keep up-to-date ('She actually still goes to the bingo at 85!').

Many people therefore expect that they will suffer some degree of dementia. Some of these people will know something of what dementia is like, but others will have a more or less distorted or incomplete view. Everybody knows that memory is lost in 'confusion' or dementia. Many indeed seem to believe that all old people lose their memories. But not many realize that true dementia involves the multiple losses described in Chapter 4. And there is a tendency to think of two conditions, one a mild memory impairment which is not a cause for concern, the other severe dementia, needing total care. The evidence suggests that this is not a proper distinction and that, unless some reversible cause is found, most people with mild impairment will, in time, become more severely impaired.

Those who think that many or all old people suffer some sort of relatively mild impairment are quite prepared for the early changes of dementia. When their memory begins to fail they are likely to say that they expected this, that it is a normal part of old age and that, therefore, there is little to worry about. They are apt to ignore the other evidence of their decline and eventually to play down the degree of their memory impairment. They continue to claim to be happy and see little need for diagnosis, help or care at the very time when they could be fully involved in planning their own future.

Experience in the family

Previous experience colours our expectations. Dementia is a common condition, so many people have at least a little exposure to it. If one member of a family develops dementia the other family members are likely to have a horror of developing it too and will fear particular behaviour problems which affected their relative, such as wandering or disinhibited behaviour. If the relative got unsatisfactory care, then family members may assume that all care is like that. They will, of course, be recalling mainly the 'outside' of their relative's dementia (p. 198) rather than thinking what the experience was like for the sufferer herself.

Inherited dementia

The family will worry even more if they consider genetic factors. In Huntington's chorea families, and in the other rare autosomal dominant forms of dementia, (p. 22) this worry becomes a realistic fear, since the child of an affected parent has a 50% chance of developing the condition (Fig. 7.1) and each child of the affected parent that is born has the same 50% risk – the risk does not reduce when an older brother or sister possesses the gene. This is a frightening prospect for each child, but they are in a still greater dilemma. The parent may develop the illness relatively early in life, even in their 30s, but it may be later, in their 50s or 60s or rarely even later that it begins. So the children may not know until they are adults themselves whether they are at risk or not. When they come to think of producing the next generation,

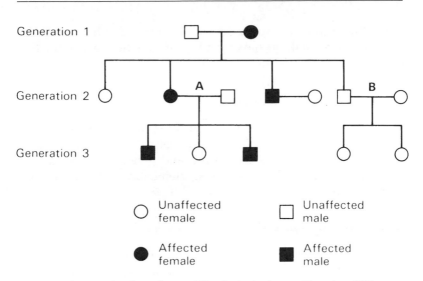

Fig. 7.1   A typical family pedigree of Huntington's chorea. There is a 50% chance *at each birth* that couple A will produce an affected child. None of Couple B's children will be affected. However, those in Generation 2 are unlikely to know whether they are in category A or category B until after they have their families.

the grandchildren, they may not know if they are passing on a 50% chance or no chance at all.

Genetic counselling services can help prospective parents come to a decision, but with such a wide variation in the risks and possibilities it must remain up to the prospective parent to make the final decision. The situation is made more difficult by the tendency of some families to conceal the illness from the next generation, making proper genetic counselling impossible, but more enlightened attitudes are gaining ground.

Recent developments in 'gene-mapping' and 'genetic markers', such as that found on chromosome number 4 for Huntington's chorea, will eventually allow much more exact genetic counselling. Diagnosis of Huntington's chorea before birth and therapeutic abortion are now available. Although there would be enormous relief for those who can be told that they do not have the gene, will not suffer the illness and will not pass it to their children, the consequences of telling someone that they do carry the gene could be tragic, since there is as yet no treatment.

Similar arguments apply to the families of inherited DAT, where it is possible to have testing for genetic markers of the disease.

'Non-inherited' DAT and VaD

There is not enough genetic risk in most cases of the common forms of dementia to merit formal genetic counselling, but it is natural that families should worry, and general advice can be given about the risk of suffering dementia and the risk of suffering other illnesses.

False expectations

All this expectation and worry is excessive and in some sense unnecessary. Individuals cannot at present predict that they will suffer DAT or VaD. They cannot predict how dementia will change them if they do develop it, what symptoms they will show and what help they will need. And their ideas of how they would react reflect more on their current state than on what their *actual* experience of dementia will be years later. Just as a child may swear that she will never marry, yet 20 years later is married and happily settled, so we look forward to old age and see its horrors as if we would experience them as we are now, not as we will be then.

People anticipating dementia may see it as a bleak, hopeless, dependent existence compared to their present active lives. They do not see the greater acceptance of old age, the blunting effects of dementia and the effects of loss of insight and memory on the sufferer's experience. So young people thinking of dementia anticipate that they would become severely depressed if they developed it, or even that they would commit suicide. Yet the suicide rate is actually remarkably low and even depression is not universal by any means.

More realistically, younger people see the burden that dementia is to the rest of a family and so think that they would inevitably need to be in institutional care. If they have negative views of care, then the outlook can seem bleak indeed.

People who are frightened by the prospect of dementia may react badly if they see evidence of its beginnings. They may imagine it is developing when they are in fact well; they may try to hide it if it does develop, or may become very distressed.

Preparing for dementia

Society

Unfortunately, there is still a social stigma associated with the diagnosis of dementia. This is related in part to the low profile it often has in society, in political, social and medical terms. Since people have such varied and often inaccurate attitudes to dementia, there is a major need to educate the public. People in general need more facts about the likelihood of any individual developing dementia, about what the illness is like, and about what can be done to help. Decision makers (such as politicians) need to have a much better understanding than they have at present about the problems related to dementia care. The media's tendency to look for scare stories and exaggerate failures in our care systems, while describing any minor advance in research as a 'breakthrough', does little service to dementia sufferers and their carers. Professionals and voluntary organizations have an uphill struggle to combat these tendencies.

The family

The families of dementing patients need to know what to expect of their relatives, in terms of the condition itself and also in terms of potential care needs. Families should be told, if they ask, about the slightly increased genetic risk, but should be reassured that the risk is still small and that there are plenty of other commoner conditions, such as heart disease, which are more likely to kill them. It is a good idea for families to discuss among themselves what help would be available from each other if it were ever needed.

The individual

The many older people who are worried by the prospect of dementia, or indeed any disability, can be helped if they have contemplated the worst and been reassured that reasonable amounts of family and other support would be at hand. They will not, however, be helped if the reassurance is false or if they try to demand impossible support or to close options saying, 'If I get confused, you must never put me in a home' or 'You'll look after me, won't you?', which merely store up difficulties for the future. Dementia is also an important subject for discussion in retirement courses and day centres. It should not be brushed under the carpet.

The subject should be raised particularly when an elderly person is planning a change in her living circumstances, to move in with her younger family or go to sheltered housing. The onset of dementia after she has moved can be disastrous, but it is worse if the patient has been misled into thinking that her place in the home is permanent no matter what happens. There *are* circumstances where families or sheltered housing schemes cannot cope. It may seem harsh to bring up the subject of an illness which only affects a minority of people. But the fact that it *has* been broached and that no unrealistic expectations have been raised can lessen the person's feeling of rejection if help has to be called in later or if she has to move to a more sheltered environment. Once the presence of early dementia is recognized, the person can be helped to make plans for the future. This could involve putting her affairs in order with a Will, granting a Power of Attorney, or making an Advance Directive (see Chapter 9).

INSIGHT

We have seen that patients come to dementia with differing personality attributes and differing expectations, attitudes and experience, and that these will influence how each individual reacts to the illness. But how strong and how appropriate their reaction is depends also on how much they understand of what is going on – their *insight*. Insight can be described as the awareness by a patient that she has changed and that the changes are due to an illness, in other words, the awareness that she is dementing. It also implies knowing the extent and severity of the illness. It does not mean knowing all about the workings of the brain or the chemistry of Alzheimer's dementia. It refers to ordinary personal experience and understanding.

At its simplest we can see that a person who realizes that she is suffering from dementia, who is aware that she is making mistakes of memory, not looking after herself properly and so on, will react in a very different way from a person who is showing the same decline but is totally unaware that anything is wrong. But insight is a complicated concept and it is difficult to be exact about it.

Stages of insight

A number of stages are involved. Let us consider a previously well-organized lady who forgets to light her gas fire when she puts it on, forgets to collect her pension or forgets appointments. There has been a slow decline in her general ability to look after herself and, to an outsider, it is clear that she is beginning to suffer from dementia. In order to realize this herself she needs first to realize that she has made these mistakes. She may not recall them or even seem unaware of them at the time they occur (see p. 115). Even if she recognizes and recalls her mistakes she must also be able to remember her *normal* way of behaving, compare with that standard and make the logical connection that there has been a change. All these abilities are likely to be impaired to a greater or lesser extent by the dementia. The frontal lobe functions of conscience and judgement are then needed for her to feel concerned about her mistakes and about the change in herself. So even before we consider how she might react to her insight, there are many reasons why insight may be imperfect or even absent. Furthermore, insight will usually begin to fail very early on in the illness.

Denial of insight

We have already seen how patients tend to assume, even if they have some insight, that their impairments are minor and an ordinary part of old age. Some of this is due to ignorance. Some is due to denial. Denial is a common defence mechanism which people employ to shield themselves from an unpleasant truth. They act as if it were not true. This self-deception or deception of others could be considered as dishonest but, as we will see, it is a normal part of the universal grief reaction to any loss (p. 238), 'It hasn't happened', protecting against the full flood of distress that might be paralysing. Dementia is both an unpleasant truth and a loss. Not only are the person's mental faculties being lost, but independence and eventually life itself are lost. It is not surprising, then, that many sufferers shield themselves against full awareness of their decline and fate.

We can be sure that patients deny their insight, at least to other people. Some patients admit that they are losing their mental abilities to one person and not to another. Others will deny insight at the beginning of a conversation but later, when they feel more secure, acknowledge that they do understand their position. The lady who hides her wet knickers is aware that she has been incontinent; she is not denying the fact to herself, but is trying to deny it to others. She is protecting herself against the ridicule and rejection which she may quite understandably expect.

But we can guess that many even deny the facts to themselves. They seem totally aware of their memory impairment and deny the consequences. They may have the evidence of a burnt pan or a neglected house in front of them and blatantly deny that the evidence exists or has anything to do with them. Both true lack of insight, due to agnosia or other impairments, and denial are involved in this reaction, though it is difficult to know in what proportions.

Estimating denial

Estimating the extent to which denial makes the patient play down her reactions either to herself or to others cannot therefore be more than guesswork. It is almost always a mistake to accuse patients of 'pretending' that they are not ill. For denial is an important defence. Attacking defences usually causes distress or makes a person defend herself more rather than less; attacking defences which we imagine are present but which do not exist is wrong.

Estimating insight

Insight, then, is a difficult concept to pin down and may be hidden by denial. In practice, the main evidence we can obtain about how much a sufferer knows of her illness is from her reactions to it. We would expect someone who had a fairly general understanding of dementia to react with distress. It would be like mourning a loss (p. 238). It would be a shock at first, and she would have some difficulty accepting that it was happening; she might feel frustrated, depressed or anxious about the future; then she would be forced to think of that future, reconsidering all her plans, her relationships with others, her ability to be independent, her finances, her will. In a way she would be preparing for her own death. She would also understand fully why other people were reacting to her differently.

As we shall see, patients' actual reactions are usually much less dramatic and far-reaching than this, though a partial grief reaction is quite common. So we must conclude that, even allowing for some denial, insight is probably limited in most people.

On the other hand, the patient who totally lacks insight is likely to be happy with herself, not realizing that anything is wrong, but completely baffled by the reactions of others. Family and strangers suggest that she needs help, even that she should leave her own home, but she can see no need for any change at all. The majority of sufferers fall somewhere between these two extremes of total insight and total lack of insight.

'Treating' lack of insight

Should we try to improve insight? In theory it is better that patients with any sort of illness should know that they are ill and learn something of the nature of their illness. This helps them to cooperate in a treatment programme and to report changes in their condition. And so it is with dementia. The patient who has complete insight will wish to discuss her problems fully and cooperate in plans to improve the quality of her life. The patient with no insight will have difficulty with cooperation, will resent intrusions in her life and see no reason for outside help.

So it is reasonable to try to improve insight. This can be done by talking with the patient about her memory impairment and other losses, naming her illness, talking realistically over how she feels about it. She may need to be reminded of some of the evidence of her failing abilities, before explaining how dementia usually progresses and helping her to realize that she will therefore need gradually increasing help. As public awareness of dementia and the possibilities of getting treatment or other help grows, as people realize more and more that dementia is not just old age, and as the stigma associated with it lessens, we can expect increasing requests from sufferers at the early stages for information.

This increase is happening already and the growth of memory clinics (p. 385) is encouraging the trend. Families and professionals who for years have assumed that 'she wouldn't want to know' or 'she is happy in her ignorance' or 'no one with dementia has insight' have had to rapidly change their mistaken attitudes and begin to learn a new set of skills, particularly the skill of discussing face-to-face with the dementia sufferer the full implications of the illness, in a way which the mentally impaired person can take in. They must deal with the person's muddled emotional reactions, and discuss in a helpful way decisions that need to be taken for the future.

The *family* should if possible be involved in all discussions. As we will see in the next chapter, families all too readily deny to themselves the evidence of dementia and are reluctant to admit to the sufferer that they know what is wrong. Many families are therefore very much against this type of open discussion. They may be fearful of causing arguments or distress to the patient, but also will find the discussion distressing to themselves. Open discussion of the diagnosis of dementia and its associated problems forces everybody in the family to treat the sufferer in a more adult way, involving her in decisions that will greatly change her life and allowing everybody's natural distress to be shared and helped.

Discussion needs to be encouraged, for it can avoid daily embarrassment as well as the tendency that many have to ignore the feelings and views of sufferers. It may be necessary to point out to the family that their lack of discussion is placing a barrier of non-communication as well as an emotional barrier between them and the sufferer. They feel they must not share with their relative the distress, problems and planning essential to the experience of dementia. This must increase the stress of living with someone with dementia.

Even with the greatest care and skill, however, attempts to help the person understand her illness will not always work, or may work only partially. For she may be *incapable* of proper insight because of her dementia. Or she may have chosen to deny insight and find moving from that position unthinkable. And in some cases insight may actually cause distress. The patient may react angrily, dismissing what is said as nonsense, or she may see the tragedy of her position and be greatly upset. All these are reasons for being extremely sensitive when trying to improve insight. It can be done to a certain extent, it can be very helpful to the patient and her family at the earlier stages of illness, but it can be distressing. Complete insight is not always a possible or reasonable goal.

Sharing the diagnosis

There are a lot of issues involved in deciding where, when and how we should tell someone that she has dementia. At present the usual clinical practice is that carers are informed, but the person with dementia is not. When asked, carers often say that they would not want their relative told, but also say that if they themselves had dementia they would rather know! The reasoning behind this is not clear, but amongst other things involves a wish to 'protect' the sufferer in some way. But is this wise?

There is an analogy to the situation in dealing with people with cancer. As late as the 1970s doctors often kept a diagnosis of cancer from the patient, often with the connivance of the relatives. The patient would be given other plausible reasons for his symptoms, and thus could have increasing distrust both of his physician and of his relatives. He was unable to properly come to terms with his illness, or discuss his feelings about it with his nearest and dearest. He was unable to plan ahead and try to put his affairs in order. We now live in more enlightened times, however, and the doctor–patient relationship is in general much better. We are able to discuss any illness and its implications as long as all parties are properly informed.

This analogy with dementia is not perfect. Often by the time dementia is diagnosed, insight and the ability to comprehend are impaired. The person with dementia may not be able to remember a conversation long enough to consider its implications. This should not, however, be used as an excuse for concealing the diagnosis.

The advent of potential treatments for dementia and the development of various support groups and specialist services mean that not divulging a diagnosis can lead to someone losing out on many valuable resources. In addition, if the person with dementia knows the diagnosis, issues such as future care needs, concerns about treatment and financial aspects can be rationally discussed with everyone involved, beginning with her, or with her at the centre of the discussion.

Anyone attending a doctor should reasonably expect to be given an early and accurate diagnosis, no matter what illness she is suffering from. Dementia is no different in this respect. Information about the illness should be made available if and when it is requested, not only for the carers, but also for the sufferer. There are of course some risks in giving a diagnosis of dementia. It should not be given until we are sure ourselves – to be told that one has a progressive, untreatable illness is a very serious matter. Different people have different ways of coping with such bad news. By the time a diagnosis is made, symptoms will have been present for some time. Many people find a sense of relief in knowing that what is wrong with them can be understood and that it has a name. Other people will react by becoming initially depressed and pessimistic – we must work through these feelings with them. Denial (p. 211) is a common reaction, that is, although a diagnosis has been given, and has been discussed, the person continues to behave and act as if it has not. This is not the same as forgetting. Rather it is a positive psychological defence, a way of coping with a situation one finds difficult. The best time to discuss diagnosis is likely to be when the person herself begins to ask questions about what is happening to her.

It is particularly important to try to avoid the situation where carers know the diagnosis but the sufferer does not. If there is a secret about it, a secret kept from the sufferer, there can be no discussion of how either feels about the illness, and no realistic discussion of future care or other plans. This air of secrecy can only increase the tension in an already tense situation.

Doctors, nurses and others will have to learn special skills if they are to be helpful to suffers in discussing this diagnosis and the future. As well as learning how to communicate with someone who has dementia (see p. 138), we have to learn how to help people who have difficulty remembering or thinking to work through the emotional turmoil of learning about dementia, to help them communicate their feelings and wishes to others, and to help them plan for the future when their ability to plan is beginning to fail.

There will have to be a lot of simple repetition of messages about the illness. Written information will help a lot in some cases, and there are now some leaflets for the purpose from various self-help groups. However, in most cases the skill is in finding just the right way to impart information to that particular person with these particular impaired abilities.

In the early stages we should expect that a dementia sufferer can grasp all the basic information about dementia, services, future plans and so on, even if some prompts and reminders are necessary to ensure that she retains that information. Later the information will have to be simplified – eventually Alzheimer's may have to be translated into 'memory problems' and a whole range of services into 'a bit of help at home'.

Mistaken insight

Finally, we should not forget the group of people who have *mistaken* insight, who believe that they are suffering from dementia but in fact are well. These include the people mentioned in Chapter 2 who suffer from physical illness and pseudodementia, and who imagine that their memory losses are permanent, as well as the ordinary elderly people who believe that the normal changes of ageing are the beginnings of dementia (p. 51), or those who have age-associated memory impairment (p. 55) and seem not to go on to develop dementia. Proper diagnosis and information to the elderly who are ill and general education about old age and dementia should reduce this problem. But there are also people who are just beginning to dement and suffer great uncertainty about whether they will get worse or better. There is little that can be done at present to reassure them. They will fear all the losses of dementia, the dependence, the disintegration of the self, the loss of control, the burden on others. These fears are powerful and difficult to cope with. They need the promise of diagnosis as soon as possible, a check for remediable causes of their mild memory loss, and honest reassurance about what help would be available if they were to go on to suffer more severe dementia.

PERSONALITY CHANGES IN DEMENTIA

We might now expect to be able to understand the individual reactions of patients to their dementia. But there is a further complication. For the person who is experiencing the dementia is being changed in herself *by* the dementia. So, except at the earliest stages, it is not the old personality with old expectations who is reacting to the illness, but a shrunken or modified personality with less understanding or mistaken ideas. Her actual reaction will be a mixture of some bits of her old ways of reacting and some bits of new ways.

Normal changes of old age

Indeed, even before the dementia begins, an older person's personality may have changed a little with age. There are enormous variations between people in how much of a change this is, but there are some general trends which have already been mentioned (p. 48). Slowness, cautiousness, rigidity, dislike of change or newness, more emotional detachment and a tendency to withdraw from involvement with activities or people (disengagement – p. 49) all occur to a greater or lesser extent in older people. In terms of our list of personality types (p. 202), people become a little more introverted and obsessional.

Effects on reactions

The reactions we expect from a dementia sufferer will be modified by these changes. An older person may not only expect dementia to happen as part of old age, but may react less emotionally and keep her feelings to herself rather than discussing them with others. She may try stoically to keep to a routine, unexciting way of life. She may react badly to sudden changes and new faces and be less inclined to mix with others than might have been the case in her earlier years. As with other older people we may feel that just a little change, such as joining a lunch club or taking up a hobby, would help matters enormously. But her rigidity, cautiousness and social withdrawal get in the way. These changes occur less in younger, early-onset patients.

Effects of changes due to dementia

Decline in personality

Chapters 4 and 5 have included many examples of how dementia affects personality and emotional reactions, by causing either a decline or a change. The decline in positive personality features and in emotional life means that most people react much more blandly to their dementia than we might expect. They are 'a shadow of their former selves'. But, as with everything else in dementia, the decline is gradual and at the beginning of the process the personality is largely intact. This explains the paradox that *reactions tend to be more troublesome in earlier, milder dementia than they are at later, more severe stages.* In severe dementia, when the emotions and personality are destroyed, the person is unable to react at all.

Changed personality

If the person's personality changes because of the development of emotional lability or because of the appearance of a completely new trait such as demandingness, obsessionality, irritability or paranoia, then we must expect completely new types of reaction. For relatives, this is one of the most distressing facets of dementia – the person reacts like a 'stranger'. And when decline and disinhibition get mixed together the reactions become a jumble. Once again, the tendency to show 'new' personality features is greatest early in dementia (p. 164). So these new and complicated reactions are most likely in mild cases.

Preserved personality

It should be recalled, however, that some patients, especially those with patchy damage in vascular dementia, may retain many of their previous personality traits until quite late in the illness. Even here, the general tendency to be more rigid and to give stereotyped responses can mean that the patient's reactions become a sort of exaggerated caricature of her previous self. It is sometimes said that in old age our worst personality characteristics become exaggerated and 'stuck'. If there is any truth in that it is even more true among sufferers from dementia.

Whether exaggerated or not, the fact that personality is often retained in VaD means that these patients tend to react more obviously to their dementia and that their reactions are more understandable. In DAT, on the other hand, it is often the case that insight declines at roughly the same rate as everything else. The result may be a vague, ill-formed regret or seeming indifference to the illness. This relative lack of reaction can be frustrating for relatives but a blessing for the patient, who accepts her declining abilities with a smile.

CONCLUSION

Despite all these modifications it is still possible in many cases to explain and understand how the individual sufferer reacts to her dementia. It is certainly very worthwhile trying to understand, using information about her previous personality, her expectations and experience and the changes in her personality with age and dementia. For if we understand, we can empathize and if we empathize, we will see ways of helping her and her family understand dementia and thus cope better with it.

TYPES OF REACTION

We will now examine some of the particular ways in which patients react to the various symptoms of dementia (Table 7.2). Obviously, one person may react differently to different symptoms. For example, since memory impairment tends to be expected, many sufferers are remarkably sanguine about its appearance and effects (if they can remember them!). On the other hand, dressing dyspraxia, which is not expected, is much more distressing. So *expectations* are important.

But it is also *easier* for a patient to be aware of some types of symptom than of others. The best example relates to the two

Table 7.2 Emotional reactions to dementia. Sufferers react either to their awareness of their failing abilities, or to the 'intruders' who try to help them when they see no need for help

Depression
Anxiety
Frustration
Guilt
Paranoid thinking
Embarrassment
Withdrawal
Covering-up and confabulation
Egocentricity and altruism

main types of dysphasia seen particularly in stroke patients. When there is a *receptive* dysphasia (p. 115) the patient has difficulty in understanding the meaning of words, her own as well as others. The result is not only that she may fail to understand what is said to her but that, when she responds with meaningless words, she does not realize what she is doing and so is not distressed by her mistakes, though she may be annoyed that her listeners do not seem to follow what she thinks is perfect sense. In *expressive* dysphasia (p. 137) on the other hand, the patient is painfully aware of the mistakes she is making and is likely to feel frustrated and distressed. It is in fact a general rule that failure of reception or understanding in any sense leads to less distress than failure of the ability to carry out actions.

DEPRESSION

Grief

Depression (Table 7.3) is the most understandable reaction to the multiple losses of dementia. It is the central emotion in the *grief reaction*, the common human response to a loss of any kind. Grief

Table 7.3   Depression and dementia

Cause of depression	Management
Reaction to losses and changed circumstances	Guide through stages of mourning Adjust circumstances if possible Reassuring, empathic, non-critical response
Chronic reactive depression	Antidepressants if managements above have failed
Disinhibited depression and consequences	Examine and adjust circumstances Tranquillizer or antidepressant
Depressive illness	Antidepressants
Depressive illness with pseudodementia	After antidepressant treatment, review mental state
Physical illness causing apparent depression	Treat the illness
Drugs causing depression	Stop the drugs
Apathy (lack of feelings) due to organic damage	Social stimulation Try antidepressants
'Face to the wall' phenomenon	Look for causes – physical illness, depression, drugs, organic apathy

reactions will be discussed more fully in Chapter 8, when we consider how families react, for the losses of dementia are usually felt much more by relatives and friends than by the patient herself. Not only is she likely to have limited awareness of her symptoms, but she may have only a patchy recollection of her normal self to compare with. If she cannot see any loss, she will not become depressed. However, in the early stages, those whose insight is good will be all too aware of their losses and will react more appropriately.

Just as with other depressed people, a patient who is depressed because of dementia needs the chance to talk about her feelings of loss to someone whom she respects and trusts. She can feel reassured and supported by knowing that someone understands, even if she does not quite grasp all that is said, or quickly forgets it.

Recovery

Recovering from a grief reaction, however, requires an eventual move from feeling and talking to a stage of planning and doing. For the best outcome will occur if the sufferer can make changes in her life which help her adjust to her new situation. This is the recovery phase of mourning (p. 239). It can be an almost impossible task for a dementing person on her own, since it requires changing attitudes, changing relationships, changing activities. She will find all these changes difficult to contemplate, never mind carry out.

Helping recovery. If we are to help the patient recover her self-esteem and feeling of well-being we need to look more closely at the causes of her depression. Often she will be more distressed by the *circumstances* she is facing (increasing dependence) than by her actual symptoms (memory impairment, dysphasia, etc.). If this is the case then there may be quite a lot of adjustment which can be made to help her. The classic example is of the lady who has to lose her independence by going to a residential home. She will mourn her loss of independence. But she can get through her depression and feel better again if she adjusts to life in the home – if she 'makes the best of it'. She must learn how to live with other residents and staff, adjust to different rules and routines and learn to get satisfaction from different activities than those that gave her satisfaction in her own home. It will take a lot of preparation, time and patience to help her make these adjustments.

If she were not dementing we could hope that she would make these changes herself. But, in dementia, family and staff will probably have to make some of the adjustments for her, changing the subject away from her depressing thoughts of loss and steering her quite actively into new interests and relationships. It is perfectly reasonable to exert pressure like this, if the alternative is that she will never get out of her depression.

Sometimes a patient feels depressed by thinking that her symptoms are affecting others. It may be that, rightly or wrongly, she feels rejected by the family because of her poor communication or because of an embarrassing decline in her habits. Or maybe she feels that she is left out of decisions and that her choices are made for her. Or she feels that she is disliked by staff. All these feelings lead to lowering of self-esteem and depression. Reassurance may help, but a change of attitude on the part of the other people involved, giving her more positive support, allowing her more say, showing that she is appreciated despite her disabilities, and talking with her about her illness and its effects, may be most reassuring of all and so help recovery.

If, however, we concentrate on the losses of dementia and disability, we do not help improve self-esteem. We must try to concentrate on those abilities which the person retains, and show her that we are working to enable her to use these to her full capacity.

Chronic depression

Some patients will manage to reach or even get through the recovery phase. Others do not and become chronically depressed. In many cases it will be difficult to tell the difference between this state of chronic depressive *feelings* as a reaction to dementia, and the state of chronic 'stuck' depressive *expression* due to disinhibition (p. 163). But, whichever the cause, the gradual decline in all aspects of emotional life in dementia will eventually lead to the disappearance of these chronic depressive states. While the depression lasts, however, it is reasonable to try treatment with a full course of antidepressant drugs.

Depressive illness

True depressive illness – that is, depression which is not readily understandable (p. 71) and which may be part of a long-standing recurrent depressive or manic-depressive illness – can occur during a dementia and will require its standard treatment with antidepressant drugs or ECT. In the later stages of dementia, this sort of depression may only be discernible by its physical symptoms, since the patient cannot explain how she feels. There will be loss of appetite, slowing of actions, a downcast look, perhaps a worsening in the mornings. The patient may be thought to have 'turned her face to the wall'. But the past history of previous depressions gives the clue that this episode should be treated and the patient may then return to her previously happy, though demented, state.

'Face to the wall'

'Turning the face to the wall' is an apparently voluntary desire to die, expressed usually by withdrawal, apathy and refusal to eat or drink. It must be distinguished not only from depressive illness but from physical illness and the effects of drugs – for it would be wrong to miss these. But that being said, we must assume that some dementing patients choose this variant of suicide. It sometimes appears to happen in very severely demented people, but they are unlikely to have enough understanding to make such a logical decision. It is then likely to be due to a severe decline in motivation caused by brain damage rather than a logical reaction to the dementia. True reactive depression and a consequent 'wish to die' are more likely to occur in people with mild dementia who also have physical disabilities and who have some insight into their condition. Refusal to eat or drink in this situation can give rise to various ethical issues (p. 145).

More active intentions of suicide are rare in dementia but not uncommon in those who fear dementia, e.g. the relatives of Huntington's chorea patients, or those who *think* they suffer it but do not, e.g. sufferers from the pseudodementia of depression.

ANXIETIES AND FEARS

Anxiety is again an understandable emotion. The patient is entering an unknown world. It is reasonable that she should be apprehensive about what will happen to her and about the changes that will come to her life.

She may have one or several specific fears – fear of missing appointments, fear of losing her keys or her money, fear of getting lost outside. Or she may be anxious about her relatives' attitudes. She may worry that she will do embarrassing things in public or that she will lose control of herself. She may even see a glimpse of the loss of her personality and identity which will occur later in dementia, and be terrified.

Expressions of anxiety

Anxiety may be expressed directly or indirectly. She may be able to talk about her fears, but if she is unwilling to talk, or can no longer communicate, then all that we can observe is restlessness (see Table 5.2, p. 172) or the physical expressions of anxiety such as tremor, sweating and a rapid pulse, muscular tension or aches and pains. We then have to guess what is causing her anxiety and what will help. Much of the restlessness that occurs in dementia may be due to anxiety, particularly fear of being lost and anxiety about forgetfulness.

Reactions to anxiety

The patient may try to do things to relieve her own anxiety. Writing down reminders on slips of paper, asking the time, asking the family for reassurance are typical reactions. But each has its problems. Reminders get lost or are illegible, causing even greater anxiety. Long-suffering neighbours are knocked up repeatedly by night and by day to be asked the time. The family get infuriated with repetitive calls for reassurance and begin to feel antagonistic towards her. Indeed, this repetitive questioning is one of the most difficult things for relatives to tolerate. It is made worse when the patient seems quite egocentric and oblivious of the distress she is causing. It is no wonder that some patients end up trying to avoid embarrassment and hostile reactions by social withdrawal (p. 229).

Management of anxiety

Listening and reassurance

We cannot stop anxious patients from trying to relieve their anxieties by themselves, but it is often better if they talk over their anxieties with others. Discussing the reality of the situation is helpful, for some fears are groundless and reassurance can easily be given. The problem in listening to and reassuring a dementing person is that she may forget that she has been reassured and return with the same anxiety again and again. Eventually, the long-suffering listener must decide whether there is any real purpose being served or whether the request for reassurance has merely become a habit which is being encouraged by the reassurance and is leading nowhere (p. 158). Reassurance will certainly not help if the 'anxiety' is not a reaction to the uncertainty of her circumstances but a manifestation of physical discomfort, a disinhibited emotion or part of a depressive illness.

Relieving tension

Reducing anxiety by techniques such as relaxation or breathing exercises is quite often only a limited help to an anxious dementing patient because these techniques require sustained effort and learning. Other people have to help her relax by using a calm tone of voice, a gentle approach, music, massage, aromatherapy or relaxing activity.

Special environments where the person gets extra sensory stimulation (such as the 'Snoezelen' room with its ever-changing lights, music and interesting shapes to touch) appear to be extremely relaxing for some restless and anxious patients. Like all 'therapies' however they are not for everyone, and even where they work for an individual the effects do not always last long. The value of such an environment for each individual should be the subject of a cautious assessment. Special environments should never be used as a form of seclusion for a 'troublesome' resident.

Removing causes of anxiety

Taking pressure off the patient will be helpful. If she is bombarded with problems to solve or is living in an over-stimulated environment (p. 167) she will become more anxious. In other words, a generally less demanding environment is best. The behavioural chart approach (see Fig. 5.1, p. 157) may help, showing in what situations she is most anxious and identifying what or who is raising the tension.

Memory aids (p. 126), used judiciously, can reassure the patient and prevent her from having to ask others for reassurance.

Anxiety about mobility or falls may be helped by physiotherapy or walking aids (p. 143). The person who is anxious needs the reassurance that gaps in her abilities are being filled. She may even feel the need of more help than is really necessary. We may have to go along with this feeling for a while if she cannot otherwise learn to regain her self-confidence. But once she has gained confidence, the extra help can gradually be dispensed with.

Drugs

Anti anxicty (or *anxiolytic*) drugs (p. 190) should only be used if anxiety is severe or 'stuck'. If they are used, it should only be for a short period, for there is a danger of dependence on them. They can, however, be very helpful. A patient who is so fretful about her inability to remember things that her anxiety actually makes her memory performance worse can be helped by an anxiolytic drug to feel more at ease and so perform better. The same can apply to a patient with expressive dysphasia who gets so anxious that she speaks worse rather than better the more she tries. Some of the antidepressant drugs (p. 191) can also be useful in treating patients who are constantly anxious, and they avoid the dangers of dependence, though they have their own different side-effects.

FRUSTRATION

This is the feeling of a person who knows what she would like to do but cannot. It tends to be most noticeable in people who were previously very competent or self-confident. The example of expressive dysphasia is typical (p. 138). But the same can apply to all expressive or physical activities, such as mobility, and tasks needing coordination, such as dressing, washing and feeding. It can also apply to memories which 'won't come' or thoughts that 'get lost'.

Sometimes patients show their frustration by expressing anger at those around them. We should be aware of this possibility and not jump to the conclusion that we are being criticized. Sometimes a frustrated patient does not cooperate with treatment or activities, knowing that she will merely get angry with herself if she cannot perform perfectly. We should not assume that she is being purposely awkward.

The person who expresses frustration is really asking for our help. She needs a realistic assessment of what her abilities are and what she can be expected to manage. Then she needs positive help with gap-filling to prevent frustration building up. Praise for small successes and avoiding comment on failures can also encourage self-confidence (but we must remember that many people find encouragement in the form of 'Well done, dear' patronizing and indeed frustrating).

GUILT

A sense of failure can lead on to self-blame. The patient feels that if she is not doing things correctly it is her own fault, or she may even blame the whole illness on herself. This feeling can be an important part of any depression, and particularly depressive illness. If it is a reaction to dementia then we should reassure that her failures are not her fault but are part of an illness which she cannot be blamed for.

PARANOID THINKING

Suspiciousness of others seems to be rather more common in dementia than guilt, though possibly it is just more obvious. If things are going wrong the patient tends to blame others. This sort of feeling arises particularly in paranoid or independent, proud personalities, but can occur in almost any patient. If a previously houseproud dementing lady leaves a pan on the cooker and it burns, she cannot believe that it was her fault, for she will not remember doing it. She believes she could never do such a thing. So she blames the lady next door. If she cannot locate the special place where she left her money, or her underclothes, or her key, she cannot believe that she has gone to look in the wrong place and so blames her home help for stealing or begins to believe that there is an intruder.

Paranoid reactions are perhaps most common in the patient who has receptive problems or agnosia. If people seem to be saying incomprehensible things to her, or if things around her seem strange, it is no wonder that she may be suspicions that someone is up to no good. Frontal lobe damage may also contribute, because testing whether the suspicions that come and go in our minds are true or not depends on our ability to compare them with the standard of reality. Between these two explanations we can perhaps see why paranoid reactions are so common in dementia.

The paranoid patient can be difficult to handle. It is important first to check whether there is any truth in her beliefs – it is, after all, not uncommon for people to steal from dementia sufferers! If there is no truth in her story, then the reality of the situation should be explained simply and calmly, and not by getting into an argument. If an argument seems likely to develop it may be best to leave the explanations for a while and try to change the subject, for she may quickly forget her accusations.

Mild suspiciousness may respond to such techniques, but the problem with paranoid thinking is that it is based on lack of trust, so the patient finds it hard to believe any reassurance we give. Repeated reassuring explanations are more likely to be used as evidence that 'something is up'. On the other hand, 'going along with' delusions merely encourages the patient to believe that she is right. Agreeing to differ is sometimes the best policy, but even this may leave the patient adamant that she is right in her suspicions.

Drug treatment is perhaps more likely to be needed for psychotic symptoms than for the other reactions to dementia. Drugs such as sulpiride and risperidone are best, but unfortunately they are not always successful.

EMBARRASSMENT

The lady who hides her wet knickers is acting out of embarrassment, the feeling that she has done something which will be ridiculed by others. Embarrassment is felt most by patients who have lost some of their self control or judgement but retain some insight. For example, a patient may lose her temper over nothing and realize how distressing this is to her family. Her embarrassment can be helped if the family reassure her that they understand that she has difficulty controlling her feelings because of her illness and that they are not offended by her anger. This will also help the family to avoid responding angrily back and so worsening the situation.

WITHDRAWAL

All these emotional reactions are distressing. It is not surprising therefore that one of the commonest reactions to dementia is to try to avoid the distress by withdrawing socially. This withdrawal can take many forms. The patient may simply be quieter than usual because of embarrassment or depression. She may drift out of her usual social activities – church, club, family visits. At the extreme, she may become completely isolated.

Effects of withdrawal

The dangers of this type of reaction are, first, that she may become detached from reality and more inclined to live in her own world of long ago. Secondly, there are physical dangers – of self-neglect, of reduced mobility and of illness due to immobility, and, thirdly, she may get insufficient treatment for all her problems because she is not asking for help. Unfortunately, withdrawal may be quietly accepted or even encouraged by friends and relatives because *they* are embarrassed, or guilty about not helping, or feel they cannot communicate with her. Other common disabilities such as poor hearing, poor eyesight and poor mobility can add to her tendency to withdraw and so compound the problem.

Stimulation

In assessing the deficits of dementia, we need to recognize that some of the person's losses may appear worse than they actually are because of this withdrawal. The person who is beginning to have a speech problem and gets no practice at speaking is at a disadvantage. So is the person whose self-care or continence is declining and who has withdrawn so that no one is around to encourage her to do better. It is these particular people who can perhaps respond best to gap-filling and retraining. The stimulation and confidence given by company and the expectation of higher standards can encourage them to use what abilities they have more fully.

Withdrawn people can even appear severely demented when their dementia is actually very mild. Someone who has had no stimulation and no practice of her skills for some time will 'come alive' when she moves from a neglected house into a residential home or hospital, or even when a visitor starts to visit on a regular basis. But in bringing people 'out of themselves' we should keep in mind that the withdrawal has occurred for a reason, being due either to feelings of embarrassment or to the reactions of others, and we should try to deal with that reason both sensitively and actively.

COVERING-UP

This is a more purposeful response to the distress of dementia than withdrawal, related to the defence of *denial* discussed earlier (p. 211). The person tries to pretend that she is not dementing. It is understandable that covering-up should happen, but it is almost impossible to discover whether it is a conscious or an unconscious action. Possibly at first there is a large conscious element, an attempt to get over the embarrassment of forgetfulness, but later some of the covering-up responses seem to become automatic.

Confabulation

It is a curious fact that people whose intellectual powers are supposed to be declining can become expert at covering-up. Yet they do, and can learn very effective and sophisticated ways of diverting and fooling others.

The classic response is called *confabulation*. This was in the past associated principally with Korsakoff's syndrome (p. 69), but it can in fact occur in those who have any sort of memory impairment. When answering questions that test her memory, instead of saying that she does not know, she gives an answer which is a guess at what might be true, often based on past life or habits. Her answer is usually delivered in a confident tone as if she was trying to fool the questioner. And, surprisingly, sometimes it does. But often her answer is very obviously untrue.

A more charitable explanation of confabulation suggests that it arises because memories are not stored in the correct time-sequence (p. 123) and so are retrieved in the wrong order. So an old memory may be recalled in place of a recent one.

Confabulation is only one form of covering up. Table 7.4 gives a few examples of other methods. The difficulty is that all of these can work very well. The result is that family or friends may not realize how severely impaired the person is. And professionals can be fooled too. We find that the patient has steered the conversation away from the questions we wished to

Table 7.4   Covering-up when the honest answer is 'I don't know'

Question	Answer
'What day is it?'	'At my age you don't bother with these things'
	'You've got me at a bad time'
	'What day is it?' – asking a relative
	'Let me look at my paper'
	'It's Wednesday' – confabulation
	'It's a lovely day' – pretending to misunderstand
	'Can't hear you'
	'Don't ask silly questions'
	'Do you not know?'
	'You're asking too many questions'

ask and on to old stories or pleasantries. Interviewing may therefore involve a lot of determination to keep her on the track. However, we should always remember that covering up and denial occur because of underlying distress and that therefore uncovering can lead to distress. If we need to know the facts of how seriously demented someone is, we may be forced to produce some of that distress for a brief period. But after that, there is little point, unless we are sure that she will eventually be able to drop her defence and be more honest without being upset.

EGOCENTRICITY AND ALTRUISM

For many dementia sufferers, the world contracts. They may lose their interests and withdraw from social activities, their ability to deal with others declines, they do not take in fully how others behave towards them, they do not see the effect of their behaviour on their family or they choose to ignore it. In general they become more egocentric and apparently uncaring. This is very distressing for relatives, who get demands for help but no thanks. Sometimes it leads to arguments between a couple, and it may tempt a carer to give up the job of caring. Considerable explanation, reassurance and support to the relative are necessary to make such ingratitude tolerable.

Other people are very aware of the effects of their dementia on their families and react, not with embarrassment at their condition (which is egocentric), but by trying to lighten the burden and distress that they themselves are causing. This more altruistic feeling can make her play down her own needs and emphasize the needs of the family for relief or support. It can be a helpful and realistic feeling, but if it is excessive it can be an all too convenient excuse for us to ignore her needs altogether. Throughout our dealings with dementia sufferers we need to keep as balanced a view as we possibly can of both the sufferer's and carers' *actual* needs, not relying only on her emotional view, their emotional view or our own prejudice.

CONCLUSION: COPING WITH DEMENTIA

As we have emphasized, all these varied reactions to the experience of dementia are understandable. What is the proper, 'normal' reaction? What does 'coping with dementia' mean? The answer is that there is no 'proper' way, there are only multitudes of individual ways. We might say that those whose reactions cause distress to themselves or others need special help but, even where no big problems arise, some distress can be expected, some withdrawal from distressing situations, some attempts to pretend that everything is normal. It would be unusual for anyone with any degree of insight to sail through dementia without feeling any distress. We should be aware of that distress, and help when necessary.

8

The experience for families

In Chapter 3 we outlined some of the home circumstances in which dementing people live. We emphasized that a large minority live alone and described some types of family set-up which are frequently found. We also indicated how factors in the family structure make it more or less likely that a patient can continue to live at home, and something of how social changes are modifying these factors and are leading to greater pressures on the helping services. In this chapter we want to concentrate more on the practical and emotional effects of having a dementia sufferer in a family, how families react and cope and how they can be helped. Two important points need stressing.

Common reactions

In the first instance it must be realized that families vary enormously in their composition, in the personalities of the individual members, how near to the affected person they live and how willing they are to help. They have differing experiences, differing family beliefs and myths and a long relationship with the affected member before her dementia began. Furthermore, they have other business on their plates as well as that of looking after the dementia sufferer. Before examining particular family structures we will look at some of the ways in which close relatives react to dementia. Although there are a multitude of individual reactions, common patterns emerge. We will describe these in terms of:

1. the dying relationship
2. the changing relationship
3. the continuing relationship.

It is interesting to compare these reactions with the common reactions of the sufferers themselves (see Chapter 7). There are some similarities but many differences.

The 'duty' to care

A second point concerns the attitudes of professionals and voluntary organizations towards families. There is a tendency to assume that families *ought* to cope with dementing relatives, even if it means considerable disruption to family life, social life or work and even though the burden of caring is stressful. This attitude fits in neatly with ideas of 'community care', particularly if institutional care is seen as anonymous, depressing or degrading. But it can be a dogmatic attitude.

It is quite wrong to *assume* that a family does not care because they feel that the sufferer would be better off in a home than living with them. It may of course be true that they really do not care, could not be bothered to think of the sufferer's needs and wishes in the matter, and do not even want to think of changing their own lives to suit someone else. But it may be that their wish not to support their relative is based on a long-standing poor relationship which will not improve because of dementia. It may be that they really do not have the skills of patience, tolerance and humour required to cope and that they are quite right to refuse. They may genuinely feel that she would be happier and healthier in residential care. Or they may believe that it is the duty of the state to provide care for those who cannot care for themselves and would wish the same for themselves if they became disabled. In Scandinavia and some other parts of the world much higher percentages of older people live in residential or hospital care than in Britain. In some other parts of the world the percentage is less than in Britain. There are no absolutes here, only opinions and customs.

Encouragement or pressure

We, as professionals dealing with individual families, have no right to cajole or coerce families into coping. We can encourage them to do so if we feel they *can* cope, asking them to consider carefully the alternatives that are available; we can urge them to consider the wishes of the sufferer and most important of all we can provide moral and practical support if they *do* wish to care. But there can be no law which states that relatives *ought* to care.

However, there *is* pressure on relatives. It may come from their own loyalty, conscience and religious beliefs. It may come from the patient's wishes or from promises given to her in the past. It may come from the expectations of other members of her family, from friends and from the community in general. Or it may come from the subtle, and sometimes not so subtle, pressures of the professions. Worst of all is the pressure that comes from lack of resources (p. 103). The common reactions of relatives seem to occur whether they are more willing or less willing to cope with caring at home. But these reactions can be harder to tolerate if the relatives feel they have been pressurized into coping. The *duty* to care may be present for many different reasons. The family sometimes continue to feel that they have this duty of care after their own physical and emotional resources are exhausted. Professionals may then have to give them *permission* to give up this duty, by accepting either temporary (respite) care or more permanent care.

THE DYING RELATIONSHIP

Dementia has been well described as a living death. As many aspects of personality disappear, as the ability to understand or respond to other people declines, as imagination, thinking and speech deteriorate, as the emotions become blunter or disappear altogether, there is little left for relatives to relate to. At the last stages there are only old memories, a few glimpses of the old personality and the body of the sufferer still intact. Relatives often, therefore, describe a profound feeling of loss which is like grief.

We describe here the phases of grief relating to a death, but similar experiences occur when someone close develops dementia.

MOURNING

Phases

The mourning process, following the *death* of someone close, has been described as a series of stages or phases, though these phases do not necessarily follow each other in orderly sequence and may overlap quite a lot.

Numbness

The immediate reaction to bereavement is usually shock or numbness, a disbelief and absence of emotion. This acts to protect relatives from the strong emotions which they can later feel in a more controlled way.

Protest

Beginning to realize the fact of death brings a mixture of feelings. Usually the relative finds himself acting to avoid these feelings and, as it were, to recover the dead person. This has been called the 'protest' phase. *Pining* and *searching* behaviour, feelings of the presence of the dead person or even hallucinations may be attempts, either conscious or unconscious, to 'put the clock back'. *Denial* of the death can persist through this phase and cause delay in coming to terms with reality.

Distress

But in order to complete the process of mourning successfully the full force of the *feelings of loss* has to be coped with in a phase of *distress*. Although sadness or depression is the commonest feeling and is often very severe, other feelings also occur. *Anxieties* about being alone or about suffering similar illness are common and may even give rise to physical symptoms similar to those of the dead relative. *Anger* towards doctors and nurses, or towards other relatives who are thought not to have responded, may be justified or unjustified but is often felt very strongly. So is the more surprising anger at the dead person for leaving the relative. And so is anger at the self, the relative feeling *guilty* that he or she has somehow been at fault in allowing or causing the death. These and other feelings, including *envy* of the dead person for dying, *gratitude* for a past good relationship, *joy* after a bad relationship, *relief* after suffering and the renewal of old feelings from the past are all mixed up together. The result is often a bewildering, disorganized experience.

Recovery

Eventually these feelings lose their strength, or are resolved, and the relative can move to the recovery phase. Now he must look at how his own life has been changed by the death and consider how to reorganize it so that he can continue to obtain satisfaction and happiness in a future bereft of someone very close.

All the phases of the mourning process must be gone through, though not necessarily in strict sequence, if the relative is to reach a satisfactory recovery. Attempts to hurry it, to avoid the feelings or to change nothing only delay or prolong the process.

Losses

It has become more and more clear since the phases of mourning were first defined that grief does not only follow death. It is in fact a universal process following the loss of any thing or person which has been important. The same phases and the same types of feeling are involved whether the loss be loss of self-esteem after a failed exam or a broken engagement, loss of a limb or loss of a front door key. So the multiple losses of dementia must cause grief in close relatives.

Factors affecting mourning

A number of factors determine the *severity* of an individual's reaction to a death or other loss and how they cope with it. The most important are the closeness and importance of the person or object lost, whether the loss was expected, the personality of the person experiencing the loss and their previous experience of loss. In assessing relatives' reactions to dementia we will see rather similar factors operating as they go through the process of grief.

Mourning in dementia

Grief for dementia differs in two important ways from grief induced by the actual death of a near relative. Firstly, the person is *still alive* and indeed may be physically very healthy. Secondly, the process stretches over *long periods of time*, usually many years.

Those who have studied grief reactions have described 'anticipatory grief', a working-through in the imagination of what it would be like to lose a close relative or friend. This naturally occurs if the relative or friend becomes ill and death is a real possibility. But many older married people think a lot about the prospect of their partner's death and prepare for it in imagination long before it is likely to happen. Some of this anticipation of actual death will go through the minds of relatives of dementia sufferers from time to time during the illness. But as well as that there is anticipatory grief for the abilities and personality traits that will be lost forever long before her bodily death.

Helping anticipatory mourning. If every loss of dementia is unexpected, then each time something changes a new shock occurs and the relatives are forced to experience a long series of severe, actual grief reactions. This is one of the most compelling reasons for proper education of relatives. They need to know roughly what to expect. Then they can think out how they will feel and how they can cope practically if changes do occur. In relatives' groups, a lot of this anticipatory grief-work can be effectively carried out in a reassuring atmosphere.

Numbness and shock

The sense of shock when the symptoms of dementia first appear can be enormous, especially when the sufferer is young and the dementia completely unexpected. There seems also to be greater shock if she has previously been active in mind and body, outgoing in personality or organized and careful. It is almost as if relatives did not expect dementia to strike such people. Shock is greater if the dementia has been covered up by the person himself or by another well-meaning relative and is suddenly discovered. And it is greater if the change in personality is sudden or considerable. The greatest shock of all, however, may be the discovery of the diagnosis, a situation not helped by the tendency of some doctors to avoid saying the actual word 'dementia' until a late stage.

Helping numbness. Time and a little privacy can help during the period of shock. The most useful active assistance that can be given to relatives is to show empathy, to say that it is *understandable* to be shocked and to give *permission*, that is, to say that it is acceptable to feel this way.

Protest and denial

But shock is usually less acute in dementia because of the slow progress of the illness. A bigger problem is *denial*. Denial can be seen as an attempt to avoid the implications of loss, both the feelings and readjustments that must be made. It is understandable except when taken to extremes. It leads relatives to deny the evidence of dementia, to explain forgetfulness or poor self-care as laziness, to cover up for the patient's lapses so well that they can ignore the evidence. It leads them to search for any diagnosis other than dementia to explain what is happening. This search is, of course, absolutely reasonable in the early stages, but later amounts to denial of the obvious. Pining and searching for the lost person are demonstrated by persisting hopes of a cure or by claiming to see fragments of her old personality long after they have disappeared. More extreme denial can cause practical and dangerous problems. A relative who believes that there is nothing wrong with a dementing person may leave her in a needlessly risky position.

Helping denial. Denial needs sensitive handling. It is, after all, a powerful defence mechanism that people use to avoid very distressing feelings. It is unlikely to be overcome by blunt confrontation with the facts, tempting though that may be. A gentle approach is much more helpful, firstly gaining the relatives' confidence, then gradually presenting the reality of the situation while preparing them for the mixed and distressing feelings that are bound to follow when reality strikes home. Denial is often based on fear, some of which may be groundless. For example, the relatives may fear that they will be left with no help, or that dementia means uncontrollable behaviour. Discussion of any such fears can ensure that denial gives way to realistic acceptance of a difficult situation.

Distress

The *feelings* which the losses of dementia arouse in close relatives depend very much on what their relationship with the sufferer was like before the illness began, and each individual relative needs to be understood in his own right. The range of possible feelings is great. As already stressed, the prolonged nature of the illness and its gradual worsening bring the relative constant reminders of his loss.

Sadness is likely to be the predominant emotion. The isolation of having to cope alone with a partner who can no longer reciprocate support or love is particularly depressing. And missed opportunities or unfinished business from the past can bring nagging regrets or bitterness. Some relatives become so depressed that they need specific counselling, or antidepressant treatment, if they are to continue to cope. Some find the depression so burdensome that they have to give up, though this can lead them to feel even more guilty that they have not stood by their nearest and dearest when they were needed most.

Anger can be directed at many targets – against fate or God for inflicting the illness on the patient, or inflicting the burden on the relative; against the patient, who may be accused of bringing it on herself, or of not trying hard enough; against other relatives or professionals who are seen as unhelpful; against the self in the form of guilt about real or imaginary actions or inaction, which have brought on or exacerbated the dementia. Anger is often a surprise in grief. Everyone expects to feel sad, not angry. Yet it is perfectly understandable that, if our whole life has been transformed by circumstances out of our control, we should feel angry and wish to lay blame.

Anxiety is another understandable reaction to a change in circumstances when there is no certainty of what will happen. It can take various forms. The relatives may have a fear of not coping, which may or may not be realistic. Or they may become anxious about their own health. They may, half-jokingly, wonder whenever they have lapses of memory, if they will 'go the same way'. Or they may become excessively worried by the genetic risk. The extreme of this anxiety is the predicament of relatives of patients with Huntington's chorea and other strongly genetic conditions, who have to live with a very real possibility of developing the illness themselves (see p. 206).

Helping distress. Helping people cope with feelings of loss is largely a matter of *listening* and giving them *permission* to speak freely about their mixed emotions. Some people need a great deal of encouragement to express their feelings because they are surprised or embarrassed by them, or expect that no one will want to hear them 'going on' about how they feel. The informal support of a good family network is the best way to help carers through this distress. For many carers, support groups are of great help in giving permission to feel and to express feelings by sharing them with others in the same position. But some relatives will also need the prolonged individual support of a 'key worker' (p. 267).

In addition, strong emotions can lead to *action*. Anger may lead to complaints against professional helpers or to arguments and even violence in the home; anxiety to attendance at the doctor for treatment of physical complaints; depression can cause relatives to feel like giving up even when they wish to go on. Workers who are giving support to carers should also be listening to these proposals for action and should spend time talking them over with the relative. They should be comparing the relative's reading of the situation with reality and, if necessary, advising delay before action.

However, there usually are realistic actions to be taken and these are the basis of the recovery phase. Listening is all very well, but it should not go on interminably. The relative should be guided towards a resolution of his feelings and on to a phase when he can deal effectively with the situation that he is in.

Recovery

For the relative of a dementia sufferer, recovery from these feelings involves coming to terms with the situation, organizing effective help and making the required decisions without being crippled by distress. It is obvious that the progressive decline of dementia, the changing situation and the multiplicity of deficits make any real resolution difficult. A new disaster comes just as the last one is being dealt with. Nevertheless, it is reasonable to attempt to get past the phase of emotional distress into a more practical phase of coping and organizing. Indeed, some relatives who have expected not to be able to cope gain considerable confidence and self-esteem by resolving their practical problems and proving that they can manage after all.

Helping recovery. Helping relatives through the recovery phase is largely a practical matter. It is best if possible solutions to practical problems are suggested by the relatives themselves.

The helper's job is then to discuss the pros and cons of different possibilities. The relatives will feel much more effective in this way and dependence on the helper can be largely avoided. For, if a relative has had a helper with a receptive ear and a sympathetic voice during her grieving, it is difficult to let go of that helper when the worst of the distress is over. He must prove that he can 'go it alone'. The helper should not be surprised, however, if some of the distress and fear of not coping returns from time to time as recovery progresses. This is understandable, though the relative will then need encouragement to get back to practical problem-solving.

Sense of relief

Each carer has to go through the process of grieving to a greater or lesser extent for each of the losses of dementia. Sometimes the loss will be very difficult, such as at the time of initial diagnosis or when the carer realizes that his emotional relationship with the person has changed for ever, or when she moves from home to residential care. Other losses will be by comparison minor. By the time long-term care is needed or when death finally comes, a great deal of grieving will have been done and all that is left is a sense of relief. That in itself can pose problems, for absence of feeling after a close relative's death can make one feel embarrassed or guilty. Reassurance may be required that the sense of relief is understandable and acceptable. And, in any case, that may not be the end of the story. Even after the patient's death old feelings of guilt, sadness, anxiety or bitterness will inevitably return from time to time. Hospitals and homes where dementia sufferers are likely to spend their last days should be ready to offer support and counselling to relatives for a period after the death. Mixed feelings that are 'left over' from the long period of illness and decline and the big adjustments that the relatives will still have to make can then be fully discussed.

Abnormal grief

There are two important ways in which the mourning process in dementia may go wrong. First, relatives may be tempted to avoid it by *denial*. Secondly, they may try to *hurry* it by giving up coping and by wishing to reject the sufferer. Many of the problems which arise as families try to cope with dementing relatives and try to work with supporting services can be seen as variants of one or other of these two problems. Denial can explain how some relatives are overoptimistic about their own or the patient's ability to cope, how some will not allow services to take over part of the burden and how others disagree with or obstruct the rest of the family who are trying to seek help.

Giving up too early to avoid distress can sometimes explain precipitate requests for long-stay care, impatience with attempts to plan gradually increasing care or pessimism about what can be achieved. We should help relatives to go through the phases of mourning the multiple losses of dementia at a rate that is reasonable for them.

THE CHANGING RELATIONSHIP

COPING WITH DEPENDENCE

If relatives are to come to terms with the many losses in intellect, self-care and personality that dementia brings then the relationship between them and the sufferer must inevitably change. The central element of this change is a move from independence to dependence on the part of the patient. Whereas she used to think independently, to look after herself, to have something to offer in conversation, to be able to fill her day with work and pastimes, she now requires someone to think for her, to look after her and to provide activities. The change will be even more striking if, before the onset of the dementia, family members were dependent on *her*. As has been stressed so often, these changes are gradual and subtle. They tend to creep up on a family, who may respond to the change almost without knowing it.

There are two aspects to the reactions of relatives to this new dependence. The first is practical, the second more to do with emotions, attitudes and roles in the family.

The practicalities of dependence

Relatives as staff

Chapter 4 indicated how family, as well as staff in home or hospital, fill the gaps in ability opened up by dementia, and Chapter 9, on decision-making, will describe other types of gap which may have to be filled by relatives. Particularly where relatives live with the patient, the distinction between staff and family becomes blurred. By carrying out practical caring the family are in a sense acting as 'staff'. Or, to put it another way, the only differences between 'formal' and 'informal' carers are that the formal carers may have had a training for their job and get paid a lot more for doing it.

Relatives are involved throughout dementia in assessing the deficits of the patient, in deciding how to fill gaps and whether to fill them, in working out who does what for the patient and in carrying out the day-to-day work. The functions of professional or volunteer advisors are to support relatives in those tasks, to 'train' them and to help decide which gaps are to be filled by the relatives and which by outsiders.

Training. Most of this training, support and decision-making tends to be carried out in a haphazard way, spread over several years as it must be and divided between different advisors, sometimes with differing ideas. Some relatives will have access to a specific educational group for 'new' relatives who are having to cope with dementia for the first time, or to one of the residential or other courses for carers which are beginning to be more common. Some relatives will have a key worker to whom they can refer throughout the illness. But for most, training consists of a mixture of learning by trial and error, chatting with other relatives in the same position, asking specific bits of advice from the health visitor, community psychiatric nurse or other staff, or reading a book. Several booklets and video guides for carers are available. They provide useful training for relatives, not only in learning the nature of dementia and getting advice on how to cope with their current problems but also in finding out what problems may occur in the future, what feelings to expect in themselves and where to go for help.

How much help?

Relatives are the providers of memory and other aids. They help with reminders of time, reminders of meals and of self-care. They help with dressing, washing, bathing and toileting. They provide stimulation and reality orientation. They decide things on the person's behalf and help with paying bills. They act as advocates for her (p. 302). How much of this should they be doing?

Realistically, how much relatives do is all too often decided by the *absence of services* as shown in the balance of care diagram (see Table 3.5, p. 103), but we should be trying to get away from that as much as possible. What relatives do should be a considered balance between what they are able to do, what they are willing to do and what can be offered in the way of outside help. We should question whether an elderly or disabled spouse is physically able to bathe and dress his or her wife or husband and whether a mentally handicapped daughter has the skill to deal with memory aids.

How much sacrifice?

Practical caring can mean having to give something else up. Is it reasonable for a daughter to give up her work, for a husband to retire prematurely, for social life to be restricted because of the need to care for a dementing relative? We should question the willingness of relatives to give support, even when they are able and seem to be offering it. Many may be offering in desperation, out of a martyred feeling of duty, out of an obligation demanded by the dementing person or out of ignorance of available services.

Much has been said about the financial sacrifices of caring. Actual figures are very difficult to estimate, though in Britain the costs borne by family carers are likely to run into billions of pounds. It is reasonable and indeed vital that willing informal carers should be repaid by society for the losses they incur in caring for relatives who would otherwise need to be in institutional care.

Present levels of financial support for families are far from adequate in many cases. But there is a danger in one or two cases of benefits being used as a 'bribe' to encourage unsuitable or reluctant carers to continue when the patient would be safer and better cared for in hospital or residential home.

How much willingness?

In general, the true willingness of relatives to cope with a dementia sufferer at home depends mainly on the strength of their previous relationship. If a relative has had a good strong relationship and feels that the patient has given him a lot over previous years together, then he will probably feel positive towards the idea of caring for her now. He will feel more sadness at the loss, but may be patient and tolerant in a way which other relatives are not. The danger, indeed, for such relatives is that they try to take on too much and resist reasonable outside help.

If the relationship has been poor, on the other hand, there is likely to be little loyalty, so caring may be half-hearted and not carefully thought out. Such relatives are likely to want to hand over the caring to others at an early stage.

Family or outsiders?

Having assessed the relatives' ability to cope and their willingness to cope, and after working out with them whether they can be trained to cope better, arranging outside help becomes a matter of filling those gaps in caring that have been reasonably left by the family.

Helping relatives fill the gaps

Intermittent help

Most of the help that people with dementia need could be described as intermittent, and most of the help relatives need is also intermittent. This consists of help with tasks that are spread over the day such as eating, toileting, dressing, getting to and from day care, etc. The sufferer needs some aids, or a person to be there to supervise her in one or more of these tasks, but only at particular times of the day or night. Providing bathing assistants, a home help or a 'tucker-in' at night helps the relatives to fill the gaps at these intermittent times but also allows them to cope better at other parts of the day.

Supervision

Even more exhausting than this intermittent dependence in daily living is the need for more general supervision. Some dementia sufferers cannot be left alone for any length of time. If they are, they may fiddle with electrical or gas appliances, attempt to smoke carelessly, wander out, let intruders in or become very distressed, going to neighbours or ringing relatives or the police for help. They need a more constant type of supervision. This is particularly stressful because the relative is not necessarily doing anything with the patient but must be constantly alert and may even feel like a jailer. It is most stressful when this sort of supervision is needed at night. The relative must stay half-awake in case she decides to go off to 'work', or to go 'home' in the middle of the night.

Most stressful of all is 'shadowing' as the anxious person feels so dependent on her carer that she follows him everywhere, perhaps continually asking for reassurance as well. Outside help that takes over supervision of the patient for some time of the day or night can ease the burden of care enormously in all these cases.

Interval dependence

A useful way to think of dependence of all sorts is called 'interval dependence' – how long a person can be left without some form of supervision. It will be seen that intermittent dependence for tasks of daily living may be for long or short intervals, but it is usually predictable. So help can be organized in a regular fashion. A more persistent need for supervision may still allow intervals of several hours during which the relative feels that he can go to the shops and leave the person quietly and contentedly at home. But it may allow only a short interval, or even none at all – in other words, constant supervision is needed. Few relatives can tolerate this, though some choose to and some have to.

Respite from caring

To deal with both intermittent and persistent dependence the relatives need regular relief for themselves – a respite from caring. Some have the ability to give themselves a break. They develop ways of 'blowing off steam' without getting at the person. The most effective appears to be *a sense of humour*. Many relatives say that they could not carry on over the long periods of caring if they did not have a good laugh at the things the patient does and the situations they get themselves into in trying to help. Relatives' meetings are therefore often surprisingly cheerful affairs despite the dreadful nature of the situations being discussed. Others get relief by *physical activity*, through a *hobby* or through *talking* to someone else either about the situation or about nothing in particular. Some, unfortunately, do get their relief by angry words or even physical aggression to the patient. But sooner or later most will need respite from outside.

Judging interval dependence helps in planning the help to be given. How long can the relative reasonably cope without a break? Some need an annual holiday, the patient going to another member of the family, a 'foster' carer, residential or hospital care for a few weeks. Some need a regular day to themselves when the patient goes to day care. Some need an hour or so when a neighbour, family member, or companion/sitter supervises the patient. Some need help at night, with a night sitter, a nurse or another family member providing the supervision. Some need most or even all of these. The judgement of what should reasonably be offered is largely up to the relatives. They will be all too aware of what has been called the '36-hour day' of caring.

The effects of dependence

A relative may be willing and able to cope with increasing dependence. But even so, changing into a 'carer' inevitably brings great changes in the relationship between relative and sufferer. People do not usually plan or choose to be carers; they have the role thrust upon them and accept it more or less willingly. And they are unlikely to foresee how it will alter their lives.

Restrictions

Firstly, there is a restriction of social life and privacy caused by caring. Even if the relative has chosen to give up some of his normal activities this can bring hidden or open resentment, to the extent of blaming the patient for ruining a good life. There is a danger that the home atmosphere becomes bitter, or even of violence towards the patient. On the other hand, a relative may adjust to the new situation by making it his 'job' to be a carer. This enables him to cope with the more distressing aspects of caring with more dispassion. The danger is that the relative becomes too business-like and emotionally detached and so neglects both his own and the patient's feelings. But in general, treating caring as a job has advantages for relatives. They do not resent the loss of their own independent life so much and can usually work with outside help more easily (unless they have become so overcompetent that they resent any outside offers of help).

Role reversal

Secondly, there is a reversal of roles. Very many relatives comment on how surprised they have been to find themselves becoming like a mother to their husband, a mother to their own mother, an intimate carer to a previously distant uncle. For many of the forms of assistance which dementia sufferers require are those required by a small child from its mother or father. Having to help with feeding, dressing, toileting, washing, having to find things to occupy time, having to keep a careful watch in case of danger, are all familiar tasks to anyone who has had the care of young children. Carers have to discover within themselves the skill to carry out these tasks. Inevitably, they find themselves tending to act in 'motherly' kinds of ways by treating the patient as if she actually was a child, using infantile forms of address, expecting childlike responses, disciplining or scolding in attempts to improve behaviour. But there are great differences between an adult dementing patient and a small child. The patient is an adult, with a past in which she has been independent and capable to a much greater degree than now. It can be hurtful to treat someone in this position like a child. She may not be aware of her deficits, or her childishness, so treating her like an infant can give offence. She will not be able to recall the reminders, advice or punishment that a mother would give to a child, and she will not learn.

Unlike a child learning the skills of everyday life, the dementing adult is losing her skills, and losing them in a disorganized fashion. So although reminders and even scolding might maintain her level of functioning temporarily, it is always a losing battle and the joy of seeing a child grow up and learn about life is missing.

The result is that treating a dementing adult like a child, while natural to some extent and helpful in a few cases, can upset her, upset a good relationship and be frustrating for the relatives. That being said, some relatives, who have lots of experience with children or strong 'maternal' instincts, love the role of parent;

and some patients, particularly if they are either apathetic or euphoric, or never were very independent personalities in the first place, love the childlike dependent position.

Dangers in role reversal

Relatives should have the chance to realize how roles have changed and to discuss the implications of this change. There are two types of situation where special help is needed.

Avoidance. There are those who do not like the idea of being 'mother'. They may find, quite reasonably, that the more intimate parts of caring – bathing, help with incontinence, dressing, putting to bed – are foreign to them. This problem is often greater for men, be they husbands, sons, brothers or nephews, but is also a problem for wives and daughters who have never imagined that they would have to do these very personal things for their husband or parent. The relatives may find the 'job' approach described above helpful in detaching themselves emotionally from the tasks they have to do. But they should also have the opportunity to talk over their embarrassment with other relatives or helpers.

Overmothering. At the other extreme are some relatives who tend to exaggerate the patient's degree of dependence, who infantilize her and overprotect her. The result is that she is allowed little independent activity, gets no practice in the tasks of daily living and is in danger of being out of touch with reality. Such relatives are often avoiding some of their feelings of loss or are dealing with guilt about some neglect they blame themselves for in the past. There is a danger for outside helpers here too. Those who overprotect and overmother may resist outside help and appear much more able to cope than they actually are. Services are let off the hook. The relative may actually feel that he is the only person who can cope with the patient. He criticizes or rejects any outside helper who treats the patient as an adult. But the relative's attitude is unrealistic. Attempts should be made to encourage him into a more adult relationship with the patient and to allow the patient a reasonable degree of independence. A gradual intrusion of outside support can help this type of situation. But, sadly, an overprotecting relative may be unshakeable.

COPING WITH NEW BEHAVIOUR

In Chapter 5 we described some examples of how dementing people behave in ways that they never did before, through loss of self control and decline of standards and judgement. To relatives, the personality that they have known for many years has changed, sometimes quite beyond recognition. Of all the changes of dementia, personality change is probably the most distressing. Furthermore, it is usually totally unexpected. The *loss* of personality characteristics, even if unexpected at first, becomes more obvious and predictable as time goes on, so that the relatives prepare themselves gradually to lose touch with the patient as a person. But *new* personality traits occur in directions and at times that are unpredictable. The most unexpected changes occur in vascular dementia when, suddenly after a stroke, even an apparently very minor one, there is a major change in the patient's behaviour. And the range of possible changes is wide – emotional lability, restlessness, disinhibited social behaviour of all kinds, coarsened habits, sexual demands.

Failure of recognition

As well as personality changes, the person with dementia may develop difficulties with recognition, or agnosia (p. 114). There are two forms of this which can cause a great deal of distress to families and in particular to spouses. The patient's familiarity with her own home may disappear. Thus she may make continual requests to return home to an address she left long ago, or she may pack her belongings or continually try to leave. Even long-loved items of furniture, and decor in the house, may be perceived as being someone else's. Failure to recognize one's own spouse, or perhaps child, can lead to many problems, particularly if it is associated with the loss of familiarity with their home. These problems put a great deal of pressure on the carer, and if not handled sensitively can be the 'straw that breaks the camel's back' in terms of providing ongoing care. Often the carer gets no thanks (or even antagonism!) as a reward for providing care, and adding a lack of recognition to their relationship may well exhaust his emotional reserves.

Automatic reactions

After the initial shock, the commonest response of relatives to disturbed behaviour is automatic – they react directly to the emotions or behaviour of the patient. If they are already treating her a bit like a child, they may scold her. If she bursts into a temper, they argue back. If she is suddenly upset, they try to console her. They may be embarrassed by her coarsened behaviour, by her apparent rudeness or by the peculiar things that she says or does. This embarrassment may lead them to try to ignore her disturbed behaviour or to avoid the public eye by keeping her in the house and away from visitors and other family members. Or they may simply feel disgusted and tend to reject her.

Search for meaning

Next the relatives will look for an explanation. They are unlikely to know much about the brain mechanism of inhibition and the frontal lobe and so may blame the wrong thing. They may blame the patient herself, thinking that she is behaving inappropriately out of malice. They may guess that she is doing things she always wanted to do and think that this is her 'real' personality emerging. Or they may blame themselves, looking for something that they have done wrongly which has offended her.

Reassurance

Relatives require a proper explanation of the damage done to control and monitoring mechanisms by dementia. They need to be reassured that the new behaviour is nobody's fault, neither the patient's nor their own. Their feelings of embarrassment, disgust, anger, anxiety or fear need to be aired. In particular their fears about how disturbed the patient may become need to be compared with the reality of the situation. Often, permission to see the funny side of the behaviour can be a great relief, though laughing directly *at* the patient should of course be discouraged.

Coping

Next, the relatives should be engaged as 'joint therapists' in attempts to modify the behaviour. They can help identify the problem clearly, look for other causes, work out what makes it worse or better, try to modify the circumstances to reduce the undesirable behaviour and help to encourage and increase more appropriate behaviour. They may need specific advice about what to say to other relatives and friends and about what to do if the behaviour occurs in public, so that their lives do not have to be restricted too much. The end result should be that the relatives are less upset by the behaviour, do not take it personally and have worked out how best to act themselves to help reduce and control it.

Learning to talk together

One of the tragedies of dementia is that two people in a close relationship with one another, coping together with the same illness, both likely to be in distress, may be unable to talk to each other about how it feels. Some manage to overcome this difficulty and share moments when they talk about the effects of dementia on each of their lives. Most, we suspect, do not. And since professional helpers are notoriously bad at allowing any such discussion there is little encouragement to relatives who may be wondering how much the patient is understanding and feeling, but may be too shy to ask. This puts a quite unnecessary barrier between the sufferer and her carers. It means that they will be emotionally distant at a time when they need all the consolation they can get from the remains of their relationship.

The key to breaking the ice lies in overcoming the taboo of saying the words 'dementia' or 'Alzheimer's' in the patient's hearing. Once we and the relatives together begin to be able to do this then it will be perfectly easy to discuss feelings more openly, deal with problems *with* the patient rather than behind her back, and so help reduce the strain of caring. Of course, at later stages talking about feelings with the sufferer will become impossible, but in early and even moderate stages we should always be reminding ourselves that abilities and insight are *being* lost, they do not suddenly disappear at the beginning of dementia. This applies to the ability to talk about feelings as much as it does to the ability to dress, eat or walk.

COPING WITH INTRUDERS

As the dementing person becomes gradually more dependent, the family will gradually need more and more outside help. As long as the relatives are not trying to cope on their own too long, or trying to reject the patient too early, this help can be organized in a gradual and agreed way (if it is available). It is important to remember that the family's relationships have previously been private, that a marriage may have been going on for 50 years without any outside help, that most people are not used to intruders in their personal business. This, of course, applies to all forms of help offered to families. But it is particularly important in dementia because the 'intruders' may have to spend a lot of time in the family house giving practical or supervisory care. And they may have to be involved in very intimate aspects of the patient's life. This can be embarrassing or disturbing to both patient and family, and needs sensitive handling. As the dementia progresses this intrusion into family life will have to increase and it may end up that outsiders are doing practically everything for the sufferer in her own house with her nearest relative almost a spectator.

Reactions to intrusion

The person who is coming in to help the situation may find himself surprisingly unwelcome because the relatives are struggling with their feelings about giving up some of the care to outsiders. The family may feel guilty about not coping enough, frustrated with the situation, possessive of their relative, more competent than the outside help. Or they may be worried that this helper is at the thin edge of a wedge whose other end is institutional care. 'Intruders' need to be alert to these possible feelings, delicate about their intrusion on the family's privacy and prepared to leave private some parts of the relationship, so that they do not seem to take over everything all at once.

Sharing care

That biggest intrusion, institutional care, should be seen in the same way. There is no need for hospitals and homes to take over every aspect of the care of their residents just because they *could* do so. Relatives, particularly spouses, should be allowed some privacy together with the patient and if possible, some continuing tasks in the patient's care. Staff who treat relatives as intruders are often missing an opportunity to share care in a constructive way. Unfortunately, some relatives are put off the idea of continuing to care by a fear that they will be asked to take over completely again. Such fears should be discussed openly and proper reassurance given.

THE CONTINUING RELATIONSHIP

Despite all the changes and disruption caused by dementia, relatives will very often wish to continue their relationship right to the end of the sufferer's life. Continuity is easier if outside help is introduced gradually and sensitively. It is sustained by good memories from the past, by imagining what the patient would have wanted in the present situation, and by loyalty. It is also sustained by clinging to those aspects of her appearance, personality and behaviour which survive the dementia. Some couples manage to maintain an affectionate relationship or even a reasonable sexual life well into dementia. One or two old habits, turns of phrase or gestures may be all that is left of a personality, but the relatives can use these as reminders of the person as she was and so continue to relate. Even after the patient seems like a stranger, loyalty, memory and imagination keep relationships good, while waiting for death of the body.

TYPES OF RELATIONSHIP AND INDIVIDUAL REACTIONS

These, then, are three 'dimensions' of reacting and coping: loss; a new relationship, which involves coping with dependence, new behaviour, the patient's feelings and intruders; and the continuing relationship. In different individual relatives, with different types of patient, there will be more of one type of reaction or more of another. We suggest that for each important relative, evidence of each of these types of reaction should be sought. Then the type of support and help needed can be worked out. Much of the variation between individual reactions depends on the actual family arrangement around the dementing person and some comments on a number of differing arrangements will show the sort of problems which can arise.

The married couple, one of whom is dementing

Whichever partner is the patient, this is, for obvious reasons, the strongest and most continuing relationship met with in dealing with dementia. Loyalty 'in sickness and in health' is taken seriously by many married couples, and accepting gradual estrangement or giving over care to others is particularly difficult. This is not, however, always the case. Where there has been a poor previous relationship the onset of dementia may be seen as just another problem and it may be ignored or lead to rejection at an early stage. On the other hand, in some previously difficult relationships, where the husband who develops dementia has been aggressive, alcoholic or unfaithful, the decline in drive that is often part of dementia can actually lead to a quieter time for his wife. So it is essential to understand both the past relationship and the changes that have occurred.

The wives of dementing men often have a particularly difficult time. They may have to cope with severe restlessness, demands for attention and irritability or aggression from a physically strong husband at a time when they may be physically frail themselves. Sexual interest may become disorganized or demanding. Attempts by the wife to calm the situation may lead to increased aggression. Furthermore, sometimes the patient fails to recognize his spouse. Life is almost impossible for a wife who is trying to remain loyal while she is being treated as an intruder in her own house. It is also particularly difficult if the dementia begins at a time when the couple were looking forward to a pleasant, active retirement, for disappointment and resentment can interfere with the spouse's willingness to cope.

Loyalty, and the feeling of a duty of care, often lead the spouse to neglect her own needs. It may be difficult for her to obtain medical or social help on her own behalf, and her own emotional needs particularly are often neglected. This may lead to resentment and will generally interfere with her ability to care.

The death of a spouse who is also a carer can obviously have a major effect on the management of the person with dementia. Often the degree of impairment has been hidden from other family members, sometimes deliberately, but more likely because the carer has met most care needs. The family has therefore suffered not only a bereavement, but also has the responsibility of providing care for the person with dementia thrust upon them.

The dementia sufferer may not necessarily understand that their carer has died, and may make constant reference to him or her. This situation can be particularly difficult to deal with, and many differing and often conflicting emotions may be involved.

As we have seen, dementia is not a rare condition. It affects as many as one in four people in older age groups. It is therefore not uncommon to see both husband and wife in a relationship develop dementia. They are often able to live in their own home for much longer than expected, as they are likely to deteriorate at different rates, and the losses due to dementia are unlikely to be the same. They may then be able to complement each other. However, they are also likely to have reduced insight, and may be unable to tolerate what they perceive as outside interference. This sort of situation will require very careful assessment of the separate problems and needs of each of the pair, and sensitive attempts to introduce help are necessary.

The dementing parent living with a married child and family

An arrangement to have 'granny' to live with the family will usually have been made before the onset of dementia. If it is considered during dementia, there should be an opportunity for the family to discuss at length the likely difficulties of the future, how much care they are prepared to give and what would happen if the situation broke down. All members of the family, including children, should be involved in this discussion. The daughter or son of the dementing parent should be strongly advised not to make the decision alone. Even decisions to accept a non-demented parent into the house should only be taken when the family have discussed what would happen if dementia or chronic physical disability occurred. And the parent must, of course, be fully involved in that discussion.

Dementia in a grandparent at home can bring a family together in sharing the tasks of caring. But often loyalty to the grandparent is not shared equally by husband and wife, or the grandchildren may not wish to become involved. The dementing person may make things more difficult by putting particular demands on her daughter or son and by becoming suspicious or critical of the spouse. And the loyalty of the son or daughter is tested to the limit by the conflicting demands of parent, spouse and children.

The dementing parent living with an unmarried child

The child who remains at home is often in a peculiar position. He retains some dependence on his parents but also develops an independent life of his own. If the child is left alone with a dementing parent he has to become 'mother' to his own mother or father and usually has to accept some loss of his own independence and some restriction of his activities. Since the balance between his dependence and independence has usually been quite delicate, this change can bring bitterness and impatience into what was previously a good relationship.

The solitary dementing patient with a visiting relative

Relatives who do not live with the patient are in a very different position to those who do. On the one hand they may have more anxiety about what she is 'up to' when no one is around. On the other hand they remain visitors who can get relief from caring simply by returning to their own homes. It is very important to assess the degree of commitment of such relatives, even if they are sons or daughters; to check on how much time they are actually giving to their patient and whether their judgement of the situation is accurate. It is all too easy for visiting relatives to *underestimate* the problems and risks, assuming that the patient is fine because she is always happy to see them and behaves normally when they are there. Neighbours and others may have a different story. It is also all too easy for them to *overestimate* the problems, dropping into the situation from time to time, seeing that it is not perfect and ringing all sorts of alarm bells. The latter mistake can arise from guilt in the relatives that they are not doing enough, from impatience or from lack of true commitment.

The large family

Large families have opportunities for real 'sharing the caring'. Some of the most effective arrangements for care are made when a number of children share the cover for a week between them, arrange meals on a rota system, have a night rota for tucking in or sitting, or take the patient to live with them in rotation. Each of these arrangements share out the burden equally, while giving everybody relief.

More often, however, one member of the family takes on the burden of care entirely. This type of arrangement can also work well as long as the rest of the family shows their appreciation of what is being done and offers the main carer some regular respite on a daily, weekly or holiday basis. Unfortunately, relationships within families are not always so neat. One 'martyr' who takes the burden of care may let the rest of the family off the hook. Or in trying to work out rotas of care some members of the family may not wish to cooperate, foreseeing possible restrictions to their own lives.

The result of having a divided family is usually an argument between those who want to support their mother at home, and those who wish her to be 'put away'. The two sides may give completely different versions of the home situation. There can be considerable value in such a family having a meeting with an outside professional, who tries to remain neutral and can help to encourage a fair sharing of burden and relief.

Family situations like this can be exacerbated by the dementing mother's expectations of one particular child, usually a daughter. And if the father lives with the dementing mother he may expect far too much of the family as a whole, saying that if he copes, they should. Very often he is not coping at all.

The other problem which arises in any family caring situation is that the burden of care falls mostly or entirely on the women in the family. It is often assumed by the family and also by society in general that a daughter, daughter-in-law or even a niece, and certainly a wife, will cope far better and longer than a son, son-in-law, nephew or husband. Besides not being true that women are always better carers, this type of attitude is unfair, and professionals should be aware of this when looking at who is available to care and what they can offer.

The younger sufferer with a family

Because dementia is relatively rare in younger people, there is almost no chance that a family will have prepared themselves for caring; the effects on the sufferer of loss of their job and of their general competence are devastating. Dementia in a 40 or 50 year old is likely to come at a time when his or her family is growing up and needing support and guidance. Instead of getting help with growing up or having the usual teenage battles, children may find themselves having to come to terms with 'mothering' their parent. Money problems are likely to increase. And the well parent will probably have to work to keep going, thus forcing the children to become carers, whether they like it or not. Such families need a lot of outside support, and one of the scandals of dementia in the past has been the absence of this support. In addition, however, the children need sensitive personal support and counselling about their understanding of dementia, their attitudes, their contribution to caring and the effects on their education and on outside relationships.

Staff as family

In any long-term institution it is not unusual for individual staff members to take on some of the aspects of being a relative. They too can feel the sense of loss and the difficulty of coping with caring. If they become attached to the patient they may feel that other staff 'do not understand' and become possessive. They may even feel that relatives are 'intruders'. The maintenance of both detachment and a caring involvement at the same time is one of the most difficult tasks for staff who are coping with dependent residents.

TYPES OF HELP NEEDED BY RELATIVES

Having described the differing types of reaction of relatives and the various family set-ups we can now see some important forms of help which are needed to enable families to cope.

Education and advice

Relatives need to know the diagnosis and the implications of that diagnosis. Neglecting to tell them is not a kindness, for without this information relatives have only their own fantasies to work on. Telling the facts can bring relief and can help the family replan their own lives and look for appropriate help. They can stop merely reacting and start working.

But they need a lot of knowledge to work with. This can be given in interview or in a small group or by learning from other families. The books listed on p. 393 are extremely helpful in introducing to relatives the stages of dementia and its associated problems, in giving advice on how to cope and in explaining about services, financial and legal matters. Used properly they are reassuring and helpful in a practical way, even though they tell a depressing story. Families need to be warned that their relative will not necessarily present all the problems mentioned. And they should be given opportunities to discuss any worry or uncertainty that comes out of their reading.

When one particular problem becomes paramount, relatives may need special education, with a chance to learn of a variety of ways to cope, or of one specific technique which may relieve the problem. In searching for residential care, a lot of information is needed about types of home, what to look for, standards of care, money matters.

Universality

Information can bring relief to relatives in another way. Very often it can seem to a carer, especially if he is isolated with the patient, that he is alone, that no one else can be going through the same type of experience. Meeting other relatives who are living with the same problems can bring enormous relief. It can also be a relief to know that others are even worse off! Indeed there are some relatives who go to only one of a series of relatives' meetings because they realize at the first meeting that the problems are universal and then feel better able to cope on their own.

Support

The greatest relief of all, however, can come from knowing that one's feelings are understood and accepted as reasonable, from knowing that there is someone to talk to about how it feels to care and from knowing that support will usually be there when needed. The feelings may be of sadness, depression, bewilderment, anxiety, fear, amusement, frustration, anger, resentment or despair. The fears may include fears about quite severe risks to the patient. The frustration and anger may reach the point of feeling like physically hitting the patient or walking out on her. All these feelings may be very powerful, and all can be distressing, especially in a previously happy relationship. Indeed, in some studies of families, more than half the closest relatives showed as much distress as typical patients going to psychiatric hospitals for treatment.

It takes a very patient and resilient listener to support a relative through such distress. A helper must be prepared to listen sometimes for long sessions, sometimes intermittently over years, encouraging the relative to talk about feelings that are painful, giving moral support and understanding the causes of distress, while keeping in mind also the need for practical action.

Relief and respite

The '36-hour day' feeling has been mentioned, but all relatives who are put in a stressful situation need some form of relief. There is an emotional relief which comes from understanding something of what is happening to the patient, from universality and from support. But relief in the sense of 'time off' or respite from caring is also essential. Respite care ranges from a neighbour or other family member looking in for a chat, through sitting services, home-care services and through day care of various kinds, to residential-care relief for short or even long periods. For some relatives it is the time to themselves that they appreciate most, for others it is the relief from tasks of caring, for others it is the chance to get right out of the situation for a while, for many it is bits of all these which help.

Relief in a crisis is equally important, though we can hope that good regular respite-care systems will reduce the need for it. Many relatives become preoccupied with the thought that if they broke down in any way, the patient would be lost. They need to know as nearly as possible exactly what would happen if they were suddenly unable to cope, because of illness, accident or even in the event of their death; and our helping arrangements are useless if they do not have the flexibility to give extra help at these difficult times.

Financial and workplace support

Carers who are also at work need their caring role recognized by their employers, in just the same way that working mothers need recognition of their dual job. Hours of work may have to be adjusted and time off in crises, or even to suit available respite dates in a home or hospital, may be necessary.

Education about available benefits and allowances is an essential part of the education of a carer, and leaving it till late in the illness is inexcusable. Those who are reluctant to claim because they see their caring as a family duty will need special encouragement. And many carers need special advice on imaginative ways to use the money for the patient's benefit and to ease their burden of care. Financial advice and support are as important as emotional or practical advice and support; all should be available by right to anyone who cares for a dementia sufferer.

PROVIDING THE HELP

Self-help by relatives

Some individual relatives, particularly elderly husbands or wives of dementing patients, are very stoical by nature. They feel they have a duty to care for their spouse, they wish to do so and pride themselves in being able to find solutions to some of the problems of dementia by themselves. They should not be decried. Presenting this type of relative with our well-thought-out programme of care for the patient is not appropriate. It may indeed be considered rather insulting. Nor should we be too critical if all the relative's techniques are not exactly what we would advise, or if some are even quite eccentric. If they work and are not distressing to the patient, then why not?

What such relatives need is some moral support and encouragement. They also need to be told which type of help would be available should they ask for it, and given some reassurance that it is not considered a weakness to have to ask for help. A watchful eye should be kept from a discreet distance in case the relative is in fact failing to cope adequately, or is shifting the load onto neighbours, friends or other family while claiming to cope, or in case the patient is suffering in some way. This type of relative usually sees care as a 'job' and appreciates very much being treated as a semi-professional or staff member when it comes to the time that they must hand over some of the caring.

Family organization

We have seen earlier (p. 260) how families can organize themselves formally to care for a dementing relative. Families are often perfectly capable of doing this without outside help. If they decide to do so, the following principles are useful. They should, if possible, hold a family meeting, so that everyone agrees together and there is a sense of a contract being made. They should seriously consider having the patient at the meeting, even if she does not fully understand or is likely to be somewhat distressed. The fact that all the family agree to a particular arrangement or course of action can have a strong influence on whether she accepts the help offered. Decisions made behind her back are likely to be less than popular. But unreasonable distress and unreasonable pressure should be avoided. The family should ensure that all the important members of the family are present, and this may extend to friends and neighbours. If such an arrangement does not work they should seek outside help as referee.

Informal support

The informal and unorganized help, advice and support that family members give each other is extremely important. And the support of friends and neighbours adds to the strength of relatives in coping with difficult problems. Again, some of the advice may seem eccentric or even negative, but outsiders should always remind themselves that these supports are normal. We should concentrate outside support on those relatives who are isolated by having few other family members to rely on, on those who are isolated from the rest of the family by the task of caring, on those who are distressed despite good family support and where the patient is posing particularly difficult problems.

Help for individual families

We have outlined some of the variety of reactions of families faced with the vast variety of problems of dementia. Each family has its own structure, its own rules and its own ways of coping. It is difficult to make general rules, therefore, about how and when to help families.

Helpers from outside can guess that they are being of use if the relatives are getting relief by talking of how they are feeling, if problems are being discussed and solutions worked out, if effective support is being organized, if preparations are being made for future changes. If these processes are not going forwards then there should be a question about whether this sort of support is needed, or whether the right topics are being discussed. It is all too easy for a professional to listen endlessly to a tale of woe without moving on to practical decisions about how to cope. It can also be too easy to keep trying to offer a nice plan of help which suits *our* system when the relatives actually want something else, for example, long-term care.

Key workers

Since dementia is a prolonged illness the best help for relatives is also prolonged. It is also rewarding and instructive for a professional helper to see a family through the long process of decline and help them cope with the varied problems that they face. General practitioners have this opportunity, though usually only intermittently. A more regular and supportive contact can be made by a community psychiatric nurse, health visitor or a volunteer from an Alzheimer's support group or other organization, acting as 'key worker'. If this supporter is welcomed in the family, is empathic and knows the local services well, so that contacts can be easily made and important information passed on, then such individual, long-term help can be invaluable. Having a key worker, the family have someone to turn to for advice when things go wrong, support when feelings run too high and help to work out what further help is needed.

It is important, though, that all other agencies involved with the patient know who that key person is and that the worker has some influence on these agencies. The concept of key worker is by no means universally accepted, but is likely to become more popular in the next few years. Without someone like this relatives have to find their way through the confusion of different organizations and professional groups unaided.

Carers' groups

Carers' groups are of several types: those for relatives of patients attending a specific facility, say a day hospital or a respite facility; those for relatives going for help from a voluntary organization such as an Alzheimer's society; those where carers of patients with a variety of illnesses attend.

Groups like these are of great importance because they can bring together all the types of help listed above (p. 262). The educational element can be increased by giving out information booklets or having specific speakers on topics such as incontinence, activities, home care, residential care, benefits or the nature of dementia. They can be used to help organize moral support, advice and relief. They give relatives a chance to share with each other their feelings and ideas. They can also be a political force, where relatives get together to press for proper services or improvements in existing services.

However, they are not a panacea. Some relatives do not like being in a group – they feel embarrassed, shy, or antagonistic to the idea of public discussion of personal problems. Although the group leaders can help to encourage reluctant people to join the group and to contribute, groups are not the answer for all. However, it is also the case that some silent attenders can gain a great deal from the group without contributing. For those who are unused to speaking in a group, the use of a guest speaker to start discussion and encouragement by group leaders can be helpful. But there is also need for individual help, for not everything can be done in the group. So the informal chat with a cup of tea after the main meeting becomes almost as important as the group itself.

Special sorts of relatives' meeting can be very helpful in certain circumstances. It is often possible to get together a group of 'new' carers and sometimes to have a group of wives of dementing husbands, the daughters of dementing parents or carers of younger sufferers. As we saw on pp. 86 and 257 there are some common problems of different family set-ups. Special relatives' meetings allow for a much more cohesive group feeling, since the members are sharing very similar experiences and can give stronger support to each other in working out the solutions to their very similar problems.

How much help?

Relatives differ in their demands for help of these various kinds. But demand is much less important than need. For some people almost never ask for help, yet they may be ignorant of the facts of dementia, isolated, distressed and burdened. Others seem to want endless support. We need to search for relatives in need.

This implies some 'case-finding', a task mainly for health visitors and other community staff who regularly visit or screen their elderly clients. It is another good reason for early referral by general practitioners of dementing people and their families to specalist old-age psychiatry services. It means publicity campaigns by Alzheimer's societies, the Health Education authorities, Age Concern and other interested groups, telling the public what help can be available and encouraging relatives to come for advice and support.

CONCLUSION

In general it can be said that all relatives need education at the beginning of their experience of dementia and continuing through it. Every carer of a dementia sufferer should have easy access to a local advice centre or support group. The need for individual support, advice and respite must be assessed in each case, and the way in which that help should be given will differ from relative to relative. There are some particular occasions and danger signs when extra help may be needed. These are:

1. When dementia is first diagnosed
2. A risky home situation
3. A sudden change in the symptoms of the patient, especially new behaviour problems arising
4. Any change in the family, especially a sudden change, such as a death or emigration
5. Distress in the relatives, especially anxiety, depression or anger towards the patient
6. A move to a new level of care, say from home to day care, or from home to hospital.

9

Decision-making

It should now be clear that during the long decline of dementia a number of major decisions have to be made. These decisions are mainly about accepting outside help, so as to reduce the problems and risks that arise in the course of the illness. Since ability to decide is likely to be included in the general failure of brain function, the patient will find it increasingly difficult to deal with such problems or risks. This chapter discusses that difficulty.

First, we will examine decision-making and how it is affected by dementia. Secondly, we will look at the types of *risk* which arise and how control of the patient's affairs can be handed over to others to avoid or lessen these risks. Thirdly, we will consider some ways of easing the problem of decision-making and the passing over of control, by better communication, group discussion and advocacy.

Types of decision

Two main areas of decision-making are important in relation to dementia. The first concerns the *financial affairs* of the patient, including the making of a will; the second concerns the *acceptance of care* by the patient in her home or in an institution, including the acceptance of medical treatment, and the related activity of taking part in medical research.

The distinction between problems of finance and problems of care is worth making because there is a separate set of laws relating to each category, though there are many overlaps in practice. Financial decisions range from the decision about who should collect the pension to major transactions such as the selling of property and the handling of large investments. *Making a will* is a particular decision which requires the maker to be fully 'capable' of appreciating what she is doing. There are risks in dementia of financial neglect by the patient, of mismanagement and of undue pressure from others. Physical risks, requiring decisions about care, include those of self-neglect, dangers in the house, maltreatment by carers and neglect of medical care. Disagreements often arise between the patient, her family and the professions about what help if any is needed to lessen these risks. Physical risks can sometimes be matters of life and death. Decisions must be arrived at somehow.

Of course decision-making is of more general importance. It affects every aspect of a patient's life – what she should eat, what she should wear, how to spend time and with whom, who does what in the house. While our discussions will centre on the major decisions, the day-by-day problems involved in making these minor decisions must not be underestimated.

Normal decision-making

Normally an adult expects to be in charge of her own affairs – her finances, where and with whom she lives, how and when she seeks help and advice from others. In practice, of course, no one makes decisions in a vacuum. Even if we *feel* independent, we are subject to all sorts of pressures from others and from within ourselves. How we decide on a particular issue will reflect our own experience, upbringing and attitudes. It will also be influenced by pressure from our family, friends and society at large, as well as by what the law says. Furthermore, some courses of action that we would like to take may not be available to us, and some forms of help not on offer.

Contracts

Nevertheless, most of us feel that we are at least *able to participate* in decision-making, that we *consent* to what is done for us or in our name, and that we could say 'no' if we wanted to. We are able to enter into agreements or *contracts* with other people, though most of these contracts are implicit rather than explicit.

If a dementia sufferer needs a home help in order to survive from day to day then a decision is required. This involves an agreement between the patient and the home care organizer that the helper should come into the home, and the patient's agreement to pay for the service. In other words, a care contract and a financial contract are made. Likewise, if medical treatment is required, a 'contract' is assumed between doctor and patient (though not actually signed unless an anesthetic is required). In this 'treatment contract' the patient, having told the doctor the problem and having been examined, is offered treatment and judges that she is prepared to accept that treatment. In going into residential care both a decision to move into care and a financial decision to pay need to be made and agreed between the prospective resident and the home.

Even in the absence of dementia the theory and practice of decision-making and contracts can be far apart. Agreements may be reached or contracts signed under pressure. The person who makes the contract may not realize the full consequences of a particular choice. Dementia sufferers are in special difficulty in making any of these important decisions and contracts.

DECISION-MAKING IN DEMENTIA

Reduced to its simplest the process of decision-making for any individual should involve the following steps:

1. Awareness that there is a problem to be solved
2. Understanding of the nature and extent of the problem
3. Consideration of possible solutions, understanding what they are and foreseeing the consequences of choosing each and of failing to choose
4. Free and informed choice of a particular solution
5. A 'contract' with whoever else is involved
6. Compliance with the implications of that contract.

In all these areas the dementing person is at a disadvantage. This disadvantage is usually said to be due to lack of *insight*, and certainly insight is important, but other changes of dementia are also involved.

Insight

We have seen earlier (p. 210) how complex a process insight is. It is the ability to appreciate that one is ill and to be aware of how severe that illness is. Loss of insight will clearly affect the first two steps in decision-making. A lady who does not think that she is ill will see no need for major changes or decisions and if she underestimates the extent of her impairment she will wonder why people are fussing so much. We have seen how denial can complicate insight and make it difficult for us to assess how much the patient really understands her position.

Understanding risks

As well as appreciating that she is ill, it is also important that the patient appreciates the risks that the illness causes. To understand a risk from leaving gas taps on or letting bogus workmen in she must be able to *perceive* the risky situation, grasp its *significance* and *remember* it. All these abilities are likely to decline in dementia, and many patients seem blissfully unaware of the dangers as they sit in a gas-filled house, fail to appreciate the risks of having a stranger in the house or, if they have understood, quickly forget the risks in these situations and refuse to discuss the problem.

Insight and understanding

Insight into illness and understanding of the risks are both important. Some patients preserve one ability but not the other. Thus many sufferers admit to failing memory but cannot see that this means that they will need outside help. They seem unaware of the evidence of neglected house, poor self-care, unpaid bills, and so, despite the evidence that *we* see, they claim to be managing well. It is possibly more startling if the patient seems fully aware of the mess yet *still* claims to be managing.

Three other deficits help to explain these situations. First, there is the loss of ability to make the *connections* between different areas of the brain that are required to think rationally. Secondly, because of frontal lobe damage, the ability to compare reality with a standard is impaired. The patient has a decline in *judgement* and *conscience*. Thirdly, the decline in *emotions* brings apathy. Even if she knows that her memory is failing badly, understands the risky situation that she is in, connects these rationally and judges the situation, she may simply not feel much about it and so ignore the risks.

Other losses

Even if insight and understanding are good, attempting the rest of the steps in the decision-making process highlights other deficits. If she suffers from *dysphasia* she may have difficulty understanding what others are saying about her problems and possible solutions, difficulty in expressing her own conclusions, or both. Her ability to formulate plans and solutions will be limited by deficits in thinking and particularly in *abstract thinking* – moving from the particular to the general becomes difficult. Indeed, she is likely to avoid working with concepts and generalizations altogether and think and talk at a *'concrete'* level, or in old, fixed ways. Thus she may be able to understand that she is not cooking safely and needs help, but be unable to generalize to the idea of having a home help, or to see the other consequences in terms of her general need for care. Indeed, she may be at the same time declaring repetitively the old platitude about 'not going into a home'. The bewildered professional who has come to assess the situation is left not knowing whether she wishes help or not. Discussion is also likely to be hampered by the problems of *attention* described in Chapter 5. She cannot focus on the decision in hand, the discussion rambles off the point continually and decisions are never reached.

Coming to a decision depends not only on insight, understanding and the ability to think, discuss and decide but it also requires *motivation*. The apathy already mentioned makes patients less inclined to bother about decisions. And, of course, difficulties with memory can sabotage any attempt at her later *compliance* with an agreement that we think she has come to. For even if we can hold her attention long enough to go through the groundwork and come to a rational decision, the whole process is dubious if she then quickly forgets and disclaims all knowledge of the discussion two minutes later.

Finally, the patient's ability to *understand things that are written down* or her ability to *write* may be impaired, so documents which we want to use as the basis of a contract and which we could come back to if she forgets the discussion may not be usable at all.

Personality change and personal reactions

For all these reasons sensible decision-making is impaired by the losses of dementia. It is also interfered with by any personality changes that occur and by the sufferer's reactions to the illness and to her situation. A decision based on delusional ideas or disturbed emotions caused by *disinhibition* must be questioned. Many patients, aware to some extent of their dementia, become more *cautious* than they were before, because they see the danger of making silly mistakes, or of being exploited. So they avoid decisions altogether and neglect their needs. Fear of making the wrong decision may lead them to hand over far too easily to others, thus actually making themselves more vulnerable to outside pressure. The opposite occurs sometimes in patients who have previously prided themselves in their *independence* (p. 203). If they retain that personality trait but lose insight, they may be adamant that they will make their own decisions for themselves, but reach completely misguided conclusions. Furthermore, they will resent any attempt by other people to make decisions for them, especially if there seems to be a threat that they would thereby become more dependent. These patients are the most difficult of all. They live on in risky situations, insisting that they have always coped, so they can cope now. They refuse all offers of help, sometimes very aggressively.

Assessing decision-making

How, then, are we to judge a dementing patient's ability to decide for herself? Assessing her 'mental capacity' – whether she is aware of her illness, whether she understands the risks it has led to and whether she can manage the steps to make a valid contract – is inevitably a complex and imprecise task. We not only need to look at the reality of the situation, what risks there are, what help 'should' be provided, we also need to know the patient's personality and her previous attitudes to outside help, and we need to know her present deficits and how much she has changed. From these we can guess what she *would* have decided if she were not ill (called 'substitute judgement'). We also need to keep in mind both the ordinary cautiousness and rigidity of old age and changes in her attitudes which are more to do with her circumstances than with her dementia. She may, for example, have good reason to mistrust her family, she may not have anyone to confide in, or she may have particular habits acquired over years of solitary living – all these affect how she will approach big decisions.

Taking over

So difficult is it to evaluate the complex process of decision-making that it is tempting to assume that from the beginning of dementia the patient cannot decide anything for herself at all. The family therefore make decisions behind her back 'in her best interests'. Care is arranged for her without discussion. Choices are not put to her. Her views are ignored. This approach is made even more tempting if she does not seem to object. The general lack of interest of the public in dementia and its problems means that there is little pressure to do otherwise.

Why not take over? There are three objections to taking over from the patient in this way. Firstly, insight and all the other functions we have discussed are *declining*, not lost. At late stages they are as good as lost, and the non-communicative, emotionally bland, severely demented lady may be difficult to engage in any sort of real contract. But at all earlier stages the losses are partial and she retains some ability to grasp, reason, draw conclusions, discuss and agree or disagree. Secondly, if she has some remaining abilities she has the same *right* to be involved in managing her affairs as anybody else and to object to others taking over from her unnecessarily. And, of course, some patients actually do object and say so. Thirdly, there are many decisions which, in order to be *legal*, require her agreement or signature, for example, many financial transactions, the making of a will, admission to a residential home, receiving an anesthetic and taking part in medical research.

Handing over

So, at the early stages of dementia, the patient should be actively involved in decision-making, either making all her own decisions or being able to agree or disagree sensibly with the decisions of others. At the end she will generally be unable to be involved. The process of handing over decisions to others would ideally be gradual, and ideally she would be involved in the decision to hand over. In practice there are six possible cases:

1. The patient has as good an understanding of the issues as she would have had before the dementia began and she retains her normal ability to judge and reason. She decides to hand over her affairs to someone else to allow them to make decisions for her.
2. She has good understanding, etc. but decides not to hand over.
3. She has good understanding, etc., but cannot communicate her views.
4. She has significantly impaired understanding, etc., and decides to hand over.
5. She has impaired understanding, etc., and decides not to hand over.
6. She has impaired understanding, etc., and cannot communicate adequately.

The possibilities are multiplied when we consider also how changeable or indecisive some individuals are, how families and professionals exert different degrees of pressure and influence, and how mental abilities in some forms of dementia may fluctuate.

Difficulties

Only case 1 actually represents a proper contract. In case 2 we ought to accept the patient's wishes, though this is not always done. Cases 1 and 2 will be common in early stages of the dementia. In cases 3 and 6, we have no idea what her wishes are. Too often her lack of communication is taken to mean agreement. We make decisions that are guided by guesswork, her previous wishes or what suits others. Compulsory powers, which should at least be considered, rarely are. In case 4 agreement is usually, quite wrongly, taken at face value. So it is only in case 5 (and occasionally, but wrongly, in case 2) that the possibility of a *compulsory* take-over is even considered, and often it is dismissed. The result is that there is very little formal discussion of decision-making. Many dementing people who would still be able to make quite rational decisions are deprived of that basic right without any formal process of law. And remarkably few dementing people who are unable to make their own decisions have proper legal protection.

RISKS

Discussions about whether the patient can decide for herself or whether others must decide for her usually concern situations of risk. Before discussing the practical aspects of decision-making, we will therefore examine these risks. There is a wide variety of risky situations that dementing people can get into. In each situation, the decision that must be made is whether, a. to leave her in charge and accept the risk, b. to persuade her to accept help to lessen the risk, or c. to take control out of her hands by compulsory means. What is actually done will depend on the degree of risk involved, which of the six categories the patient is in, the feelings of everybody else involved in the situation and the compulsory powers available. As emphasized in Chapter 3, availability of help may actually be more important than any of these in deciding what is done. If a lady needs a hospital bed, and does not want it, but it is not available anyway, then she will stay at home whether we like it or not. We should not use this reality as an excuse for not carrying out an assessment of the situation.

FINANCIAL RISKS

The dementing person is likely to *neglect* to collect her pension or neglect to pay bills for gas, electricity, rent, insurance policies, taxes, etc. She may *miscalculate* how much money she has in the house. She may make mistakes in shops. Simple *memory impairment* and loss of the ability to calculate (*dyscalculia*) are not the only problems, however. If memory impairment is linked with some *loss of judgement* the patient may withdraw money repeatedly from the bank, pay the same bills again and again, or hand out large sums of money to others. Loss of concern and carefulness, together with *poor understanding* of the value of money and possessions, leave the patient open to *exploitation* by bogus workmen who charge excessively or by bogus salesmen who offer tiny sums for valuable furniture or clothes. Relatives or 'friends' may also exploit her by getting her to sign cheques for them, give them money, change her will in their favour or sell her house, when she has little idea of what she is doing. *Hoarding* of large sums of money and *miserliness* over bills are common. These habits probably arise early in dementia when the patient realizes that something is wrong and wants to protect herself against making mistakes or being exploited (compare p. 168). Memory impairment and *paranoid thinking* can lead to mistaken ideas that the home help, the family or others are stealing from her. Telling the difference between real and imaginary stealing is often very difficult indeed and such situations need to be handled very sensitively.

The risks of neglect, mismanagement and exploitation are obvious. In some ways richer people are more at risk, for they have more complicated financial affairs and are more tempting targets for exploitation. But people with little money run exactly the same types of risk. They deserve just as much protection.

Reducing financial risks

How can the patient or others take decisions which will reduce these risks and ensure the protection and proper management of her financial affairs and property?

Informal arrangements

Anybody who cannot get to the post office herself can sign over the right to collect her pension to a relative or friend. She should of course be able to understand that this is happening. If she is unable to arrange to pay her bills, perhaps because she can no longer manage to sign cheques, the bank manager may be prepared to arrange informally for their payment if a relative sends them in. Standing orders or direct debit arrangements allow regular payments to continue. For couples, joint accounts can usually overcome many potential problems. But informal arrangements to hand over to others (called *mandates*) are sometimes dangerous. Unscrupulous relatives or friends can apply undue pressure or manipulate the arrangement for their own ends.

Department of Social Security (DSS) appointeeship

If a person is incapable of collecting and managing her benefits the DSS can appoint a relative or friend to take these tasks over. Appointeeship only covers DSS benefits. There are no systems to check that the appointee is acting in the interests of the incapable person.

Institutional arrangements

The staff of a residential home can help manage the day-to-day financial affairs of residents and have a duty to ensure that they have a certain amount of 'pocket-money' each week. In hospital, pension books can be taken over and the patient's finances can be run by the hospital management. Continuity of family relationships (p. 257) can often be maintained better, however, if relatives are allowed to go on managing the finances of the patient after admission to care, though they may need to be reminded of the regular clothing and comfort needs of a long-stay resident and the need for regular pocket-money.

Most of these arrangements assume at least the passive consent of the patient. It is assumed that she cannot manage her own affairs but can *instruct* others in their management (category 1 on p. 278). Theoretically, she has instructed the family or the institution to manage her affairs for her.

Power of attorney

This same theory applies to power of attorney, invented originally to cover temporary physical illness, where the person was unable to conduct her financial business and needed someone to stand in for her. She could make the other person her 'attorney' with full or limited powers over her financial affairs by signing a legal document to this effect. When well again she would take back control.

Validity. In order to sign a valid contract the patient clearly has to be able to understand what she is doing, what her 'affairs' consist of and who she is granting them to; and she must *continue to understand* if she is to be able to revoke it. As a general rule, therefore, people who are dementing would be unable to sign power of attorney. But many have done so and the vast majority of these arrangements have worked well and have not been challenged. But they are open to challenge as the patient becomes more and more mentally impaired. Families and solicitors are wise to ask the doctor about the person's mental capacity before proposing to someone with dementia that she sign over financial control to them.

Enduring powers. This problem has now been overcome to a considerable extent by the development of 'enduring' powers of attorney. A patient, *as long as she is legally competent when she signs,* can grant power of attorney which lasts throughout her dementia, even after she can no longer understand her affairs. But the dangers of exploitation could be even greater in this type of arrangement, so it is most important that they are only signed by people who are entirely competent, that is before dementia begins to cloud judgement, and that each use of such powers is carefully and regularly scrutinized by the Court of Protection or similar bodies.

Compulsory powers

A patient who can neither manage her affairs nor instruct someone else to manage them is in danger of mismanaging her money herself and of exploitation by others. She needs protection. And if she is unwilling or unable to give her affairs over to someone else voluntarily this must be done compulsorily.

Court of Protection and Curator bonis. In England and Wales this is done by an application with medical evidence to the Court of Protection, a branch of the High Court. Normally the Court passes the power to a relative, accountant or lawyer who acts as 'Receiver' on behalf of the Court. Or the Court may manage the affairs itself. 'Visitors' from the Court visit Receivers on a regular basis to check that the patient's affairs are being managed correctly. In Scotland the Court, following an application and the medical evidence of two doctors, appoints a 'Curator bonis' who has to report annually to the Accountant of Court on their management of the patient's affairs.

In both cases, the main aims are the protection of the patient's estate intact, as well as providing for her needs. So Receivers and Curators are expected not to invest the patient's money in risky ventures or make major changes in its use. For example, selling her house because she no longer needs it is a major decision which requires special consideration.

Limitations. There are two main problems with these procedures. Firstly they are expensive. If the patient has capital of less than a certain amount (maybe £20 000) the costs of protection will eat gradually into her estate, defeating the purpose. Legal aid may be available to cover some but not necessarily all of the expenses. It is unfair if the less well off are thus excluded from proper financial protection.

The other problem is that the powers apply purely to financial decisions. It is therefore wrong if they are used to make a patient sell her house against her will in order to force her to enter residential care. Despite these drawbacks, protection of this sort is most important for people with dementia and, if anything, could be more widely used.

Making and changing wills

Since dementia leads to the death of the sufferer, it is important that she has made her will. If she has done so before the dementia began, and if there are no big changes in her circumstances during the illness, there is no problem.

Problems arise in two ways. First, if no will exists the patient may, during the course of dementia, herself decide to make a will or she may want to change a previous will. Secondly, the solicitor, family or friends may suggest the need for a will or the need to change her existing will. Is she able to make the judgements required to make or change her will? Is she vulnerable to pressure and suggestions because of her dementia? Unfortunately, these questions are sometimes only asked after the patient's death. Then the will can be contested on the grounds that she did not have 'testamentary capacity', that is, she made or altered a will while legally incapable of doing so.

To make a legally binding will, one must know roughly the size and nature of the estate and who are the possible beneficiaries. One must also be able to make judgements for oneself, not be abnormally suggestible, and one must be free from undue pressure. Testamentary capacity may be lost relatively early in dementia, at a time when other types of decision can still be left entirely up to the sufferer. As a general rule it is better to dissuade dementing people from making or changing wills and to question any attempt to do so. To some extent it is a solicitor's task to know whether his clients are capable enough, but where there is any doubt an examination of the patient's mental state by a psychiatrist and an opinion on her capacity should be recorded. Later disputes can thus be lessened.

The worst problems arise when an old lady has already got into the habit of will-changing or has been open to a number of pressures from a warring family. Solicitors and professional carers must protect anyone whose judgement is impaired from undue pressure from others and from their own dithering.

PHYSICAL RISKS

The many different impairments of dementia and the decline in personal standards mean that many patients are at risk of self-neglect and forgetfulness. Malnutrition, unnoticed constipation, poor mobility, untreated incontinence, undeclared physical illness are all common results of self-neglect. Forgetfulness around the house brings particular risks – leaving the gas on unlit, forgetting to turn electric appliances off, leaving water running, leaving the door open. Forgetfulness, together with loss of self-concern and loss of the ability or motivation to react or complain put the patient at risk from muggers, intruders in the house, family violence and occasionally from sexual abuse. Family violence may be provoked by the patient's changed behaviour and, as with violence to children, or indeed all domestic violence, is often concealed. As well as mugging, other risks can occur outside the house. Wandering can put patients at risk, especially, of course, in winter or at night. Road sense may be lost. Or a dementing person may still be driving her car with considerable impairments in reaction time, spatial sense, memory and judgement (p. 290).

Such risks are not confined to the patient living at home. An institution where standards of care or staff morale are low may put its residents at risk of neglect or even of physical abuse.

Reducing physical risk

Consent by the patient

Many patients accept that they need extra help as their dementia progresses or do not object to others taking decisions about care or treatment for them. They are in categories 1, 3, 4 or 6 of the list on p. 278. Such patients will likely (if they are able) say they agree to the decisions made, or will sign contracts which accept care or supervision in the home, day care or residential care or for medical treatment. There are possible dangers of coercion and of false contracts being made, but if the patient goes along with what is decided without protest there is little likelihood of any challenge. The result is that much care and treatment is given 'in good faith'.

It is possible to defend much that is done in this way even when consent has not been given by the patient. Relatives who arrange, without asking the patient, for the gas mains to be turned off when the home help is not present, relatives who lock the front door at night to prevent wandering, relatives who bring patients to day care by telling white lies, and hospital wards or homes which have locked doors or complicated devices to prevent aimless wanderers wandering are all in somewhat the same position legally. They may be restricting the rights of a patient without her consent. But they can claim that they do these things in her best interest. And few will complain as long as the restrictions are not excessive, they are carried out in a kindly way and are not resisted by the patient.

The *common law* (that is, law not based on Act of Parliament – which is called statute law – but based on cases and judgements both past and recent) gives some protection to people in these situations. Even quite intrusive or restrictive actions may be seen as legal, as long as there are very clear advantages to the patient's welfare and safety. Indeed the opposite also holds true. Professionals who are looking after vulnerable patients may be seen as negligent if they do not provide sufficient protection for their charges.

Consent by others

Legally speaking, consent cannot be given by anyone other than the person herself, except in the case of a child or a person who has a legal guardian of some kind or where a court has made decisions for the patient. The agreement of a relative or someone in charge of a patient's care may, however, be helpful to those who feel they must act without the patient's consent in her best interests. It may be used, for example, when a patient needs a surgical operation which requires consent for an anesthetic. It may be used when alterations have to be made to a house to improve safety. Perhaps wrongly, many admissions to hospital, be it to general, geriatric or old-age psychiatry wards, are of this general kind, where the decision is not really made by the patient but by doctors with the agreement of relatives acting informally on her behalf. But we should not be complacent about doing things to other people in their best interest. We may be well-meaning, but we may not always be acting in the patient's true best interest. The 'rightness' of each situation must be considered individually. And the law gives no protection to anybody, relative or otherwise, who makes a harmful decision which is clearly against the patient's best interest.

The patient who refuses help or treatment

If risks are present and the patient is in categories 2 or 5, that is, she is refusing help, then compulsory powers may be considered. But these should really only apply in category 5, for in category 2 the patient, who seems to understand the situation, has decided to refuse offers of help and this decision is entirely up to her, even if we think it unwise. This particularly applies to medical decisions, when a patient may see that she has not long to live, knows that her mental powers are failing and is really expressing a wish to die. She may then refuse treatment or care. But other possible reasons for a negative response should always be sought. Is the patient suffering from depression? Is her pessimism due to discomfort caused by physical illness? And we should also consider how the decision will affect others. If her decision means staying at home, does it put others at risk? Do relatives agree? Further, how major the treatment would be may be important. It may be reasonable to avoid very complex treatments which have some risk attached, while pressure may be put on the patient to accept simple treatments which would improve her comfort or quality of life considerably.

The wish to die. There are some patients who 'turn their faces to the wall', (see p. 224) but they deserve a full assessment of their situation before the decision is reached that this wish to die is rational. The position of a person who, *before her dementia began*, expressed a clear wish not to be treated for life-threatening conditions if she became demented is different (the written and witnessed form of this wish has been called an 'advance directive' or less appropriately, a 'living will'). Some assessment needs to be made of whether we would expect her still to feel the same way now that she is suffering from dementia. If it is thought that she would, then her wishes must be taken into consideration as an important factor (thought not the only one) in deciding whether to treat or not.

Positive euthanasia is not a possible option in dementia, even if a sufferer wanted to plan it for themselves. For by the time the option would be taken up they would be no longer able to give consent, so effectively it would be another's decision. It would be very dangerous if society gave the power to decide about euthanasia for this helpless and vulnerable group to doctors, or even to doctors supported by other advisors and relatives.

Those who express the view that dementia sufferers should be 'put down' are usually expressing their own impatience with 'caring' or a distaste of people who are dependent. They misunderstand the subjective experience of dementia for the sufferer.

But the *decision not to treat* (sometimes called 'negative euthanasia') is often taken by doctors and nurses. For a patient who is severely demented and unable to express a wish (category 6) it can be reasonable and humane to consider that a chest infection or the like is evidence of the body's failing ability to survive. It may then be decided, but only after consulting all concerned in the patient's care and the relatives, that treatment would not enhance the quality of her life and would needlessly prolong suffering in a terminal illness. There should be no general rules about this in a ward or a home. A decision should be made, after consultation, about each patient as an individual.

Compulsory medical treatment

If the patient is at home and neglecting herself badly, the compulsory power in Section 47 of the National Assistance Act may apply. This allows a person who is infirm (which could mean either physically or mentally), living in 'insanitary conditions' and refusing all necessary treatment or care to be removed to a suitable place for a limited period. This power could occasionally apply to dementia but is very rarely used. Apart from this, medical treatment of a dementia sufferer when she has refused or is unable to give consent, has to be based on a common law duty to save life and to protect people from unnecessary injury or danger, and on the informal but not legally binding agreement given by relatives. Where the patient's treatment is very major, irreversible, risky or disputed, decisions may have to be taken by a court (in Scotland a *tutor dative* may be appointed by the court to give consent for the patient).

All other treatment given without proper consent is given 'in good faith'. Where this is done team decisions are always better than individual decisions, and it is very important that all 'good faith' decisions are recorded, for they usurp the patient's right to decide for herself. This way, if things go wrong, the motives and reasons for whatever treatment was given (or not given) are not hidden.

Compulsory psychiatric treatment

The laws about psychiatric treatment are much clearer. If a patient suffers from a 'mental illness' (which can include dementia) *and* there is concern about her health or safety, or about the health and safety of others due to that illness, *and* if she requires or would benefit from psychiatric treatment in hospital (which can include psychiatric nursing care) *and* she refuses this treatment, then certain compulsory powers can be used. These are laid down in Sections 2, 3, 4 and 5 of the Mental Health Act (Sections 18, Act (Sections 18, 24 and 26 in Scotland), which cover admission for observation or assessment and detention for short-term and longer-term treatment. Planned admission follows an application to the courts by a relative or a specialist social worker (called an approved social worker in England and Wales and a mental health officer in Scotland) supported by two medical recommendations. The emergency or short-term orders require fewer formalities but must be reviewed very quickly. If necessary, an application can then be made for a longer-term order.

Safeguards. The powers in the Mental Health Act are great. But they are surrounded by a complicated system of reviews and appeals and by the general supervision of an independent body called the Mental Health Act Commission (Mental Welfare Commission in Scotland). These powers take away some of the rights of the patient to independence, but at the same time protect her right to proper care and attention.

Limited use. In practice, although these powers are often considered for dementing patients, they are rarely used. Although many dementia sufferers are at risk because of their dementia and refuse help, often the care they need is not psychiatric treatment or nursing; it is a more general form of care which does not quite seem to justify the very wide and formal powers of the Mental Health Act. This attitude may be mistaken, for the alternative is that decisions are often made behind the patient's back, subterfuges used to get her into care, or else that the risky situation at home is allowed to continue.

Another argument against using the Mental Health Act is that many patients who protest about being asked to go to hospital settle remarkably well once they are through the door of the hospital. However, while this has been used as a reason for not bothering to use compulsory powers, it can also be used as an argument for their brief use to get the patient out of the risky situation into a safer hospital situation.

Guardianship

The 'admission' sections of the Mental Health Act cannot properly be used to ensure treatment of medical conditions unless they are the direct cause of the dementia. Nor can they be used to ensure proper supervisory care at home or to admit someone into a residential home or an ordinary nursing home. However, in Sections 7 and 8 (Section 37 in Scotland) the power of 'Guardianship' is described. This can be of use in organizing proper general care for the patient. The procedure is similar to that for Section 3 (Section 18) but in this case the court, instead of arranging admission, arranges for the appointment of a 'Guardian'. This can be anybody who is deemed suitable to act in this way, but is often a social worker.

Powers of the Guardian. The Guardian has powers to insist that the patient allows entry to professionals who are giving or supervising her care and treatment. The Guardian also has the power to insist that she lives in a particular place. This power has, therefore, sometimes been used to arrange admission into residential homes. It should, however, only be used in this way after all other avenues have been considered and in practice it is much more often thought of than actually applied for. Its effectiveness depends on cooperation between the relatives, the Guardian and the services which are trying to provide help for the patient. It also depends on the patient being persuaded by the Guardian to go along with what is required. If she does not understand who the Guardian is or what their legal powers are she may refuse the help just as effectively as she did before she had a Guardian, making the procedure powerless. For a few patients Guardianship is lifesaving, or can prevent them having to go into care prematurely.

Non-accidental injury and other abuse

There is at present no law in most parts of the world that gives protection to people who are the victims of 'granny bashing', except the criminal law. Families and professionals are reluctant to call in the police, even when quite serious injury is occurring, and the police are sometimes reluctant to act, especially if the abuser is also elderly. The development of appropriate adult schemes and improved training for the police are helping change attitudes slowly.

Dementia sufferers are particularly at risk of abuse, for their care can be extremely stressful, their behaviour may be irritating to their carers and carer and patient may be stuck together in the house for long periods. Whenever bruising or falls seem to be happening repeatedly the possibility of abuse should be considered, though only with great caution, since there are so many different reasons why an elderly person with dementia could injure herself. Other forms of abuse such as regular verbal insults and rows, neglect of physical care, deprivation or over-use of medicines, confinement in a small room, confinement in a chair or sexual abuse can all occur in dementia.

Proper multi-agency procedures need to be developed, but in their absence the model of child abuse registers and case conference procedures should be followed. In extreme cases the patient may need to be removed, and the Mental Health Act can be used, since the patient is at risk if she has been maltreated because of her illness. But in many cases helpful services, such as day care, sitting services or respite care, and providing someone to both oversee the situation and help the relative 'blow off steam', will avoid problems.

Abuse does not only occur at the hands of close relatives and carers. Dementia sufferers may suffer at the hands of intolerant neighbours, bogus workmen, muggers, abusive children and many others. And they may be abused by the staff who are supposed to be caring for them, especially if the staff are not properly trained, do not know enough about the patient as a person and are not well supervised.

Nor should we forget the other side of abuse; that carers are sometimes abused by sufferers who are disinhibited or paranoid. Such abuse may be played down by loyal relatives desperate to continue coping and anxious to avoid overmedication. But it can be just as serious and systematic as abuse by a cruel carer.

Driving and dementia

A common problem which can arise is when someone who is a car driver develops dementia. The sufferer may be unaware of any difficulty, and may resent any advice to stop. All licence holders have a responsibility to inform the licensing authority (DVLA) if they develop a condition which may affect their fitness to drive, but where there is significant impairment of reasoning, the driver may not understand the obligation to do this.

The number of older drivers is increasing rapidly; between 1965 and 1985 the number of older male drivers increased three-fold, and the number of older female drivers seven-fold. Thus the number of drivers with dementia is increasing accordingly. Often a man is the only driver in a household, and the car has become necessary for shopping and to maintain social contacts, so loss of driving ability can isolate a spouse as well as the driver.

There are no clear guidelines on when someone's driving becomes impaired, or at what stage dementia should be reported to the DVLA. Recommendations are given in Box 9.1.

Where someone's driving is becoming a danger, relatives or friends should make a notification to the DVLA on her behalf. The DVLA will then be able to make further enquiries, and if necessary revoke her licence. It is doing no favour to allow a driver to 'remain on the road' where she has become a danger to herself, to other passengers and to other road users. This situation is also one where a doctor may have to breach confidentiality about a patient; he may decide to inform the DVLA himself.

Research

Another increasingly important issue is that of research. Some research does not require the patient's consent and there is little problem. But much research into the causes and treatments of

---

Box 9.1   Adapted from Medical Aspects of Fitness to Drive.

Dementia – Organic Brain Disorders, e.g. Alzheimer's disease et alia *NB*: There is no single marker to determine fitness to drive, but it is likely that driving may be permitted if there is retention of ability to cope with the general day-to-day needs of living, together with adequate levels of insight and judgement.

In early dementia, driving may be permitted if there is no significant disorientation in time and space, and there is adequate retention of insight and judgement. Annual medical review required. Licence likely to be recommended to be refused or revoked if disorientated in time and space, and especially if insight has been lost or judgement is impaired.

dementia involves some degree of intrusion into the life of the sufferer and therefore requires her consent. The intrusion can be as little as asking her a few not very personal questions, or may be very great, as when injections are given, potentially dangerous drugs are administered or scanning with radioactive substances is used. Some research can claim to be potentially therapeutic for the individual who is taking part, some is not at all therapeutic and some can be said to have benefits for sufferers in general but not necessarily for this individual. And not all research is medical. Nursing, psychological, occupational and other assessments and therapies all need to be properly tested, and proper consent is required before that testing can begin.

At early stages of dementia consent may be quite easily and properly obtained from the patient. But how can a severely demented lady give consent to receiving a hazardous drug for research purposes when she has no understanding of what is being asked of her? She cannot. Yet, if we are to improve our treatments and eventually find cures for dementia, research must proceed. Can relatives give consent for research? The answer is that they are often asked to, and it would be very unwise to proceed to do intrusive research on a dementia sufferer without the relative's knowledge and agreement but, in common law, such consent has no real legal standing during the patient's life.

At present there is no clear way out of this dilemma. Some form of representative or independent body, as suggested on p. 302, is needed to act in the patient's interest, as her advocate. This would not only protect her rights in a very vulnerable situation but also protect the position of the researchers, who need to get on with necessary work but must not put themselves, or be put into a position where they could be accused of 'assaulting' patients without their consent.

THE PRACTICE OF DECISION-MAKING

We have now seen a number of circumstances where decisions must be or may be taken away from a dementing person. On the other hand we have seen that most patients retain, for a time, their ability to make reasoned and reasonable decisions. Between these two extremes there are considerable difficulties.

For financial decisions, power of attorney often bridges the gap and enduring power of attorney can be continued beyond the stage of incompetence in decision-making. But, of course, not everybody has arranged this. For other decisions, either the patient is theoretically in charge or else she is incapable, in which case the decision ought to be taken away from her by legal means. The gap is in practice filled by the goodwill and good judgement of those around the patient. They make up for her loss of reason and judgement just as memory aids fill the gaps in her memory.

This may look good on paper but there are many occasions when it is unsatisfactory. What if it means that unscrupulous relatives are making decisions against the patient's interest behind her back? What if the patient sees things differently from relatives or staff and wishes to argue? What if there are no relatives of goodwill around? What if the relatives disagree with each other or if professionals and relatives disagree? Who is to judge what is right? Who is to make sure that the patient's interests are protected? Who is to ensure that decisions that need to be made are made?

On the other hand, it should surely be unnecessary to go to the extent of taking legal powers over the majority of day-to-day decisions. It should usually be possible to trust husbands or wives, children and professionals to act in the patient's best interest on most occasions. What follows applies mainly to those cases and points of decision where there is doubt or disagreement.

Communication

Making decisions for the patient

A relative who judges on his own how much a patient can decide and then either makes decisions for her or leaves her to look after her own decisions can be vulnerable on either count. At the one extreme he may be accused of usurping the rights of the patient. At the other he may be accused of putting her at risk by neglect. The same vulnerability applies to a professional who makes judgements about the patient's ability to decide things.

As far as possible we would like to leave decisions to the patient, even if this means taking some risks. But where do we draw the line? Some staff choose to be very protective and 'look after' their charges, avoiding risks where possible. But this can mean restraining their activities, and in the USA, for example, led in the recent past to many a dementing patient spending her days confined to a chair and sometimes even tied into it. Others have gone to the other extreme and always want to allow the patient to decide for herself, even if she is putting herself at risk of wandering through an unlocked door onto a busy road or is neglecting herself in squalid conditions at home.

Relatives or staff 'get away' with any of these judgments for a variety of reasons. First, and most importantly, dementing patients do not usually complain about someone else deciding for them because they are losing the ability to perceive their situation and the ability to state clear opinions, or because they forget what has happened. Secondly, the goodwill of relatives or staff is very often assumed. Thirdly, and unfortunately, other relatives or professionals may be careless about the rights of the dementing and feel that it is not worth questioning decisions that are made.

Usually, therefore, difficulties only arise when there is a major disagreement between some of the parties concerned – the patient, relatives, staff. In fact we should *always* be aware of the problems that can arise if others make decisions on behalf of the patient, even if the person involved is a husband who appears to have his wife's best interests at heart, or a highly respected staff member, or even if the patient herself appears not to be complaining. The decisions we are talking about may have major implications for the health, welfare or safety of a human being who may be neglected, put at risk or exploited by those nearest to her.

Talking together

The simplest way to get around this problem is to communicate, both with the patient and with other people concerned. The basic question is 'Do you agree with my judgement?'. If all the people concerned are in agreement about something, then they can work together better and accusations of self-interest or dogma are much less likely. So, when we see that a decision has to be made, or is being made, either by the patient or by someone else on her behalf the best thing to do is to *discuss it*. But what if there is disagreement? Simply asking 'why are we disagreeing?' may resolve the issue, but if there are more fundamental or persistent disagreements a formal meeting of those involved, a *case conference*, is justified.

Case conferences

A case conference is advisable in three circumstances:

1. Where there are disagreements about the patient's care or about whether she is able to decide for herself
2. Where there is uncertainty or dispute about who should be responsible for different aspects of her care
3. Where a major decision has to be made about her future, because of a change of circumstances or increased risk, and she is not able to decide completely by herself.

Who attends?

A clear decision should be made beforehand about whether the patient herself should attend all or part of the meeting. Whatever happens, she should always be informed that it is happening and of any decisions made.

A case conference will be limited in its value if some important people are missing. It can be worth expending some effort to find all the people who regularly visit the patient or are closely involved with her, including not only the nearest relatives, home help, health visitor, GP, social worker and hospital staff but remembering also close friends, neighbours, more distant but important relatives, clergy and church visitors, voluntary workers and solicitors, if any of these are closely involved in her day-to-day life. Small decisions may justify only a small meeting, or contact by phone. But important decisions deserve the formal collaboration of all concerned.

That being said, the most important consideration about such a meeting, which will take a number of people from their work to spend a considerable time in discussion, is whether there is adequate reason for having it at all. Case conferences get a bad name if they are used for trivial decisions or are indecisive. Whoever calls such a conference should formulate clearly what has to be decided and why it needs the time of so many people. In these ways meetings can be shortened and made more effective.

The agenda

This should consist of:

1. Introductions and explanations of who is present and what the meeting is for and apologies for absence
2. Formulation of the problems, each participant getting a chance to present his/her views

3. Clear description of the options for action (or inaction) and their likely consequences
4. Decision-making
5. Summary by the chairman.

The chairman's role

It is the chairman's task to ensure that these five stages are gone through fully, kept separate from each other and limited in time. He has a special task in helping relatives and the patient (if she is involved) for they are often not used to speaking in a group and may feel embarrassed. Relatives are also likely to be more emotionally involved in the problems being discussed and need protection from feeling that they are being pressurized when vulnerable, or exposed to ridicule. They need to feel that their voices are being heard amid those of more sophisticated professionals. On the other hand, the outcome should balance the views of *all* parties concerned and no one should be allowed to 'bulldoze' others into a particular course of action by emotional pressure. Finally, the chairman should arrange for a clear account of the proceedings to be made, sending copies to all concerned, including the relatives, and even the patient, or at least communicating the decisions to her. It will be seen that such conferences will only work if the coordinator can be relatively unbiased and clear-thinking. Flexibility is also required, for in practice it may be necessary to move more freely between the different stages of the process as participants recall more of the experience or feelings or try to move on to decision-making too early.

The outcome

A number of types of decision can emerge from such conferences.

1. Often no change is made – nevertheless, there can be great benefit if the relatives feel that their concerns have been understood or shared by professionals and if there is a feeling of solidarity in allowing a somewhat risky situation to continue.

2. Lines of responsibility may be clarified, communications improved and limits set on how long the present arrangements should continue or in what circumstances further changes need

to be made – one way of ensuring a good outcome in this respect is the appointment of a 'key worker' (see also p. 267). This can be anyone who is in regular contact with the patient and who takes the responsibility of monitoring the situation – checking that services are provided and that supervisory care is maintained, continually assessing the risks of allowing the present situation to continue, looking for any change in that situation, if necessary contacting other people to review it and eventually recalling a case conference to renegotiate the decisions made.

3. A change in the level of support may be organized – this may involve relatives offering more time or it may mean that they are able to withdraw more. It may mean the start or increase of home help, sitting, nursing or medical supervision, day attendance or respite care. It may mean the supply of aids in the home or of incontinence services. Or it may mean major decisions about a move from home to residential care or hospital, or from institutional care to home.

4. If there is uncompromising disagreement between the patient and everybody else, with regard to financial matters or major decisions about care, then the conference may have to consider compulsory measures – usually the idea of compulsion can be considered and rejected. Relatives or others who feel that 'something must be done' see the consequences and limitations of compulsion and can consider alternatives. But when compulsion is necessary, then a conference decision gives confidence to those involved in carrying it into action and allows coordinated preparation if, say, a place in residential care or hospital is to be sought.

5. In most cases the important final decision is to *meet again*, either at a definite date to review continuing risks and see if the care plan is working, or at any time when the situation warrants it.

The value of conferences

Much of the purpose of the case conference is to smooth out disagreements. The worries of those who think that not enough is being done may be lessened if they see that the other participants are agreed on a particular course of action and most especially if arrangements are made to review the decisions of the conference at a later date, or to set limits on acceptable risks. The worries of those (including the patient) who may think that decisions are being made against her interests can be lessened by the open agreement of the participants that the action taken is necessary and that there will be safeguards and review. Often relatives have been unhappy about explaining their fears to the patient. Although it can be very upsetting, a clear statement of concern by an important person in the patient's world and the fact that she is being involved in the decision-making process can have great influence.

A case conference should never be used to pressurize a patient into a decision for the convenience of others. If disagreements persist, compromise and later review may be the only course open.

HEARING THE PATIENT'S VOICE

In all that has been said so far, the greatest danger is that the patient's voice will not be heard, or will be overridden in argument. In many cases the patient is not directly consulted at all. Who, then, is to speak up for her?

The patient herself

In early dementia it will in most cases be perfectly possible for the sufferer to state clearly what she wants to do. There is a danger that no one listens, particularly if she has difficulties in communication, and this can be very frustrating for her. Both relatives and staff need constant reminders that a dementia sufferer can express choice, can be involved in decisions and generally can be an active participant in her own life. They need to be reminded that participation can bring enormous satisfaction to someone who fears that her competence is failing. They need to be reminded that rational disagreement is perfectly possible.

Guessing the patient's view

In later stages, and if there are severe communication difficulties, it becomes difficult to perceive what view the patient is expressing. Often a look at her past decisions and preferences will show quite clearly what she would wish to happen now, a further example of how essential it is to know about her past life.

On the other hand, such judgment from past to present can be dangerous. We have seen the awful position of a daughter who has been forced to promise never to 'put me in home' (p. 261). We have also seen the difficulties posed by patients who in the past have asked to be allowed to die or even to be 'put to sleep' if they develop dementia (p. 286). We should always remember that no one can anticipate how they will feel in the future. In particular one can have little idea what the experience of dementia will be like. And the needs and wishes of those around the person are also important. So the present situation is the most important consideration, involving a balance between the needs and the present and past wishes of the patient, the needs and wishes of those around her and the judgement of professional services involved.

In severe dementia, it is almost impossible to guess at the patient's present wishes. If she has in the past formally stated her wishes in an *advance directive* we can be clearer about her attitudes and avoid guesswork. But even so it becomes more and more important that someone speaks wisely on her behalf.

Relatives

Relatives are in a special position with regard to a dementing person. They know what she was like before the illness and are therefore likely to understand the changes in her abilities and personality far better than professionals can, and often better than the sufferer herself. They also have greater or lesser degrees of loyalty to their ill relative. They may, therefore, feel with considerable justification that they can understand what the patient's interests require and can act on her behalf – as her *advocates*.

Conflicting interests

Their own interests, the disturbance to their lives and the stress of caring can, however, lead relatives into decisions which conflict with the needs of the patient. It is possible for relatives to imagine that they are acting on the patient's behalf when in fact they are pursuing their own ends. We should not exaggerate the importance of this but it needs to be noted for it can put relatives in a difficult position.

Conflicting relatives

Sometimes there is conflict between two sets of relatives, each claiming to act in the best interest of the patient. This type of conflict is likely to be greater when the stress on the relatives, or one particular member of the family, is very great, where some of the family have high expectations of health or social services or where the patient cannot express her own needs clearly. In these cases, professionals need to pay special attention to the separate needs of the patient herself and must emphasize to the relatives that the correct course of action is likely to be a compromise.

Relatives as advocates

It would be wrong, however, to dismiss the role of relatives as advocates. In reality, they constantly act in this way. It is they who usually bring the patient to medical attention, who ask for services, who complain when things go wrong, who assess changes in the situation, who demand action when the patient is at risk. The existence of Alzheimer's societies, many initiatives for day, sitting or other care services and much general political pressure depend entirely on the advocacy of relatives who care about obtaining proper respect and care for dementia sufferers. Advocacy from outside need only be considered when advocacy by a relative is absent because there is no one available, when the relatives appear to have negative views of the patient, where they do not understand her condition, or when the relatives disagree among themselves.

Professionals

Most people who work with older people are committed to this work. Their interest and expertise tell them where help is needed, where improvements could be made, where abuses are occurring. On behalf of dementia sufferers they are advocates within their professions and organizations. Most of the pressure to improve resources for dementia in the health and social services and the drive to improve standards of care comes from those who work day-to-day with dementia sufferers. This general advocacy will gradually lead to a greater concern for the rights and needs of individual patients, though at present the fact that the amount of resources rarely meets the size of the problem is a more pressing issue.

Professionals as advocates

On the individual level professionals and voluntary workers are often advocates for sufferers. They are advocates when they point out to relatives that the mildly demented person can still express her wishes and can be involved in decisions; when they encourage a 'personalized' approach to care, with choice, privacy and as normal an environment as possible; when they highlight the existence of problems and stimulate the necessary action; when, on the other hand, they resist rushing prematurely into 'doing something' in a crisis without due consideration. In all these cases a professional or volunteer can be seen to emphasize the importance of the sufferer's rights when she cannot do this herself and when there are other, opposing influences – the wishes of relatives, the tendency in institutions to have convenient but depersonalizing routine and the pessimism and lack of imagination that is 'ageism'.

Conflicting interests

The compulsory powers discussed above have similar aims – in financial matters ensuring the protection of the person's money, in Mental Health Act matters ensuring proper care and treatment on her behalf. In these formal cases, there are safeguards against abuse. But as with relatives, the professional or volunteer acting as informal advocate may have conflicting interests or attitudes, or be in conflict with his colleagues and others. Institutionalizing attitudes, laziness, impatience or lack of understanding can all interfere with impartial decisions about 'what a patient would like', 'what her best interests are', or 'what is good for her'.

Conflicting theories

Furthermore, theoretical stances can lead to conflict. An attitude which stresses the rights of the individual, though it is much-needed on behalf of dementia sufferers, can tempt one into playing down the wishes of relatives or the strain they are feeling. The same can be true of those who have a theoretical objection to institutional care. Those who campaign for burdened relatives are in danger of playing down the rights of the sufferer. Those whose loyalty is to their own institution may pay too little attention to the right of both patients and relatives. Steering an unbiased course through this minefield and still being decisive is difficult.

Advocates

Because of these difficulties many have been considering whether some form of outside advocacy system might be useful. We could hope that between relatives and professionals the true interests of the patients would be preserved, but sadly this is not always true. There are circumstances where there are particular dangers. First, there is the dementing lady living alone, in an increasingly risky situation, with worried neighbours and a not-too-close family. Secondly, there is the lady with few or no relatives, especially if she is in a large institution or in a private sector residential or nursing home. Thirdly, there are cases where the patient's voice may not be 'heard', for example the lady living with a family who may be neglecting or abusing her. In these situations the dementing patient is vulnerable to neglect, poor standards of care, physical abuse or exploitation and she is often unable to complain. If she *is* able to complain, her complaints may be ignored.

The following possibilities have been considered:

1. A type of 'Ombudsman' who would be available to look into complaints of neglect or maltreatment – someone would still, however, have to be prepared to initiate the complaint on the patient's behalf, unless the Ombudsman had a right to enter the patient's home and make enquiries about what was happening. The Mental Health Commission (or Mental Welfare Commission) has this sort of power in hospitals, particularly with regard to detained patients. Their powers need to be extended or duplicated for residential and nursing homes, and more widely in the community. Some nursing homes in the USA have access to an Ombudsman system.

2. An extension of the type of provision suggested in the Disabled Persons Bill to allow the appointment of

'representatives' to act on behalf of dementing patients who are unable to appoint someone themselves – such a representative would have to be in a position to assess the situation properly and to ensure that necessary help was provided. This idea begs the questions of who would appoint such representatives and how they would have any power.

3. An extension of Guardianship to allow Guardians to act in more varied ways on the patient's behalf – this would necessitate a much more widespread use of this compulsory power and might be seen by some as lessening the patient's right to decide, rather than protecting her.

4. Advocates could be made available on a voluntary 'lay' basis, perhaps through an Alzheimer's society – such advocates would need to know whether they were to act as befrienders, representatives to ensure that the patient's needs were assessed, agents for the patient who could make decisions or sign documents on her behalf (i.e. guardians), or all these. Whatever their role, there is the same difficulty of knowing how to appoint an advocate for the patient who sees no need for one, even though she is at great risk. Advocates would need to be experienced and well-trained and would need to know a lot about the patient's previous life and attitude, as well as her present state, before they could speak authoritatively for her. The relationship between the advocate and professionals who would be asked to provide for the patient's needs, or might be criticized, would have to be very clear. But if it was then such a system could work well.

CONCLUSION

None of these suggestions is a reality in the UK, though some of the ideas have been tried in other countries. Unless some change in this type of direction occurs, many dementing people will remain vulnerable to neglect, abuse and exploitation. We must continue in most cases to trust the goodwill of relatives and the wisdom of professionals. Thankfully, that goodwill and that wisdom do exist in most cases and in many places. When they are absent or when the patient is not heard, advocacy and proper legal protection are needed.

Assessment and management

We have discussed a wide variety of problems that relate to dementia; wide because the brain is a very complicated organ, and wide because people and families are of many different types, reacting in different ways to a dreadful illness. How are we to collect together all the facts about a particular patient and her situation in a way that is *concise, comprehensive* and *useful*? This is the job of assessment.

Assessment

The word 'assessment' has developed something of an aura around it. To some it has become the magic answer to difficult situations. But, to be worthwhile, every assessment should have a reason behind it – it should be *assessment for a purpose*. Some *action* should follow logically from it and that action should *benefit* the patient. It is, for example, useless to diagnose which type of dementia a patient has if making the diagnosis has no helpful consequences for her. We should question the use of expensive diagnostic tests if they lead to diagnosis but no treatment. In a similar way, knowing the severity of dementia may not be very important in deciding placement or management of the patient (p. 96). So we should always question the time and energy that is spent on assessment rather than on

Table 10.1 Diagnosis and assessment of dementia – an outline of the stages of diagnosis and the methods of assessment. A '+' shows which methods contribute to each stage of assessment

Stages	History from patient	History from relatives	Mental state	Physical state	Rating scales	Screening and special tests	ADL assessment
Baseline (before dementia began)	+	+					
Diagnosis of dementia	+	+	+		+	+	+
Cause of dementia	+	+	+	+		+	
Severity of dementia	+	+	+		+		+
Problem list	+	+	+	+	+		+
Cause of a particular problem	+	+	+	+			+
Problems not due to dementia	+	+	+	+		+	

doing things with the patient. In this chapter we will look at what is being assessed, and the various stages of assessment (Table 10.1). This leads on logically to a summary of *management techniques*.

What is being assessed

Assessment of dementia involves much more than looking at the sufferer. It involves making a diagnosis of dementia, trying to make some sort of statement about its severity, and about the effects it may have on the sufferer. It also involves looking at the problems caused by the various losses due to the illness. As we have seen, behaviour and personality changes can cause major problems. So too can changes to the ability to look after oneself, or *activities of daily living*.

We must look at the effect dementia has on others. This means the effect on carers, on neighbours, on fellow residents of a care setting, and on society in general. Availability and acceptability of help from family and voluntary or professional carers must be taken into account. Recent legislation gives carers, as well as the disabled person, a right to assessment.

There are many issues which we can call *environmental* which must form part of any assessment. We must look at the suitability of the current living placement, whether this be the person's own home, a nursing home, residential hospital or hospital care.

THE STAGES OF ASSESSMENT

Background information

The person's life before the illness

This is the *baseline* from which all other information is judged. We cannot say that someone is changing unless we know what they were like before. We cannot expect to rehabilitate a patient to a better level of function than she started with – whether in breadth of interests, activities, level of self-care or intellectual ability. Our standards should be set not by our own ideas of cleanliness, activity, sociability or intelligence but by the patient's previous standard. Thus, an untidy person is not dementing just because her house is untidy; there must be evidence of a definite and gradual decline. On the other hand, the evidence of a change is very obvious in someone who previously was very tidy and obsessional.

Background information continues to be relevant in other ways throughout the illness. For the less severely impaired the past is an anchor of reality that they can cling to. For both patients and families, past relationships and attitudes determine their present reactions. For the more severely impaired, fragments of past interests, attitudes, habits and relationships emerge from time to time. For families and professionals, the past is a constant reminder that this patient is a person with long experience behind her, not a child.

In order that staff can have a meaningful personal relationship with the dementing person, they need to have as much background information as possible. This allows them to be able to encourage reminiscence, remind her of her past interests and important relationships, and help her to share her past experiences with others.

The person's history

A large amount of information about the past can of course be obtained from the person herself. Older and more important memories may be maintained late in dementia, partly because they have been rehearsed so often over the years that they are very fixed, and partly because the person returns to these memories when the present and recent past are fading. She will be able to give us some idea about her childhood and early family relationships, together with some glimpses of her jobs, her marriage, her children. In the earliest stages she will be able to give quite a full account of her life up to recent times. But this information must always be checked, for memories become incomplete and time sequences muddled. The generations of the family may get mixed up in her mind and recent memories get put too far in the past, or vice versa. However, even these more or less muddled memories are very important in understanding how the patient reacts to her illness. For example, do resentments about the past sour her judgement of the present? Does pride in the past make her reluctant to accept her present dependence on others?

The relatives' history

We can obtain a great deal of information from relatives about a sufferer's previous personality, attitudes, level of activity, interests, social functioning and self-care. It is important to help the relatives separate recent events from events that happened before the dementia began (and since the beginning is vague that is a difficult task). Such information will provide clear evidence of how much change has occurred. And this helps us to understand what new problems the family is having to cope with and explains their reactions.

Background information gives the essential baseline in assessing what support the patient can expect from family and friends, what interests and activities she might continue to engage in and what her living conditions are. A simple *list of the family*, with an indication of how near they live, how often they visit and their commitment can be helpful. Alternatively, a *timetable of regular visitors and activities* in the patient's normal way of life shows what can reasonably be expected. More detailed investigations of the relationships in the family and the attitude of family members (Chapter 8) is also required. We need to know whether a good supportive relationship has existed in the past or whether there was animosity or indifference.

Life-story work

An ideal way of understanding the person with dementia is producing a life-story book. This involves the patient, with the help of others, pulling together information from her past life. The contents of the book depend entirely on whom it is about, and collecting the anecdotes, biographical information, photographs and objects for it can be a therapy in itself. It can help everyone involved to see the person with dementia as a person, with her own individuality. Reminders of the past are usually a great comfort to those who are losing the ability to make sense of the present.

It is not always necessary to produce a book as such. The important thing is to allow insight into the personality and past experience of the person that the life-story work is about. However, a book can prompt future work, and also act as a continuing reminder of who the person was. This is invaluable as, when dementia progresses, new carers become involved. In the later stages of the illness it may provide the only available information on this person, especially if no relatives are available.

Diagnosing dementia

We have seen in Chapters 1 and 2 that we need to make a clear diagnosis as early as possible, in order to plan appropriate care. We need to reassure those who are not suffering from dementia, and to organize later reassessment where there is doubt. We must recognize and treat those illnesses which may affect the dementia, or which may even look like dementia (such as thyroid disease or depression). If there is evidence for another diagnosis, that illness should be treated and the patient then reassessed.

Dementia should be a positive diagnosis, not simply the exclusion of other illnesses. To make a firm diagnosis of dementia we must show that:

1. There is significant impairment of memory but also of other aspects of brain function, to a degree which affects the person's ability to carry out activities of daily living
2. Impairments are chronic or progressive and represent a decline from previous functioning
3. Other diagnoses have been ruled out.

Detecting losses

Looking at the losses described in Chapter 4 we can see that much information can be gained from interviewing and examining the patient and by observing her carrying out her daily tasks: by observing, in effect, how she 'uses her brain'. In an interview it is possible to assess orientation, detect memory impairments and other intellectual failure, observe speech difficulties and test special functions such as those of the parietal lobe. Information from any available relatives or other informants helps clarify these impairments.

The patient's appearance and behaviour give useful information about poor self-care, lost social skills, disinhibition and poor attention or concentration. Her attitude to the losses that are revealed is most important. Is she upset or apathetic? Does she try to cover up (see Table 7.4, p. 232)? Are her emotions stable or labile? Does she have good insight? In the course of an interview, evidence that she has mistaken beliefs or hallucinations can be obtained, though sometimes very direct questioning is required.

Rating scales. Some of the information about intellectual impairment is summarized in the standard *intellectual rating scales* (Box 10.1), but strictly speaking these were not invented to make the diagnosis and are certainly not enough in themselves. Other deficits or illnesses may cause a person to perform poorly on these scales (Box 10.2), so they can only be part of our assessment. The same argument applies to observations that are used in *behaviour rating scales* (Table 10.2). Both are better used to indicate *degree of dementia* or *degree of dependence*.

Box 10.1   Cambridge Assessment Procedure for the Elderly (CAPE) information orientation scale (adapted from Pattie AH, Gilleard C J 1976 British Journal of Psychiatry 129: 68)

1 point for each correct answer:

Name	Day
Address	Month
Date of Birth	Year
Age	Prime Minister
Place (e.g. building, ward)	USA President
Town	Colours of Union Jack

Box 10.2   Some causes of poor performance in an intellectual rating scale

Deafness
Dysphasia
Low intelligence
Lack of interest
Antagonism to the tester
Poor concentration
Dementia
Delirium
Pseudodementia
Korsakoff's syndrome

Showing progressive decline

All this information put together indicates what losses have occurred, but it must always be remembered that an interview or an observation represents how the patient is at one particular time; it must always be put in the perspective of the *course* of the changes.

Evidence from the patient. Dementia sufferers can almost never answer the question, 'How long has your memory been poor?'. Indeed, it is almost a nonsense question. For the difficulty of putting memories in the right order means that, even if she has some recollection of the recent past, the memories will probably be mixed up in time. Because of this we can only get very indirect evidence from the patient herself. For example, if she does have some very accurate recent memories, then her memory cannot have been too bad when they were laid down. If we see that she has been neglecting her appearance for many months then it may be that the dementia has lasted at least that long.

Table 10.2 A behaviour rating scale – the Modified Crichton Geriatric Behaviour Rating Scale (originally devised by R. A. Robinson)

Dimension	Description	Score
Mobility	Fully ambulant including stairs	0
	Usually independent	1
	Walks with minimal supervision	2
	Walks only with physical assistance	3
	Bed-fast or chair-fast	4
Orientation	Complete	0
	Orientated in ward, identifies persons correctly	1
	Misidentifies persons but can find way about	2
	Cannot find way to bed or toilet without assistance	3
	Completely lost	4
Communication	Always clear, retains information	0
	Can indicate needs, understands verbal directions, can deal with simple information	1
	Understands simple information, cannot indicate needs	2
	Cannot understand information, retains some expressive ability	3
	No effective contact	4
Cooperation	Actively cooperative, i.e. initiates helpful activity	0
	Passively cooperative	1
	Requires frequent encouragement or persuasion	2
	Rejects assistance, shows independent but ill-directed activity	3
	Completely resistive or withdrawn	4
Restlessness	None	0
	Intermittent	1
	Persistent by day	2
	Persistent by day, with frequent nocturnal restlessness	3
	Constant	4
Dressing	Correct	0
	Imperfect but adequate	1
	Adequate with minimum supervision	2
	Inadequate unless continually supervised	3
	Unable to dress or retain clothing	4
Feeding	Correct, unaided at appropriate times	0
	Adequate, with minimum supervision	1
	Inadequate unless continually supervised	2
	Needs to be fed	3
Continence	Full control	0
	Occasional accidents	1
	Continent by day only if regularly toileted	2
	Urinary incontinence in spite of regular toileting	3
	Regular or frequent double incontinence	4

Evidence from relatives. Relatives will be able to fill in many more details. In fact, only the relatives, or someone who has known the patient well over the recent past, will be able to tell us of the course of the illness. They will need guidance in giving their account. They will need to be reminded of the many different types of brain function that might be declining (see Chapter 4), and the criteria, that there must be both a change from normal and a continuing decline, should be applied to each loss separately.

Because a particular close relative is likely to have strong feelings about the patient, or because the relative may not be with the patient all the time, it is often necessary to have more than one account. Other relatives, the sheltered-house warden, the home help, friends and neighbours, shopkeepers, police, lawyers, clergy – all may have bits of information which complete the picture or correct a biased account of how the patient has deteriorated mentally. In many cases the combination of a history from the patient and other informants, together with a good examination of the mental state of the patient and some observation of her behaviour, will be enough to ensure a proper diagnosis of dementia.

Ruling out other causes

However, in some cases there are doubts that remain. These are cases of early dementia, possible pseudodementias and cases where there is another potential diagnosis, e.g. a thyroid problem. A history of depression in the past and of depressive symptoms which began before the onset of the 'dementia' can help in diagnosing a pseudodementia. Interview and observation may hint that the correct diagnosis is depression rather than dementia.

We might expect shrinkage of the brain to show up on a CT scan in a case of dementia, but not in a case of depression. But among elderly people there are many false positives (patients who do not have dementia but show shrinkage) and false negatives (those who do have dementia but no obvious shrinkage). In younger patients this is not the case and for them scans are an essential part of diagnosis.

Slowing of the regular rhythms of the electroencephalogram (EEG) and changes in the electrical activity of the temporal lobe are often found in dementia, so this can add to the certainty of diagnosis. Again this type of evidence is not very specific. A search is going on for tests which will distinguish dementia from pseudodementia or from normality. For example, two developments of the EEG, called the auditory evoked potential and visual evoked potential tests, may help. These add together the tiny electrical brain responses that can be detected over the auditory or visual cortex when a sound or light is repeated many times. In dementia, some parts of the response are delayed. At present this is not an accurate diagnostic test, but from this type of development useful tests may eventually come.

Newer developments in scanning, such as magnetic resonance imaging (MRI) positron emission tomography (PET) and single photon emission computed tomography (SPECT) will offer more sophisticated pictures of brain damage, and in the case of PET and the easier, cheaper SPECT can show aspects of the activity of the brain such as blood flow and the metabolism of essential chemicals. These are helping to increase the accuracy of diagnosis significantly.

In the last 10 years attempts have been made to define the diagnosis of dementia much more closely and researchers have developed elaborate questionnaires which will ensure proper diagnosis of this and other psychiatric disorders in elderly people. Examples are the Geriatric Mental State Examination (GMS) and the Cambridge Mental Disorders of the Elderly Examination (CAMDEX). These have computerized versions which help to ensure standardization in diagnosis. They are not for everyday use as yet. We need shorter versions of these tests which can both positively establish the diagnosis of dementia and rule out other possibilities.

Diagnosing dementia has momentous consequences for the patient and her family. As a wrong diagnosis is equally momentous, every patient deserves proper investigation to ensure that the diagnosis is accurate and that other causes have been excluded. This means that all younger cases and most older cases should be referred to a geriatrician, old-age psychiatrist or neurologist as early as possible after the telltale changes begin. Unfortunately, older people are often subjected to ageist negligence in this respect.

The type of dementia

The best test of which type of dementia a patient suffers from would be a brain biopsy, which involves taking a tiny sample of

Table 10.3   Screening tests in the diagnosis of dementia

Test	Diagnosis
Full blood count, vitamin B_{12} and folate	Vitamin B_{12} deficiency Folate deficiency
VDRL and TPHA tests	General paralysis of the insane
HIV test	AIDS–dementia complex
Thyroid function tests	Hypo- or hyperthyroidism
Blood calcium level	Parathyroid disorder
Blood urea and electrolyte levels	Renal failure
CT, MRI and SPECT scan	Brain tumour, normal pressure hydrocephalus, VaD, DAT, Huntington's chorea

the patient's brain during life, by operation, and seeing the pathology of the dementia. However, because of the risks of the operation, the fact that there is as yet no curative treatment for the common dementias and the enormous problem of getting proper consent, this test is rarely carried out. In deciding how far to go with tests that are currently available to differentiate the various types of dementia, we need to consider two age groups.

Patients whose dementia begins after the age of 70

The older a patient is at the beginning of dementia, the less likely are the rarer and the reversible types of dementia relative to DAT, VaD and DLBT. These disorders increase in frequency with age. Some illnesses, such as Huntington's chorea and AIDS, are more likely to affect younger people. So the most likely other diagnoses in an older person are normal pressure hydrocephalus (NPH) and brain tumour, both of which are quite uncommon. The general feeling among specialists is that it is not worthwhile going to great lengths to find these conditions unless there are suggestive symptoms: for NPH, unexplained early incontinence, gait dyspraxia and a history of head injury, etc. (p. 36); for a tumour, signs or symptoms of very local damage to an area of the brain out of proportion to the severity of the dementia (*localizing signs*), signs of raised fluid pressure within the skull due to the growth of the tumour within a confined space (raised intracranial pressure) or, since most brain tumours are secondary growths spread from primary tumours elsewhere in the body, evidence of a primary growth.

Other types of reversible dementia due to physical illnesses can be detected more easily. The blood screening tests in Table 10.3 are therefore worth carrying out in all patients.

Patients whose dementia begins before the age of 70

The chances of a diagnosis other than DAT or VaD increase the younger the onset of the dementia. Since many of these other causes have some treatment, investigation is important. Everyone who is thought to be suffering from dementia should have the screening tests mentioned above, and a CT or other scan test. It must be stressed that the fact that older patients are not quite so extensively investigated is not a sign of ageism. It is entirely justified by the relative incidence of the various treatable causes of dementia.

DAT or VaD?

How important is it to know which of the two common causes a patient (of any age) has? Until now the only practical value has been to warn the relatives that the prognosis might be different. In DAT we expect a slow gradual decline, with death probably occurring gently after a mild chest infection. In VaD we cannot predict the course so well, but we can warn the relatives of possible sudden changes, periods of stability, patchy losses of function and the quite likely occurrence of other illnesses due to arteriosclerosis. Death is more likely to be sudden. It is not worth spending money on expensive and sometimes disturbing tests for this benefit. The Hachinski score (see Table 1.9, p. 29), using background information from relatives about other arteriosclerotic problems and present evidence of multiple small strokes, gives a rough diagnostic guide, though it is not entirely reliable. The CT scan, and more successfully the MRI scan, can show strokes in the brain, but using these more expensive tests simply to tell DAT from VaD is not justified at present. Many patients seem to have both conditions at the same time (p. 32). However, the time is coming when it will be very important to distinguish the two conditions as clearly as possible. Treatments (p. 188) are going to be available for one or other illness and it would be wrong to give a treatment that might have serious side-effects to the wrong patient. The very characteristic appearance of DAT on CT scan (p. 340) will help. And there have been a number of attempts to find a blood test (which might reflect the changes in the brain), lumbar puncture test (looking at the cerebrospinal fluid which surrounds the brain) or even biopsy of the olfactory nerve in the nose (which can given an indication of what pathological changes there are in the brain), which will eventually lead to a definitive and simple test for DAT.

The severity of dementia

How can we define severity? There is a complex interrelationship between activities of daily living, degree of cognitive impairment, extent of behavioural changes and a loss in self-care skills. Severity is often taken to mean the level of decline as measured by tests such as Mini Mental State Examination (MMSE), (Box 10.3), but some people with minimal decline show very severe behaviour problems or vice versa. This can apply to all of the aspects of dementia. So, we can define severity by a score on a test; or perhaps more appropriately, by the difficulties which the person (or their carer) may have as a result of the dementing process.

Rating scales

Scales such as the MMSE or the CAPE Information and Orientation Scale (Box 10.1) do make some attempt to measure the level of impairment, and to some extent when repeated over a period of time can measure change. The lower the score the more severely demented the person is. We must keep in mind that these scales are not linear; a change of 4 points from 26 to 22, for example, does not represent the same change as a drop from 18 to 14. Beyond a moderate level of dementia, patients are likely to score zero or 1 on these tests for the rest of their life. So these tests are only helpful in the early stages, where they are undoubtedly useful in charting the progress of the cognitive decline in dementia. The main use of such scales, however, is in screening for the presence of dementia. A score of 23 or under in the MMSE, for example, is an indication that the person *may* have

---

Box 10.3 Mini Mental State Examination (adapted from Folstein MF et al 1975 Journal of Psychiatric Research 12: 189)

1a. What date/month/year/day/season is it?
   Maximum score 5
1b. What town/county/country/building/floor is this?
   Maximum score 5

2. Remember three objects, e.g. apple/table/penny
   Maximum score 3

3. Serial sevens: Keep subtracting 7 from 100, i.e. 100 ... 93 ... 86 ... 79 ... 72 ... 65
   Maximum score 5

4. Repeat words from 2
   Maximum score 3

5. Name two objects, e.g. watch and pencil
   Repeat sentence 'No ifs, ands or buts'
   Maximum score 3

6. Read and obey, 'close your eyes'
   Write a sentence
   Maximum score 2

7. Obey verbal instruction, 'Take this paper in your right hand, fold it in half, put in on the floor'
   Maximum score 3

8. Copy this simple drawing (intersecting pentagons)
   Maximum score 1

---

dementia. It is important, however, not to use a score in a rating scale in isolation. Much more information is required before a diagnosis can be made with confidence.

The clock-drawing test

One simple test that can reveal a lot about how the brain is functioning is the clock test. There are many variations of this test. One method involves drawing a circle and asking the patient to draw the numbers on a clock face. If this is reasonably accurate, she should then be asked to draw the hands at 3 o'clock. The test looks at the ability to plan, as well as visio-spatial skills. It is a sensitive test, and has in some research been shown to demonstrate the presence of dementia well. It can also be used to show change. Fig. 10.1 shows some such abnormal clocks.

Behaviour rating scales

Because of the limitations of intellectual rating scales, behaviour rating scales have been devised (Table 10.2). Much of the information on these scales refers to the losses of dementia and will continue to change right through the later stages of dementia. It is important to extract this information if we wish to gauge the severity of the dementia, for the overall score on a behaviour scale indicates the severity *plus* disturbance of the patient. This overall score gives an indication of how much help she will need and so can predict the best *placement* for her, but it is wrong to use total scores on these scales as evidence of *severity*. Like intellectual scales, behaviour scales are best used to chart progress, particularly when attempts are being made to improve the patient's behaviour.

Knowing the score in tests of impairment, such as the MMSE, and on behaviour scales is of limited value. It can tell us roughly how dependent a patient is, and allows us to chart any decline. It can help to emphasize that a particular symptom such as

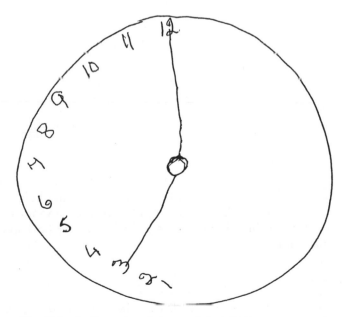

Fig. 10.1a–f Examples of abnormal clock faces.

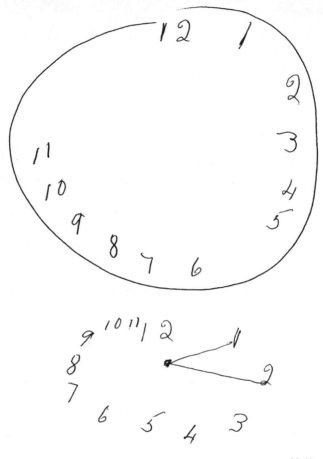

10.1b

incontinence is occurring at an inappropriate point in the progress of a dementing illness. However, it does not help us to say what kind of care the patient ought to receive, and it cannot predict future decline. It also gives no indication of how long a dementia will last.

Staging dementia

Box 10.4 shows one attempt to classify the stages of dementia. It is useful as a general guide to what we should call mild,

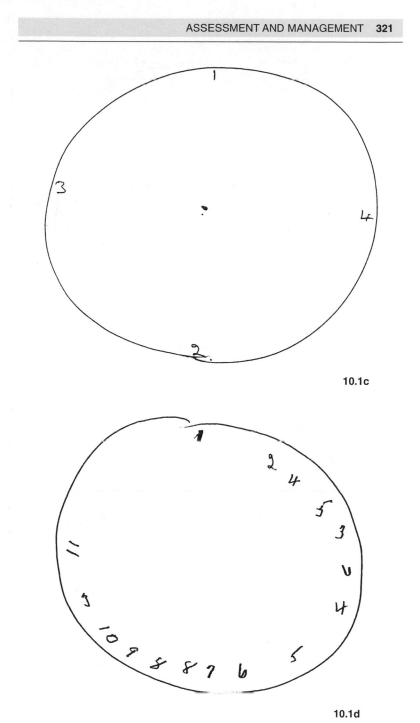

10.1c

10.1d

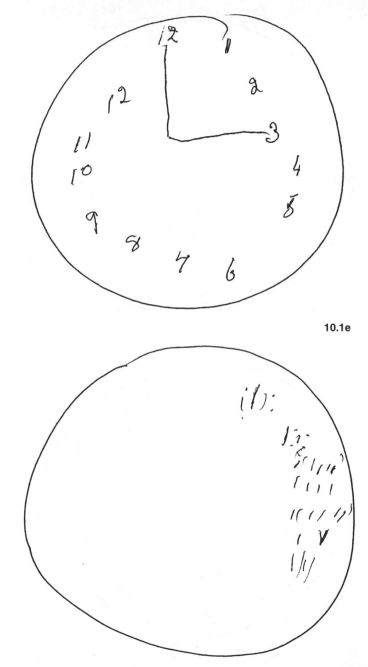

10.1e

10.1f

Box 10.4   The stages of dementia (loosely based on Hughes C P et al 1982 British Journal of Psychiatry 140: 566)

Healthy
No memory loss, orientated, solves problems, has outside interests, independent in home and in self-care

Questionable dementia
Mild forgetfulness, but orientated, doubtful impairment of problem-solving and general interest outside and inside the home, independent in self-care

Mild dementia
Moderate recent memory loss affecting daily life, some disorientation in time, may be disorientated in place in strange surroundings, difficulty handling any complex problems, cannot maintain outside interests, abandons complicated tasks at home, needs some prompting in self-care

Moderate dementia
Severe memory loss, retains only highly learnt material, disorientated in time and often in place, cannot handle problems or make judgements, unable to function independently away from home, only does the simplest chores at home, needs some assistance in dressing, hygiene, etc.

Severe dementia
Severe memory loss, fragmentary mental activity, completely disorientated except as to own identity, unable to solve any problems or make judgements, unable to care for self or to function at home or outside, often incontinent

---

moderate and severe, so that we all use the same language; people who are unused to dementia are likely to call a mild case 'severe'. But these stages are not rigid in any way and mean little for an individual patient, except as a very rough guide. They help tell us, for example, what symptoms should surprise us if they happen in 'mild' rather than 'severe' patients.

Problems

In practice, once the diagnosis of dementia has been made, the most helpful approach is to look at *problems*, rather than severity. It is these specific problems which burden relatives and require special attention and treatment, rather than the severity of the illness. This goes a long way to explaining why some mildly demented people are in hospitals and some severely demented are at home (p. 97).

We can only examine a patient's problems properly when we have made the diagnosis, got a full history, examined and observed her extensively and know a considerable amount about her background. But right from the beginning the list of problems will be emerging, for it is likely to be one specific problem which has made the patient and her carers come for help. It is unlikely that the main problem at the time of referral is simply the gradual decline, unless we have detected the patient by screening or case-finding.

The problem-orientated approach

What is a *problem*? It is a title, in as few words as possible (or one, preferably), which describes some aspects of the experience or behaviour of the patient which she, her relatives or others around her find distressing or difficult to cope with. There will be many stories or anecdotes of what the patient feels or does. In working out a problem list, our aim is to simplify these stories into the smallest number of problem titles which will be comprehensive. We need to use two problem titles only when one will not suffice. If a patient wanders and is unsteady on her feet when out wandering, then there are two problem titles – 'wandering' and 'unsteadiness' – even though the two things happen at the same time. If she wanders by day and by night but the consequences of both are the same, namely that she is at risk of being mugged, then there is one problem title. In practice it is up to each individual or team to decide how much they are going to join problems together and how much they separate them into smaller problems. However, for a general assessment we suggest that somewhere between five and ten problems is plenty to be both comprehensive and to plan for effective action. Fig. 10.2 shows a typical problem list.

Behaviour rating scales can be useful in working out what problems a patient has, because they can act as a checklist, but the full checklist of potential problems is endless (see Table 3.4, p. 98). The purpose of a problem list like this is to be a starting point for action, but it is also describes the patient in a simple and effective way. It can, for example, be used in talking to relatives. After the relatives have given their account the interviewer can feed back the list of problems he has been compiling, asking, 'Does that sum up all the difficulties as you see them?'. Relatives can then feel

Name	Mrs. J. McK.
Date of birth	25 - 8 - 12
Address	15 Castle Grove
Date admitted	17 - 5 - 97
Proposed length of stay	Medium
Purpose(s) of attendance	Assessment and relief for relatives
Number of days attending	2
Family supports	Lives with daughter and family
Support services	Health visitor
	Sitter service

Date	Problem	Action	By whom	Date of roviow	Outcome
5·97	Restlessness in house	Physical assessment	Doctor	6·97	Constipated
		Organised activity	Sitter and daughter OT	6·97	Slight improvement
		Treat constipation (6·97)	Doctor and nursing staff	7·97	Much improved Still some present
		Thioridazine 20 mg. (7·97)	GP	8·97	Much better
5·97	Sleep disturbance	More activity by day	as above	6·97	Improved
5·97	Bathing	Assessment	OT	6·97	Aids provided
5·97	Accuses daughter of stealing	Reassurance	Nursing staff	6·97	No better
		Thioridazine 20mg (7·97)	GP	8.97	Slightly better
5·97	Daughter depressed and anxious	Information booklet	Day hospital	5·97	
		See CPN	CPN	6·97	Little improvement
		Family meeting	All staff	7·97	For respite admission (8·97)

Fig. 10.2 A problem list for a day-hospital patient.

that they have got their message across and that it is understood (or not) and have the opportunity to add extra details.

Causes of problems

Having made our problem list, the next step is to try to work out *why* a problem is occurring. This is *not* the time to rush into action. It is a time for thought and further assessment if needed. Chapters 4, 5 and 7 have explained how we can think about causes. We can almost always explain the causes of a particular problem under one or more of the headings of Loss, Loss of self control, Personal reaction and Family reaction (Table 10.4). As we have gone through these types of causes we have seen a number of examples (e.g. Tables 5.1, 5.2, 5.3 and 7.3) of problems and their analysis. The importance of discovering the *different types of cause* is that they require *completely different management*. Of course, things are rarely

Table 10.4 The causes of problems in dementia and possible styles of management

Cause of the problem	Management
Decline in function	Encourage the use of remaining function Fill gaps Retrain
Disinhibition	Encourage what is normal External control Behaviour management Drug treatment
Reactions to the experience of dementia	Listening with empathy Counselling and reassuring support Drug treatment
Reactions of relatives	Education Universality Support Counselling Respite from caring
Decision-making	Conference on rights and risks Patient keeps control Advocacy on patient's behalf Hand-over by patient Compulsory take-over of decisions
Physical disability, physical illness, delirium	Ensure proper medical investigation, treatment and rehabilitation Nursing care when necessary

simple in dementia. It is not always possible to define problems as clearly as we might like, the causes may be obscure or multiple and the whole assessment is rather subjective – what one person sees as a problem, another may think not worth bothering about. Group discussion of problems and their causes is the best system.

Priorities

The value of a problem-orientated approach is that it leads logically to action once the cause or causes of the problem have been identified. The most pressing problem must obviously take precedence. We can quickly see how a crisis has arisen and how to prevent the patient from losing her independence if we describe *crucial* problems. 'If that problem was solved, the family would cope', for example. Some of the problems will be inactive rather than active ones, and some of the active ones may not need very urgent attention, but this comprehensive shorthand description of the patient is practical and easy to recall.

Problems not due to dementia

It is important to try to separate off any problems that are not due to dementia. There is a great temptation to lump together everything that is wrong with the patient and blame it on the dementia. But other illnesses, loss of sight or hearing, mobility problems, drug side-effects and family troubles may have nothing at all to do with it, though they will have an influence on the patient's management and treatment. They will not, however, follow the typical course of the problems of dementia itself.

METHODS OF ASSESSMENT

Talking to the patient

Some people seem to have the knack of talking with dementing people. Others have to learn it slowly. Some, who probably were not interested anyway, never learn. In Chapters 4, 5 and 7 we have described a number of important ways of compensating for the patient's disabilities in an interview, and discussed how to deal with disinhibition and the patient's reactions to the illness. Here we bring together some general principles which can help in assessment and, indeed, can make any type of conversation with a sufferer easier.

1. Explain what is happening – introduce yourself and explain why you want to talk to the patient, in a way that she is likely to understand. Say what is going to happen in the interview. This information may well have to be repeated several times.

2. Give of yourself – as much as possible, the interview should be like an ordinary conversation. Replying to her answer with an empathic comment can help build up a rapport. For example, when a patient answers the question 'Where were you born?', the interviewer might well reply, 'Oh that is near such and such', or even, 'there have been a lot of changes there'. Discussing a common knowledge of football, of places, of illnesses or of events helps with this.

3. Find out how she feels about the interview – she may be unable to understand what is happening, or may not wish to know; she may object, believing that she does not need your help; she may think something completely different is happening, for example, that she is in a shop. All these reactions are bound to affect the quality of information that one gets.

4. Don't spend too long – poor attention and fatigue can make the patient muddled or emotionally upset. Come back again later. Within the interview, intersperse questions or mental 'work' with general talk, reminiscence, etc.

5. Allow for sight, hearing and speech problems – help the patient who has expressive problems by guessing what she means; do not leave her to try desperately to get her message across.

6. For all patients, not only those with communication problems, use simple speech, not complicated sentences – this does not mean treating the patient like a child.

7. Use non-verbal communication – a smile, a friendly touch, a firm handshake can help the patient feel more at ease. Once again do not treat her like a child.

8. Go at the patient's pace – this will always be slower than our pace. The correct pace has to be worked out at the time. With severely demented people there may have to be long gaps and silences, and very few words need to be spoken.

9. Do not change the subject too quickly – remember perseveration, the difficulty in moving from one subject to another.

10. Repeat messages, not in a way that puts the patient under pressure but in a way that helps the message get across – saying the same thing in differing ways may help. Cues help her to get more answers.

11. Expect and look for emotional changes in the interview – if a particular line of questions is upsetting, take the pressure off, sympathize with her feelings and then change the subject for a while.

12. Allow for any uncontrolled reactions of inexplicable tears, laughter, anger, over-affection or the catastrophic reaction – again, give the patient a rest. If she is distressed by her reaction, reassure her. Never respond spontaneously to such reactions – decide what response will be most helpful.

13. It can be useful, however, to find out how she does cope under pressure by asking a quick series of questions or changing the subject quickly – this can help us to guess how he would cope at home if something went wrong, if someone was trying to exploit her or if he was in a strange situation.

14. Talking to a dementing person should seem natural and relaxed to her – we need to be flexible and modify our approach, depending on her personality and what she expects. Some patients prefer a formal approach, others less formal. Some cope with physical contact better than others, some appreciate more sympathy than others. We will get more information if the patient feels that we are on her side.

15. Information from interviews does not come in an orderly sequence – we may have interviewed the patient to help diagnosis, assess problems, discuss plans of management or talk of going into care. As far as possible we should try to stick to the purpose of the interview. But other things will happen in the interview which tell us of speech problems, of how the patient is feeling, about family relationships, attitudes or completely new difficulties that we had not known of. Always keep an open mind and an observant eye. Review what has been learned afterwards.

16. End on a positive and friendly note, even if some of the interview has been upsetting – summarize simply what has been said so that the patient can have some memory of what went on. If the summary is upsetting, end with a very general chatty conversation and then a formal farewell, preferably with a handshake.

17. Do not base judgements on one interview – the patient may perform very differently in other settings or at other times. Find out about these other times.

Talking with relatives

We have emphasized that family members have as much if not more information to offer than the patient. Indeed, the problem is usually that they have too much to say. It is most important, therefore, to decide what is required from a family interview beforehand by preparing an *agenda*. The interviewer then has the task of ensuring that all the items of the agenda are discussed in the time available. Inevitably, the relatives will want to introduce other subjects, and some of these have to be put to one side for discussion at another time. But what the relatives want to talk about is important to them. It may be that they have come to the interview with one message, or one strong feeling ('She can't stay at home any longer', 'We are anxious about her safety'). If these strong messages are not listened to and acknowledged the family will feel dissatisfied and may not cooperate in giving information or agreeing to plans.

Therefore, in proceeding with an interview the interviewer should be aware not only of the agenda that he has brought along but of the relatives' agenda. The interviewer should make sure that he understands these feelings and messages and should say so clearly. There may have to be a compromise between the two agendas.

In making an 'agenda' the problem-orientated approach works best. This allows discussion to fall under a number of headings. It also allows other problems to be raised at the end. If the interviewer is skilful, there will not be much that has been left out. The problem list is very helpful also for further meetings. Progress on each problem and the action taken can be discussed separately and efficiently.

While talking with relatives it is important to realize that they bring along feelings which are inevitably stronger than ours and these feelings may bias or cloud their judgement. Part of the interviewer's job is to empathize or 'be with' those feelings, but he should not let his judgement be clouded or his decisions biased by sympathy for the relatives. He also has to keep clearly in mind the reality of the situation, the patient's views, the professional assessments. The relatives' feelings are another factor, indeed one of the most important, but not the only one to be considered in making decisions.

We should also be on the lookout for gaps in education and knowledge of services, which make it difficult for the family to come to wise decisions. Some part of most interviews will be spent in filling these gaps. The most important knowledge families must have is that their relative suffers from dementia and that this is progressive. As soon as it is possible to be sure about this, the family should be told. We can hope that then, after the initial shock, staff and family will be able to work on the same wavelength.

The relatives also need to know why all the information we ask for is necessary. We need to explain to them the importance of a baseline and the necessity of identifying problems and looking for their causes if we are to help the patient effectively.

Families are not, however, simple organizations. In making a list of the family and their involvement (p. 309), the relationships in the family should become apparent. Some families have a head or spokesperson and the rest will agree with his or her judgement. But most are much more diffuse, so that talking to one member is not sufficient. We should be aware of false spokespersons who want their view to prevail in the family; often they are temporary visitors and not the real carers. We should be particularly aware of quieter members who may not be getting their views across. We are often dealing with several generations – the patient's brothers or sisters, spouse, children, grandchildren or great-grandchildren and in-laws. Sometimes friendships are more important to the patient than family ties, a lover's views more important than those of the children. The differing needs of all these people must be considered in working out what 'the family' feels.

Relatives and the patient

In talking to relatives we should be continually aware that the patient is the patient. Her permission should always be asked before seeing them, and we should explain to her why we want to see them.

Some relatives are happy to talk with the sufferer present, others find this very difficult. We should encourage openness between relative and patient unless it is causing major distress to either. If, however, a relative refuses to talk with the patient present, ask why this is, but go along with the request for a private talk (after asking the patient's permission), for such a relative will be unlikely to give the whole story otherwise. Indeed, it is useful to offer the opportunity of even a short private word with the relative, for there may be just one or two things which they feel unable to say in the sufferer's hearing. Seeing a professional carer can be an intimidating experience for many people. This can lead to thoughts being left out, even things which may prove important. We should also make sure there is a way of getting back to us at a later date, perhaps by leaving a telephone number or a card, or by simply saying when we will be available again.

Remember that the patient also may wish to talk to you without her relatives present, perhaps not wishing to show up her difficulties in front of them. It is sometimes tempting to listen only to the relatives' story. Instead, it can be very useful to use the information we get from them to ask more questions of the patient, about her background, her relationships, her present feelings. The result is a better understanding of both relatives and patient.

OBSERVING THE PATIENT

Observation

Much useful information is gained simply by observing how a patient spends her time. Does she engage in activities or sit quietly? Are her activities purposeful or meaningless? Can she concentrate and persist in activity? Is she easily distracted? How much does she talk to other people and is she talking sense? Is he restless? Does she seem happy or otherwise? Is there any odd behaviour? All these can help in assessing the severity of dementia, show changes in the patient's state, indicate problems and suggest solutions.

Dementia care mapping

This is a means of describing the care which a patient receives, how it is received and how the patient reacts to it. It is rather labour-intensive, but can give useful insights not only into the activities carried out by the person, but also to many aspects of her day-to-day life. It involves someone acting as an observer, watching the person and recording how she acts and reacts, for long periods of time. This allows some assessment of the person's quality of life over this period.

Activities of daily living (ADL)

It is often helpful to look specifically at the things that each of us needs to do to manage from day to day. These include dressing and undressing (including remembering to change clothes), washing and bathing, toileting, getting about the house and outside, shopping for food and cooking it, eating, heating the house correctly, coping with laundry, dealing with bills, leisure activities, going to bed and sleeping. Many different losses of dementia can affect the patient's performance in these tasks. They show up the *practical* effects of dementia. Impairments in these functions are more crucial to the patient's independent survival than whether she can recall a name and address. They will therefore be high on any problem list.

Accurate and specialized assessment of daily living tasks is required. This is the special responsibility of the occupational therapist, as well as being part of the wider job of all care staff. A few important points need to be made in relation to such assessments:

1. Remember the baseline – if people vary a great deal in their intelligence and interests, they vary even more in their standards of hygiene, pattern of daily living, styles of cooking and shopping. The standard for judging the patient's performance is her own, not ours.

2. Assess what she *needs* to be able to do now – the amount of independence in self-care that is needed by a dementing person varies depending on who she is, but also on her situation. A dementing man with a willing wife at home may get away with quite severe impairments in self-care without the wife feeling that the burden is too great. Unfortunately, the opposite is not always the case. A patient who lives alone and refuses help needs all her daily living skills if she is to survive. To survive in residential care, only a few basic skills of dressing, washing and toileting are required, and many get away with less.

3. Assessment should take place in the patient's home if possible. Much of our ability in daily tasks is based on routines with familiar objects and equipment. Although it is useful to see how a patient deals with new equipment or a new environment (and this can be important if she is to move from her old home), testing in a special 'ADL suite' does not always give an accurate indication of how she would cope at home. There is no substitute for a visit home. If a patient has been in care for more than a few days, the return home may be difficult, for she may be confused by the move or have quickly got out of practice. More than one visit may therefore be required in order to make an accurate assessment.

4. Assessment should not be like a 'test' – inevitably there is pressure on the patient to perform well and inevitably the person assessing is an 'intruder' in her home. But the skill of the assessor lies in making the situation feel as natural as possible to the patient. Acting like a friendly visitor, avoiding standing over the patient, not giving too many instructions, avoiding hurry and ensuring that the activities are done as nearly as possible in the way the patient would normally do them can all be of help. Positive encouragement and praise without pressure is helpful, so that she is able to relax and enjoy what she is doing.

5. As with interviews, it may nevertheless be useful once or twice to test the effects of pressure or hurry – for some patients, it is only when they are under pressure or things do not go along their usual routines that they make mistakes and get muddled.

6. In carrying out any assessment, the *purpose* should always be kept in mind – the assessment should lead to action. The action may be to improve the safety of the home, to recommend aids, to retrain the patient, to suggest ways in which the family could fill gaps, or to come to a decision about whether the patient can stay at home.

A proper ADL assessment requires a good knowledge of the particular patient, of possible aids and adjustments in the house and especially of the deficits that lead to practical difficulties. Understanding of sight, hearing and smell disorders, mobility problems, memory problems, agnosia, spatial problems, dyspraxia, attention problems, poor motivation and emotional lability are all needed, and useful information about all these types of deficit can be fed back to other staff who care for the patient as well as to the patient and her family.

Box 10.5 shows one example of an ADL checklist. This comprehensive look at the patient's abilities can be of the greatest value in determining what help is needed and where the patient can live. As with interviewing, it is vital, however, that one ADL assessment should not be used as the sole evidence of how the patient is coping. She may behave differently at different times or

---

Box 10.5 Information to be obtained from a home assessment, including activities of daily living

Description of accommodation
Access, including stairs
General care of house, including warmth
Rooms and equipment
    kitchen, bathroom, toilet, living room, bedrooms
Heating and lighting
Telephone, alarm system

Supports
Informal
Alone or not
Visiting family, friends and neighbours
Formal
Home help
Sitting service
Meals on wheels
Laundry service
District nurse
Health visitor, CPN
Social worker
General practitioner

Outings
Shopping, pension, other regular outings
Lunch club
Day care

Timetable of regular visitors and outings

Mobility
Standing, walking, stairs
Getting in and out of chair, bed, bath and on and off toilet
Orientation around house
Aids used

Other physical disabilities
Sight, hearing, smell
Physical symptoms or signs

Box 10.5 Information to be obtained from a home assessment, including activities of daily living (*Cont'd*)

Personal care
General appearance and interest
Dressing and undressing
Washing and grooming
Bathing or showering
Toileting, including incontinence
Reminders needed
Aids used

Food preparation
Planning
Shopping
Food in store
Assessment of making tea, a snack and a full meal
Safety with kettle and cooker
Eating and aids used

Household chores
Dishes
Dusting and cleaning
Laundry

Safety
Road safety
Keys and entry
Checking strangers
Fire from cigarettes, cooker, heating
Flooding
Rubbish and food waste disposal

Managing finances
Understanding money and prices
Pension, bank
Shopping
Bills, rent, taxes, etc.
Money in the house
Help with finances

Managing medication
Need for reminders
Accuracy

Mental state during visit
Attention and concentration
Restlessness
Abnormal behaviour
Orientation in time, place and person
Communication
Memory
Agnosias and dyspraxia
Emotions and motivation
Abnormal beliefs
Insight

with different people. If the ADL assessment does not fit with other evidence, then both should be questioned.

Psychological testing

In the past it was customary for clinical psychologists to be involved in tests of intellectual capacity, learning and memory to make the diagnosis of dementia. Nowadays it is realized that as a general rule the history, mental state examination and information about daily living activities are sufficient for diagnosis, so that special tests have not much to add. However, they still occasionally have their uses in diagnosis and assessment. The tests which psychologists use include standard intelligence tests and some modified ones, memory tests, tests of the ability to learn new material, and tests of parietal lobe function (p. 116), or frontal lobe function. So they are of more use in defining specific areas of brain damage than in making the overall diagnosis. They may be useful, for example, when a patient is not doing as well as might be expected with a particular daily activity.

The development of computerized testing is likely to alter the position of psychological testing. Using a simple push button, touch or lever response, computer programs have been devised which include elements of intelligence testing, the ability to learn new materials, speed tests and memory tests. Eventually these tests will be of value in the early detection of dementia, for they are easier to standardize than interviews and they remove the personal influence of the tester on the results. But like every method, the results have to be interpreted sensibly and in context. They only tell how the patient performs at that time and not at other times of day or in other situations. Such techniques will not be useful for later stages of dementia. We also have to remember that the next generation of elderly people, as well as the present one, will not be able to handle any more complicated computer materials, since they will not have become 'computer literate' early in life.

Rating scales

As we have seen, the two types of rating scale in regular use – the intellectual (Box 10.3) and the behaviour (Table 10.2) – have tended to be overused in diagnosis and have a limited value in identifying problems. They are most informative when they are used to measure the progression of impairments over time and to predict the future care needs of the patient. They should not be a lazy person's substitute for good history-taking, intelligent observation and full mental testing, which alone can show the vast range of deficits and disturbances caused by dementia.

In using these rating scales, some points are worth remembering:

1. Decide what the scale is to be used for *before* using it – what action will follow from its results. Routine testing of everybody in a ward, home or in day-care might be useful for research purposes but is unlikely to be useful in practice.

2. Decide how often it needs to be used in order to show up the changes that are being measured.

3. Try to standardize the use of the scales by having practice sessions with all staff involved.

4. The use of rating scales should help improve sharpness of our observations rather than leading to sloppiness – try to ensure that the information is accurate, not just hearsay or one individual's biased report.

5. The difficulty of getting accurate and reliable information for rating scales reminds us just how variable a dementing person's performance can be – try to check that the information is valid for the whole day, not just the good times or the bad times.

6. Interpret the results intelligently – remember how physical illness and drugs (Ch. 6), as well as poor attention, poor hearing, dysphasias, restlessness and poor motivation can interfere with intellectual testing; how losses interact (p. 112); and how loss of control can produce contrary effects (e.g. emotions, p. 160). No rating scale tells *why* the patient acts in one particular way. That question must be asked, but must be asked separately.

7. Remember that total scores only give a very general guide to the level of impairment or dependence – look closely at individual scores and the changes that occur in them. Then rating scales can help enormously in the day-to-day care of dementia sufferers.

It might be better if we devised individual ratings for each of the problems of each patient, and sometimes this can be done, but the popular scales offer a useful shorthand way of recording some of the commonest problems of dementia.

Medical examination

Medical examination is necessary at the time of diagnosis, to exclude other causes of apparent impairment, to determine the cause of the dementia and to look for quite separate physical illnesses.

We have already pointed out (p. 60) that a dementing patient may be unable to give a good account of the physical complaints of any illness. Even severe pain may be forgotten quickly or not described clearly. We have seen that delirium, emotional distress or restlessness may be the only signs that the patient is ill. Every dementing patient, therefore, deserves a regular (though not too frequent) medical check.

In general terms dementia is a slowly progressive illness. Sudden changes in behaviour are thus unlikely to be due to the dementia alone, and are more often due to treatable difficulties such as an infection or other illness. A medical check is therefore also called for if there is a sudden change in the patient's condition or if a symptom or sign develops which does not fit into the usual pattern of dementia.

Obviously there is special emphasis on neurological examination, and this is particularly difficult in dementing patients because much of it depends on carrying out orders – 'move your leg', 'touch your nose' – and on reporting sensations – 'did you see that?', 'did you feel that?'. Particularly in VaD there will, however, be widespread neurological damage. Strokes often have very minor or no observable neurological effects or they may have unusual or mixed effects. General physicians need to be reminded of these facts. It is far too easy to say that a stroke has not occurred just because there is no paralysis or other physical sign. Yet both the stepwise and the gradual changes of VaD may be due to a series of dozens of separate stroke events.

The doctor needs to be particularly painstaking in examining dementing patients, for he may not have the guidance of a good history from the patient, and in older patients there could, of course, be several different diagnoses. It is worth spending the time, however. It is remarkable, for example, how often a rectal examination reveals *constipation* as the cause of restlessness. It is also remarkable how many illnesses are neglected for many months by patients, and even by their families, who may think the symptoms or signs are part of the dementia, or 'just old age'.

Special tests

The arguments which justify good diagnostic examination and routine physical check-ups for dementia sufferers also justify the use of the special tests in Table 10.3. All these tests will lead to clear and useful action either in trying to reverse a dementia, or treating associated illnesses.

In choosing tests and interpreting them, we should note:

1. It saves time, energy and expense to realize that, since many older people have multiple medical problems, some or all of the investigations may have already been carried out by another doctor – a little detective work can help enormously.

2. We should take into account how disturbing each test may be to the patient – simple blood tests are a temporary nuisance only, whereas urine testing requires a little cooperation and is of course difficult in an incontinent patient. The more time and cooperation required for a test the more difficult it will be for the patient and the more we should question its necessity. A good CT scan, SPECT scan or EEG test requires that the patient keeps quite still for up to 15 minutes; MRI scanning requires longer and PET scanning longer still.

3. It is important to know that the normal values of many tests change as people grow older.

4. For several tests we have emphasized the problem of 'false-positive' and 'false-negative' results (see, for example, p. 32).

5. A diagnostic test is only justified if it is likely to give a conclusive result – however, a combination of tests may increase the confidence of our diagnosis.

6. Some tests are more expensive than others – in particular, a PET scanning facility costs several million pounds and this technique will only be available for research purposes, and only in one or two places. All the more usual tests of dementia, if justifiable for proper diagnosis or care, are worth the expense.

New tests

It remains difficult to be sure of the diagnosis of any dementia very early in its course. Indeed, we cannot be one hundred percent sure of the diagnosis until postmortem in most cases. There is therefore a great need for tests that can be used during life and at the earliest possible stage of the dementia. We mentioned a few possible ways forward earlier (p. 316). The most conclusive test of all, brain biopsy, cannot be justified in the absence of effective treatments for VaD or DAT. This area is one where great development is likely to happen in the next few years. We may even see the development of tests which will show up telltale signs of dementia before it has any observable effects on the sufferer.

MANAGEMENT OF DEMENTIA

In the 'management' column of Table 10.4, we have summarized the various approaches which we discussed fully in previous chapters. A little more needs to be said about curative treatments, and some comments are needed on the carrying out of management plans.

Reversing dementia

Table 1.5 (p. 12) lists the causes of potentially treatable dementia. In these conditions, if the damage has not been severe, the patient has a good chance of regaining a reasonable level of function. If there has been severe damage to the brain and many nerve cells have died, then he will be left with permanent impairment after some gradual improvement. It should go without saying that all patients with treatable dementias deserve that treatment, and therefore need to be examined and investigated very thoroughly. Although investigations are likely to be more extensive in a younger patient the age of the patient is not relevant as far as treatment is concerned.

The main purpose of research into Alzheimer-type dementia and vascular dementia is to move them into the group of treatable dementias (see Chapters 1 and 6).

Alzheimer-type dementia

There are five possible approaches to treatment:

1. The lost *neurotransmitters* may be replaced – as we have seen, part of the deficit in DAT is due to lack of acetylcholine. Drugs are now available which slow down the natural breakdown of acetylcholine (anticholinesterases such as tacrine and donepezil) (see p. 188).

2. The damaged brain could be encouraged to function more effectively – we have discussed, in dealing with the losses of dementia, external aids to fill memory and other gaps, stimulation of abilities that the patient has not been using and retraining. But there is no evidence as yet of any day-to-day management technique which will reverse the decline of dementia and bring lost faculties back. We can encourage a patient to use her failing memory in the most effective way possible, but can still not actually improve her basic memory function.

3. If the loss of function in the brain of DAT patients is largely due to damage and loss of the connections between nerve cells, there might eventually be a drug treatment which could reverse that process – there is even some evidence that a very stimulating environment can encourage nerves to connect with each other, but how much this might help the actual functioning of the brain is unclear. The discovery of *nerve growth factors* (p. 189), has brought hope of effective treatments for damaged cells. But there is little chance of a treatment which could make completely dead nerve cells grow again. For this reason it will be important, whenever treatment is devised, to treat the patients at the earliest possible stage.

4. Whatever is causing the damage and death of cells could be attacked – if, for example, it was aluminium or another metal poison, the levels of aluminium reaching the brain could be reduced. If it is a more complex form of chemical damage, then more complicated treatments might be necessary.

5. Genetic causes lead to the possibility of genetic counselling for those rare families in which there is a strong genetic component – the finding of any responsible gene brings the possibility of pinning down the abnormal protein which this gene is producing and this could lead on to future treatments. Alternatively, the genetic information may be most useful in

detecting people who are *at risk* of developing DAT. They could then be given a treatment to slow the progress of damage or replace lost transmitters.

When curative treatments are available, and it surely is a 'when' rather than an 'if', they cannot be expected to reverse major brain damage. The most important task will then be to learn how to detect cases in the earliest stages, to prevent worsening or, better still, to detect illness before it is having any obvious effects. It is probably the case that, because of the cerebral reserve (p. 7), changes of DAT are occurring in the brain several years before the first signs of decline show themselves.

Except in treatment which actually deals with the cause, the damage may still go on occurring despite treatment, but delayed perhaps by a year or two. Such benefits will nevertheless temporarily transform the lives of dementia sufferers. They raise many interesting ethical issues for the future.

Vascular dementia

The most effective treatment in VaD would be prevention. As VaD is related to arteriosclerosis and hypertension it can be hoped that dietary and other changes which are already reducing the incidence of these conditions would also have an impact on dementia. Treatment of hypertension, if it is present, may help, though lowering the patient's blood pressure too far can be counter-productive.

A more specific preventative treatment is the use of drugs which reduce clot formation by affecting the blood platelets which are involved in the steps that lead to clotting. Drugs such as aspirin and dipyridamole have been used in this way and shown to have some useful effect. It remains to be seen whether these or similar drugs will prevent the deterioration of VaD.

Researchers are also looking at ways of preventing neuronal damage that is due to vascular difficulties. It may be possible to prevent secondary damage following a stroke, or even damage from other vascular problems. A wide variety of drugs has been used in attempts to improve blood flow to the brain in VaD. These are unlikely to be effective because in most cases the reduction in blood flow happens as a *result* of the brain damage and not as a *cause* of it. So increasing blood flow would not improve function.

A number of so-called 'cerebral activators' have also been used. It is not always clear what such drugs are supposed to do, and drug trials show varied or equivocal results. It is safest to assume that there is, as yet, no drug of this type which has proved effective in improving the function of the damaged brain in either VaD or DAT.

Carrying through management plans

Our aim in this book is to show that, despite the lack of curative treatments, we can approach the care and treatment of dementing people rationally, with some hopes of alleviating the problems experienced by sufferers and their families. In Chapters 4–9 we discussed specific ways of managing a wide variety of problems. If such managements are to be effective in lessening distress and improving the quality of life of patients and relatives, a few general principles need to be applied:

1. Set reasonable goals

What is reasonable must be judged by reference to the patient's pre-illness baseline and our assessment of the present deficits and changes. The further away from her norm the patient has moved, the more unlikely does it become that she will be able to get back to normal. Thus, although we should always refer back to her previous life as a baseline, we should not raise our hopes and those of her family unnecessarily. Drug treatments for dementia will only work for some, and may only help a little bit for a short while. Remember that none of the techniques described in Chapter 4 will replace lost functions. Only occasionally will retraining have any impact at all. Otherwise we can only try to fill gaps from outside, keep encouraging the patient to use her abilities to the full, and help her cope with the losses. We can hope to have some impact on symptoms that are due to poor self control and emotional reactions, but even here we have emphasized the limitations of treatment. Furthermore, we have seen many examples of how losses and other problems interact and make helping more difficult. Overoptimism leads to disappointment just as underoptimism leads to poor morale.

2. Establish priorities

Since every patient has multiple problems we could invent a long list of possible management programmes in every case. What we actually choose to do should be guided by deciding what are the crucial problems (p. 326), what are the biggest problems, which cause most distress to the patient or her family, which are the easiest to treat. From this we should be able to make a list of priorities and start working down that list. Attempting too many treatments at once can be confusing, for it may be impossible to know which has helped, so relatives may have to be warned that we will be trying to deal with only one or two problems at a time. We will all need considerable patience.

3. Decide who is to carry out the management

There is not much use in assessing problems and formulating elaborate management plans if no one is prepared to do the donkey work of actual management. Team or conference decision-making can help the fair sharing of work. As we shall see in Chapter 11, only certain jobs are anybody's specific responsibility in dementia; many jobs can be carried out by any one of a number of workers. Enthusiasm and willingness usually have to be complemented with patience if any of these techniques are to work. If a person is delegating to another worker or teaching the family how to help, he has a responsibility to continue to support the worker or family and to inject his own energy and enthusiasm into the programme. This is particularly true of group activities, slow retraining, reality orientation and behavioural programmes.

4. Call in expert help where necessary

As there are so many different types of problem in dementia, it is most unlikely that one person or even one team can manage all aspects of the care of a patient. We should never be ashamed to have to ask for an expert assessment or for expert help in management. Of course we hope that the expert will teach us something that we can use again with other sufferers, but no one is an expert in everything. There is still some nihilism about dementia treatment – a lack of belief that any treatment or management can be helpful. Partly because of this, and partly because of ageism, primary care teams may be reluctant to seek specialist advice. This inevitably leads to patients and their carers missing out on various sources of help. Community teams and residential homes should have no hesitation in calling in expert nursing, physiotherapy, speech therapy or medical help. Hospital teams may need the advice of other specialists, and should ensure that they are not ignoring the expertise that exists in the community.

5. Tell the patient what is happening

A dementing person may not be able to understand fully what is happening around her. But she will have difficulty coping with changes, new faces and new styles of treatment. As far as possible, we should explain to her what we propose to do, and why. There is no excuse for ignoring her.

6. Engage the family in treatment plans

Relatives not only need to be told what our plans are, but are often important members of the treatment team. We have seen this particularly in relation to managing behaviour problems. But they also need to be taught gap-filling techniques, told how best to cope with emotional disturbance and how to deal practically with physical problems such as incontinence, immobility, dressing problems and fits. They must learn the side-effects of the drugs they are supervising and many other aspects of management. Continuing contact and cooperation with the family throughout is therefore essential.

7. Set a time scale

Treatment plans should not drift on without reassessment. For each problem that is being assessed we should have a rough idea of how long the management will take, so that whoever is taking on the job can plan ahead, and a date for reassessment can be set.

8. Record what is decided

A problem sheet such as Figure 10.2 (there are many variants of this) allows an accurate record of decisions, reminds people of the responsibilities they have taken on and allows clear reassessment.

9. Assess success or failure

When the time for review comes, or when difficulties occur in the programme, the status of the problem should be reassessed. If the goals are not reached, the problem needs to be reassessed and, if possible, a different strategy tried. Failure can be due to a mistaken assessment of the problem, overoptimistic (or underoptimistic) goals, imperfect carrying out of the programme or a change in the whole situation (a further decline in the patient, for example), as well as all sorts of extraneous factors. The reasons for failures need to be recorded under 'outcome'. This leads on to a reformulation of the management plan.

CONCLUSION

Problem-orientated working is simple to organize. It requires that all the people involved sit down together regularly to plan and reassess the patient's care. There are many advantages in using proper multidisciplinary teamwork. It leads to good communication between professions and with families and wider education about the variety of management techniques available. A patient who is dealt with by one or two people in isolation misses out on a lot of possibilities for help.

However, often the possible ways of helping her are not as available as they should be. It would be difficult to make all the conceivable environmental changes necessary for hard-pressed staff to spend the time they might wish to support relatives or to keep patients engaged in activities, so management often has to be rationed. And while this is so there is still a 'political' task of ensuring that resources of money, people and places are available to help in the proper management that dementing patients deserve. In the meantime, we have to provide care as comprehensively as we can with the resources available, focusing on the worst problems, using family as staff, setting realistic goals, giving treatment in groups where possible.

Nevertheless, the whole problem-orientated approach can transform the attitudes of those working with dementing people from a pessimistic despair to an optimistic but realistic commitment. For, at all stages of the decline, it shows how 'success' that is limited, but no less real, can be achieved, even if the outcome always includes decline and eventual death.

11

Organizing help

Defining responsibilities
Organizations involved in dementia
  The family
  The 'community'
  The primary care team
  The local social services department
  Voluntary services
  The care environment and dementia
  Sheltered housing
  Day centres
  Private care
  Local authority and voluntary sector residential care
  Homes for the elderly mentally infirm (EMI)

  General hospitals
  The geriatric service
  General psychiatric services
  The old-age psychiatry service
Segregation or integration
  Coordinating care
  Education
  Contact point
  Communication between services
  Towards a dementia team
  Towards a dementia resource centre
Planning services
  Norms
  New developments

As we have examined the many and changing problems of dementia, we have seen a variety of ways of helping individual sufferers and their families. As dementia has a multitude of effects on the patient and her family, organizing help can be a complicated matter. In this chapter we shall look at the organizations involved and at the different professional groups and their responsibilities, before looking at how coordination of care and planning could be improved.

As people in the different professions and organizations have gradually realized that a new problem exists, they have, to a greater or lesser degree and more or less willingly, accepted dementia as *part* of their responsibility. No one in any area of the world has accepted complete responsibility for all aspects and stages of dementia. This is in part an accident of history, but it is also inevitable and desirable. The different types of care required are very unlikely to be all available from one source in high quality. Various agencies provide multiple services and so offer some choice. But the complexity of the system can be a nightmare for a newcomer.

Defining responsibilities

The responsibilities of professionals

Core. Each profession will attempt to define its role in relation to a condition like dementia. But as we try to define our individual roles we can see that there are some responsibilities that are clear, some not so clear. The clearest of these make up the 'core' responsibilities of our job.

Thus, doctors are the only people who can write a prescription and they have special training in diagnosis and special access to facilities which help in diagnosis. Social workers have specific roles in arranging admission to care homes and in relation to the Mental Health Act (p. 288). They are responsible for community care assessments and management, and they act as *budget holders* on behalf of local authorities. District nurses have special training and responsibility in carrying out nursing tasks in the patient's own home.

Overlap. A professional who tried to keep only to the core of his job would have a narrow and unsatisfied life. He would have to spend much of his energy in passing patients on to other professionals. To work together we must accept considerable *overlapping* of roles. Many tasks can be handled by any one of a variety of groups.

Mutual advice. Between these two types of responsibility, the core and the overlapping, there are areas where one professional will be able to *advise* another how to do a job which is close to his own core responsibility. Thus a physiotherapist may help nursing staff in techniques of lifting and in passive and active exercising. A clinical psychologist visiting a home may teach staff how to carry out a behavioural programme. A community psychiatric nurse may teach a home help to look out for particular side-effects of drugs. Families may be taught by a variety of professionals to become 'amateur therapists'.

Job satisfaction. It could be said that professionals tend to feel satisfied in their work if they feel that they have clear responsibilities in their core job and that others respect that core without trying to tell them how to do their work; secondly, if they can freely overlap with others in the more general aspects of helping, not keeping exclusively to their core but avoiding rivalry over who does what in these shared areas; and thirdly, if they can pass on their special skills and knowledge to others without meeting a hostile reaction. Of course, there are some who prefer the overlapped areas of work, or even someone else's core to their own core responsibility! They are, as it were, in the wrong job, and it is up to others who work with them to decide how to react to this.

In any team the proper sharing of work between different professions depends on balances between the different cores and a fair division of labour. Communication is the key to good collaboration. Individuals should decide their roles and tasks not in a vacuum but in discussion and negotiation with their colleagues, thus ensuring that every client who needs help is covered fairly and that all the team have satisfying work to do.

Care of older people in general, and of those with dementia in particular, is often seen as the 'Cinderella' of care, with low status both in terms of payment and of job satisfaction. We can hope that these attitudes are slowly changing, with more and more people making a positive choice to work in this field, rather than drifting into it because of a lack of alternatives.

The responsibilities of organizations

Each organization involved with dementia, whether it be a complicated one like an old-age psychiatry service or a simple one like a family-run nursing home, can be viewed in a somewhat similar way. Each has a core responsibility for particular types of dementing patient but also accepts, and has to accept, overlapping areas of responsibility for people who do not fit neatly into a 'hospital' category or a 'nursing home' category. The staff of any organization can easily feel hard done by if they have to look after more of the overlap patients than they themselves think should be in their care. And sometimes, of course, there are differing views from inside and outside about what that organization's responsibility should be.

For example, residential homes traditionally looked after only mildly-demented people, or provided continuing care for people who demented while in their care; they tended to look for them to be moved if they became disturbed. Inevitably they are now taking far more of the severely demented population and keeping some they think should be in hospital. Many home managers are facing up to these problems and are considering how they should adjust to accommodate the 'rising tide' of dementia sufferers by, for example, developing specialist units. In the meantime, there is limited job satisfaction for those who stick to outdated ideas or dogmas about their responsibility.

At the extreme, the two biggest problems which can arise for patients in this world of core and overlap are, first, that interesting patients get all the services while less exciting ones are left uncared for, and secondly, that suspicion and 'institutional paranoia' develop between services. Only better communication and real joint planning of services and policies can avoid or overcome these problems.

ORGANIZATIONS INVOLVED IN DEMENTIA

Let us look at each of the different organizations and see where their core responsibilities lie.

The family

We have emphasized previously both the difficulties that face families and the ways in which they can be active in managing the problems of dementia. From their own experience, family members learn not only how to cope with their feelings about the illness but also how to cope in a practical way with memory impairments by inventing memory aids, with restlessness by engaging the patient in useful activity and with poor self-care by filling gaps. Altogether they may become more skilled than many professionals.

Apart from dealing with how they feel and the change in relationship with the sufferer, carers have no role that is specifically laid down as their 'job'. There is no law which states that families must look after elderly or sick relatives, no equivalent to child-care laws. What they take on in the way of care is entirely their *own* choice, and in this they differ from all the professions. Naturally, we hope that families will be loyal and continue to wish to care, but we cannot insist on this. It is tempting for professionals who have chosen the job of caring to criticize those families who decide not to care, even when there are perfectly good reasons for the decision. And it is tempting for the professionals to be so relieved when families *do* choose to cope with the less pleasant aspects of dementia that we let them get on with it without adequate outside help. We should guard against letting families willingly take on unreasonable burdens. Furthermore, we should also be aware that many families feel that they have *not* been given the choice of how much help to provide. The choice has been made for them because of the lack of appropriate outside help. These families need our special attention.

On the other hand, we can be mistaken if we interfere with families who choose to care in rather eccentric ways. Some have rather 'unprofessional' methods of preventing wandering or getting the patient into the bath. Remember that families have no professional training or rules and so make up their own style and rules about how to care. Only if the patient is in danger of being neglected or of coming to harm should we be concerned enough to interfere.

Sharing care

The family's chosen role will overlap with the roles of outside helpers and they should therefore be seen as part of the treatment team. They must be involved in all decisions about how the work of caring is to be divided. In the same way, if they are discussing the division of labour among themselves it is helpful if they bring professionals into the discussions. Sometimes a family will see itself as a team, and share the responsibilities between family members just as a professional team does.

Working together and negotiating responsibilities allows better planning of care and avoids sudden decisions to abdicate responsibility for no good reason. If the family members feel that their responsibilities are too much for them they should be perfectly at liberty to renegotiate their roles.

Remember that if relatives feel that they are as competent as the professionals they may well be critical of what we do and they may not be quite so restrained and unemotional as we are when we criticize our professional colleagues. Sharing care is not always a comfortable experience.

Financial help for carers

Families need more than just recognition by outsiders to enable them to continue in their job of coping. There are inevitable expenses in caring and there may be loss of income if a relative has to give up or cut down hours of work. More and more families are having to pay for services from a variety of agencies if they choose to care at home, though some services continue to be provided free. And an individual situation can be made worse by a sufferer who is outraged at having to pay modern prices when she has forgotten 20 years of inflation.

Attendance allowance or disability living allowance should be granted for any patient who requires regular care. This allowance is in theory given to the patient, who can sometimes mislead the assessor into thinking that she gets and requires no help, so it is important that the family are present at the assessment. An appeal should be made if the application is turned down. *Invalid care allowance*, paid to women who have lost the chance of working because they have chosen to be a carer, and other benefits can also help. *A discount from council tax payments* is also available to dementia sufferers. A benefits advice worker is an essential part of the care team for people with dementia. In some areas there are benefits advice workers specializing in work with families of dementia sufferers; they have discovered many hundreds of thousands of pounds of underpaid and unpaid benefits.

But all of this is small compared to the money that has been spent supporting residents in institutional care. In gradually increasing areas social services funding, which would otherwise have gone towards private residential or nursing home care, has been available for families to buy appropriate care at home, but there is still a general tendency to use money to move people into care. The *Disabled Living Fund* has also provided this type of help on a limited scale, sometimes giving younger individuals large sums to help them survive at home rather than go into care.

There is no guarantee that enough money will ever be made available for the tens of thousands of dementia sufferers who live at home. At the time of writing, the deliberations of a UK Royal Commission on the funding of long-term care for older people have just been published. The Commission recommends that the more 'nursing' aspects of care for those with dementia should be free and paid for by taxes. It remains to be seen whether this approach will be acceptable to government and whether it will shift the balance of care to true care at home.

In Chapter 3 we emphasized changes in family structure which will slowly lessen the number of fit relatives available to help dementia sufferers directly. Planners will have to take this into account in estimating how many families will be able to cope and how many patients can stay 'in the community'.

In recent years various 'charters' have been published – for example for NHS users, for energy users, transport users and the like. We would like to suggest a *Charter for Carers*, outlining what those caring for someone with dementia should be entitled to (Box 11.1).

Box 11.1

Carers have a right to:
- easy access to services
- diagnosis and explanation
- respite care
- full involvement in decision-making
- assessment of the needs of the carer as well as those of the sufferer
- flexibility of care

The 'community'

It is now almost an article of faith in some quarters to say that community care is always better than institutional care. This is dangerous, for some caring institutions have extremely high standards and can avoid the risks of neglect, isolation, abuse and unnecessary distress which are features of bad community care. Anyone who knows anything of what life was like for so-called 'lunatics' before the advent of the 'asylum era' in the 19th century will pause a little before assuming too much about the community and its willingness or ability to care. Nevertheless, there is no doubt that, given the choice, many if not most dementia sufferers would elect to stay in their own homes with support, rather than live in a hospital or care home. If we pay any attention to the wishes of sufferers we must try to support their choice to stay at home, as long as it is not dangerous for them to do so.

In practice the community has usually meant the family, or more precisely the female members of the family, supported to a greater or lesser extent by the primary care team and the home-help service. Gradually, however, voluntary and private organizations with a special interest in dementia are developing. There are also informal community supports which largely go unrecognized. Friends and neighbours of a solitary dementing lady may play a major role in her care by checking that she is safe, by helping with shopping and meals, even sometimes with more intimate aspects of care. If they are heavily involved they deserve recognition just as families do, with the respect of professionals and with financial support if appropriate.

The shopkeeper who keeps a dementing lady's money right for her or prevents her from repeatedly buying the same thing is also involved in her care, as is the policeman who brings her back home when she is lost. They should all be in communication with the more formal carers, so that everybody learns what the true situation is. Churches have a special role to play in visiting, stimulating, providing meetings and clubs. Unfortunately, some churches do not maintain their loyalty to old members who may have stopped attending some years previously or may have fallen out over a new clergyman or unfamiliar music. Neighbourhood wardens and other 'checking-up' schemes are more formal arrangements which can provide reliable community supervision for dementing people at home.

The informal and voluntary network of care is very important, but we cannot expect the amount of care offered informally to increase greatly as the numbers of dementing people increase in the community, and we cannot dictate to informal carers how much help they provide. So, if there is to be a shift from institutional forms of care to more care 'in the community', families and other informal carers who are already stretched to the limit will have to be relieved to a much greater extent by well organized voluntary or professional community supports.

The primary care team

The primary health care team of general practitioner, health visitor and practice nurse, often with other professionals, has a number of responsibilities through the course of dementia. They should be involved in case-finding and accurate diagnosis; in planning care in liaison with family, social services and hospital services; in the support of families; and in the provision of medical and nursing care for patients who live at home.

The GP is the commonest route of referral to hospital services and to community psychiatric nurses. Indeed, some old-age psychiatry services only accept referrals from this source.

Due to a lack of understanding of dementia, or a feeling that it is 'just old age', general practitioners or health visitors may be reluctant to be too involved in case-finding, diagnosis and planning. If this occurs, families are left feeling unsupported and floundering as they try to organize services by themselves. The requirement that GPs (or their representative, often their health visitor) visit all their over 75 year old patients annually will help *that group*, though sadly an assessment does not always include screening tests for dementia.

Many primary care teams have introduced age-sex registers or at-risk registers of the people in their care who are most likely to have problems. Regular visiting, perhaps monthly, and proper assessment of the patients on these registers can go a long way towards foreseeing and preparing suitable care and towards helping families to see where they are going instead of having to 'wait for a crisis'.

General practitioners

It is, unfortunately, true that some carers are disappointed by the service that they get from their GP. Some GPs have not yet realized how important it is that the *diagnosis* of dementia is made and clearly explained. Carers say that the diagnosis helps them by explaining all the changes which they could not understand; they stop blaming old age, they stop blaming the patient and they stop blaming themselves. Furthermore, they see diagnosis as a 'gateway' to services. They may also complain that the GP does not listen to the actual *practical problems* they are coping with and therefore does not understand how desperately they need help.

Some GPs, particularly if they have been qualified for many years, have not had much training about dementia, some do not seem to like referring on to social services or voluntary agencies and a few are still reluctant to see the importance of good communication and liaison between the services. There is urgent need for better education and for continuing education for GPs, and this is quickly being developed. Since most GPs do not have enough time to spend explaining all about dementia to families they should have access to educational literature (p. 262) to give to relatives. Remember that each general practitioner is likely to have no more than 20 elderly dementing patients in his practice (a few of whom will be in care) and no more than one or two younger dementing people. He will see perhaps only three or four *new* sufferers each year.

Health visitors

The health visitor is uniquely placed to find cases of dementia, assist in diagnosis by getting background information, plan services and support families. Ideally the health visitor can be a 'key worker' (p. 267), a contact point for relatives and other professionals. Despite an increasing move towards working with elderly people, many health visitors still see their core job as being with young children and their families, and may have limited training in psychiatry or geriatric medicine. A vigorous campaign of retraining and persuasion is needed to help health visitors fulfil a potentially very useful role.

Nursing services

The district nurse or practice nurse is likely to be involved with specific nursing tasks such as dealing with incontinence, dressings, supervision of medicines or injections. They may be involved with bathing, or there may be specific bathing aides, and they may offer a 'tucking-in' service or, for the severely ill patient, a night nursing service.

The local social services department

Home help

Out of all the helping agencies, the home-care department gives the most valuable help to patients who live at home. Home helps have long included in their 'core' jobs a number of tasks that can help the dementing person – help with shopping, care of the house, cooking, dressing, some laundry. In the past, however, their main job has been with physically disabled people, so supervision, social stimulation, reminiscence and recreation with dementing people have been seen as marginal interests. Now, more and more home helps are being trained and given responsibilities for dementing people and their problems. There is an increasing trend to replace home helps with home-care workers, who as well as carrying out some home-help duties, have a wider role in providing support to those with dementia. Also, in many parts of the country it is being recognized that regular help only in the mornings is insufficient for many patients. A much more flexible home-help service is required, offering evening visits or weekend cover and with the ability to increase cover suddenly in an emergency, if the patient is ill or a relative goes away. Special 'augmented care' schemes with a nursing contribution combined with the home-help service could go a long way towards coping with some of the crises of dementia (see Table 1.4, p. 8).

Social workers

The social worker is often the first point of contact when specific problems arise.

Care managers are involved in assessing the needs of individuals who are identified as requiring community care and who may need financial assessment to provide it. It is most likely that the primary health care team will be the main identifiers, but there is no guarantee that everybody with dementia will be brought to their attention. The numbers of sufferers are so great, and the tendency to deny or hide the condition still so strong among both sufferers and carers, that we would be right to remain sceptical. And, if funds are limited, there will have to be some selection of who gets the help, even if it is available. Despite these problems, the care management responsibility creates a clearer core to social workers' roles with older people. There is anyway a growing trend of *specialization* within social-work departments, and workers with a special interest in the elderly are more likely to develop a clear 'core' job and gain more satisfaction, as well as providing a much better quality of service. In departments which do not have such specialization, emergencies such as child-abuse cases and legal problems often relegate the problems of older people to a poor second best.

Social workers deal with problems of finance, housing, benefits, family problems (including complaints of poor care or abuse) and the organization and planning of care in the community or in residential or nursing homes. Specialized, *approved social workers* or *mental health officers* have a specific job in relation to the arrangements for compulsory guardianship or hospital admission under the Mental Health Act. Any developments of 'advocacy' (p. 302) for the dementing would be likely to create a further specific role, as would the transfer of child-abuse practices to the elderly who are being abused (p. 290).

Unfortunately, the subject of dementia is absent or underplayed in many social work training courses. This is an unforgivable gap which needs to be filled urgently. Qualified social workers also need to gain more knowledge and understanding of dementia through in-service training.

Occupational therapists

The core responsibility of the community OT is mainly concerned with the assessment of 'activities of daily living', including dressing, washing, bathing, toileting, as well as recreational activities, and with the provision of suitable aids and adaptations. Occupational therapists need training with regard to dementia, for they must assess the patient's mental state as well as her physical deficits in order to know whether she will be able to make proper use of any aids.

Voluntary services

The title 'voluntary body' covers a vast range of different types of service. Some are small local organizations running one specific service, some are nationwide bodies offering a wide range of services, others lie between these extremes. Some are involved with the care of patients, others with the support of relatives, others act as pressure groups. Some use paid staff to provide their services, some use volunteers and some use both. Some are partially funded by the health or social services, some are completely self-financing. Some run in parallel, offering identical types of service to those offered by health or social services, some offer completely different or innovative services.

Filling gaps. For dementia sufferers and their families the voluntary bodies come into their own when they fill the gaps left by the public services, either a gap of quantity in a service or the complete absence of a particular sort of service. Voluntary groups, being less stuck in a world of cash limits and the bureaucratic delays of large organizations, can often bring new ideas into practice more quickly. Thus many of the gaps in community care, such as in transport services, sitting services, night cover, small day centres for dementia sufferers, counselling services, helplines, relatives' support groups and public education have been filled locally by the initiative of voluntary bodies.

Finance. Most of these projects need considerable sums of money, because a paid organizer and payments for staff are needed to keep them going, and to pay for premises. This, unfortunately, means that organizations have to spend much of their effort on fund-raising, be it in making applications to charitable trusts, local social work or health service funds, government agencies or industry, or even from street collections.

Continuity of support. The greatest problem for small voluntary community care projects is to keep up the impetus, especially if volunteer helpers are being used. Support, training and even supervision by established social work or health service teams, or individual professionals, can help considerably as long as it is not seen as interference – above all, voluntary bodies value, and need, their independence.

Counselling and relatives' support groups

Voluntary organizations are increasingly providing help to individual carers who are struggling with the burden of their task. An experienced carer can help a 'new' carer in many ways that are not available to even the best trained social worker or community psychiatric nurse. They may become the key worker for a family, and in the future it is likely that this type of role will be extended, so that a representative of the voluntary organization could act as the patient's or relative's *advocate*.

Support groups are usually run by local branches of national organizations such as the Alzheimer's Society, Age Concern and the Huntington's Chorea Society, or they may be organized by a local voluntary organization. They can be specially useful because more time can be given than most professionals can offer, because special understanding and knowledge is built up, because other relatives share experience (p. 263) and because the organizations are seen to be independent of health and social services. Voluntary organizations can thus both know and keep in good communication with the statutory services, while at the same time listening to complaints or disappointments about services and giving advice about how to get a better deal. Such groups can become quite 'political' at times, campaigning effectively for improvements in local services or providing a local 'carers' panel' which can look at and comment on health or social-service plans.

Helplines

Carers often feel that they need to talk to someone when the strain of caring is greatest. They may feel shy of asking for help from their GP or social services department for a variety of reasons. They may not even know what help they could be asking for. For these and other reasons a *Helpline*, organized by the local Alzheimer's association and manned by volunteers, if possible offering a 24-hour service, can be invaluable. It can also help by bringing together the nucleus of a new neighbourhood support group.

Education

Carers' guides and explanatory information leaflets on local services are invaluable to anybody who is trying to find their way through complicated systems of care. Helplines or local Alzheimer's groups point callers to where this information can be found. Television, radio and newspaper advertising bring the information to wider attention. Specific carer education groups may be provided.

Meals on wheels

This service is of great importance for dementing people whose time sense is faulty and who are in danger of neglecting themselves. A little extra supervision is required, however, since all too often the meal is forgotten about, stored in a cupboard, thrown away or given to the cat.

Transport services

Transport services are vital in the care of dementia, because of the patient's lack of motivation, poor geographical sense and poor sense of time. Voluntary transport to outpatient clinics, to day-care centres or for outings and visiting relatives contributes towards helping dementing people keep in touch with the outside world.

Sitting services

A volunteer or paid sitter stays with the patient for a few hours to offer stimulation, companionship and activity and to allow relatives a break for shopping or recreation. The sitter gives supervision but not a home-help service. Sitting services can also provide useful stimulation and orientation for dementing people who live alone. *Night sitting* can be very helpful if the patient tends to be restless, though, as in day sitting, the presence of a stranger in the house can occasionally be disturbing. *Tucking-in* refers to a visit to the patient during the evening to ensure that she goes to bed safely and at an appropriate time.

Day centres

Local specialist day-centre provision for dementia sufferers is an ideal project for a voluntary organization. Centres like this are very popular with patients and carers alike and are now multiplying very rapidly. The day centre may be open for anything from one to seven days each week, perhaps including evenings, and usually six to ten patients attend at a time. One or two paid organizers with volunteers can run an effective service and may be able to provide one-to-one attention to the attenders. This allows the centre to offer a very imaginative and personalized range of activities which is usually not available in a large day centre or day hospital. Being local, the problems of transport are lessened and patients may be less reluctant to attend.

Respite and residential care

Some of the older established voluntary organizations have provided residential care for many years, but in recent times there has been a steady growth of interest in specialist residential care for dementia sufferers, including respite care. Again, voluntary organizations are in a good position to experiment and be innovative, as well as filling the gaps left by health and social services.

The care environment and dementia

Ideally, as we have seen, someone with dementia should be looked after in the place most familiar to her. In other words, she should be in her own home where she wishes to be so, and where it is possible. Often, because of increasing dependence, behavioural problems, lack of available carers, or for other reasons another care setting must be utilized. There is no *ideal* model of care. Often a particular setting may be appropriate for one person but totally unsuitable for another. Thankfully the old days of massive and non-personal institutions are largely behind us.

Many different factors must be taken into account in deciding where someone's needs can best be met, particularly since it is likely that the nursing home or other placement is where she will spend the rest of her life. Choosing the best place is a process which should involve all those concerned with care. As well as the person herself, this means that family, other carers, the local social services department and anyone else involved should be consulted. It is also good practice for the carers from any proposed establishment to meet with the person with dementia as well as with her family prior to any move, to make sure the person's needs can be met by them, and to get to know her.

Behaviour difficulties, as we have seen, are related to the environment as well as to the effects of dementia itself (p. 166). The care environment should strive to be such that it minimizes problems for the patient. There are a number of issues which must be addressed.

Size of establishment

There is no ideal number of places in a group-living setting. Traditional hospital wards often have around 30 places, and many units are built with this figure in mind, with larger placements subdivided to reach this number. In general it is probably better to look after people in small groups of about six. This allows the person with dementia to develop familiarity with the layout, with her fellow-residents, and with the carers (this works both ways). Rooms such as the dining area and toilet should be easily accessible and easily identified.

Residents should ideally have their own bedrooms. This allows greater use of their own furniture, and also allows private space for themselves and for visitors. Where possible, residents should have their own keys, emphasizing *ownership*. Having name plates on doors and using different colours of doors also increases the sense of personal ownership.

Site

Residential and nursing homes should not be isolated from the rest of the world. A resident with mental impairment will value continuing contact with her old home, neighbourhood, family and acquaintances. This will only be possible if her new home is within her local community, with a view onto familiar scenes if possible, and easy access to local and familiar roads and shops, etc. The idea that residents are more in danger of 'wandering' if they have access to familiar scenes is the opposite of good care.

Staffing levels

Much care of older people is run as a business. This applies not only to homes in the private sector, but also to local authority and health service facilities. Budgets are tight and staff costs are the major financial outlay. For these reasons the levels of staffing are usually determined by resources rather than by need. Lower-paid care assistants often have a difficult and demanding job, and may be on short-term contracts. This often leads to poor morale and therefore high staff turnover, which then impinges on the quality of care. Training of staff, conducted in a regular and continuing way, can help increase morale and job satisfaction, as does good management support.

Noise and light

Unexplained background noise can upset any of us, and can cause us to become agitated. The person with dementia is no different in this respect, except that noise is more likely to be inexplicable because of mental impairment. Door alarms and various buzzers can produce much unsettling noise, as can the background noise from television or radio. It is, unfortunately, still all too common to see residents grouped round a television, on at high volume, with no one actually watching or listening to it. This stilts normal conversation, and staff and visitors as well as residents may need to speak with raised voices to make themselves heard, adding to the din. It often seems that in modern society if an area is empty of noise, we must fill it!

Likewise, it is important to have adequate lighting levels in a unit, but this does not mean having very brightly lit, clinical-looking areas. As near as possible the lighting should be that of a well-lit family home.

Activities

The attention span and interest level of someone with dementia are often reduced. However, this is no excuse for failing to engage people in some form of appropriate activity, for example, discussion groups, games, singing or even simply sitting chatting. Involving people in activities such as these can often reduce boredom and agitation in all members of the community – not only residents.

Locked doors

In looking after people with dementia, a balance must always be struck between independence and choice on the one hand, and risks on the other. Some facilities have a locked-door policy so that residents are unable to come and go as they choose. People who wander, especially where the wandering is aimless or searching, will often be found trying to leave a building. Where this is a deliberate attempt to get out, there are issues around the use of restraint such as locked doors – should Mental Health legislation be utilized? (p. 288). Many people who are described as being aggressive in fact only become agitated when attempts are made to stop them leaving.

Exit doors to premises should not be at the end of a corridor. If they are, we see situations, all too commonly, where someone stands constantly at a door rattling the handle. Doors in the middle of a wall are less likely to be recognized as being the 'way out'. 'Baffle locks' (e.g. where two handles must be turned to allow opening) or electronic means of unlocking, allow access to those who are able, but at the same time are difficult to go through for people with cognitive impairment. On the other hand, use of doors locked by a key can make staff appear as jailers to residents and indeed to visitors, and we must think about whether residents are being detained without considering their rights.

Institutionalization

As long ago as 1961 a man called Goffman described the main features of institutions which looked after long-stay psychiatric patients. These were:

1. All social functions carried out in the one environment ('batch living')
2. A highly regulated daily routine
3. Loss of usual social roles
4. Rigid rules of social distance between staff and patients
5. Nurses as gatekeepers of access to care and to all other aspects of life
6. Progressive loss of autonomy (independence and choice).

These features result in institutionalization, with residents' time being spent staring blankly into space or lying in bed, avoiding any form of stimulating activity, and general apathy.

Sadly, some of these features are still present today in many hospitals and care homes. We must make care settings as homely and care as personalized and engaging as possible, to avoid these *secondary handicaps*.

Sheltered housing

The core responsibilities of sheltered housing schemes usually have little or no link with dementia. Yet, inevitably, there are a few dementia sufferers in each scheme. Wardens need to know how to cope with their problems and how to educate other residents to help. Dementing residents should not as a rule be segregated from 'normal' people. So the non-demented also need training and advice in how to communicate with and help their dementing neighbours, who may be forgetful, disorientated in time, wandering or distressed. Dementia will, however, inevitably mean for some that they must leave sheltered housing. Contracts of tenancy and collaboration with social work and health services should be such that a transfer to fuller care is relatively easy if it becomes necessary, but such that residents are not put out just because they are beginning to develop mild dementia. In general, sheltered housing schemes have to accept more dementia in their residents than is assumed in the 'core' job.

Options

Some organizations have their own residential or nursing homes to which people can be transferred, some even on the same site (a 'geriatric campus'). Others are developing *extra care housing* for more disabled people, including dementing patients. Here a small group of residents, maybe six or eight, lives in a unit with individual bed-sitting rooms and communal living space supervised more closely than in ordinary sheltered housing, in a design which allows good observation and an enclosed 'wandering' space in a garden or courtyard. The concept is not far from that of a good 'EMI' home (p. 373), yet the patient still has her 'own house'. Staff for such a unit may come from the housing agency or may be jointly funded from health, social services or other agencies.

Day centres

These are usually run by the social services department or by a voluntary organization. We have already mentioned small local day centres organized especially for dementing patients. These have been developed partly because larger day centres are not usually organized to cope with dementia. The core of the large day centre's work concerns older people who wish to meet other people and engage in activities. It is assumed that they will be able to select their friends and select their activities, will take an active part in what goes on and, in most cases, make their own way to and from the centre.

Dementia

As in every other service, day centres have had to take more than their fair share of dementia sufferers and their functions overlap with those of the day hospitals. There is a danger that non-demented attenders ostracize or ignore the dementing, and this is made worse if staff do not have time to break the ice, encourage dementing members to get involved and encourage the non-dementing to learn how to cope with forgetfulness and not be frightened by it. Although it is true that, with good supervision, a day centre can cope with a minority of mildly demented attenders, most find that it is not possible for them to cope with a large number, or even with more than one or two severely demented people.

On the other hand, day *hospital* care is not necessary for patients who have been assessed and whose main needs are now relief for the relative and stimulation and activity for the patient. Thus the need for specialist *day centres* to cater for dementia sufferers. In country districts such specialization is more difficult. A more all-embracing approach to day care is needed, with the fit, the physically disabled and the mentally impaired attending together, and involving a mix of services.

Private care

Care at home

Like the voluntary sector, the private sector of care has, to some extent, grown to fill gaps left by the public services. Private help in the house, including domestic help, sitting services, nursing services, bathing services and live-in help, can maintain a dementing person at home for long periods and has always been a possibility for rich people. In the new community care legislation in Britain it is hoped that providing grants to allow the less well-off to buy such private care will go a long way to allowing dementia sufferers and other disabled people to stay in their own homes and so lessen the load on the public service institutions. However, it should be remembered that many of the helpers involved in private care are untrained and unsupervised, though proper supervision is possible in larger organizations. Registration and inspection of organizations which provide private help at home are vital in order to protect both the vulnerable dementing clients and the organizations.

Residential and nursing-home care

The number of private homes has greatly increased in the past 10 years or so. Though there has been some increase in the number of private *residential* homes, by far the larger increase has been in private *nursing* homes. This is very much a growth industry, and in common with other industries there is a tendency for bigger and more efficient companies to buy over others. Not so long ago most homes were small or family-run homes. However, more and more homes are part of large companies. These companies often own homes throughout the country and there are now many organizations which run 50 or more homes. The advantages of this are of standardized care, in providing staff training and providing modern purpose-built premises; but as with any large organization it is easier to lose sight of the individual staff member or individual resident.

Planning the site and size of homes tends to be left to discussion between the home owners and the local authority planning committees. There is all too rarely coordination with the health and social services. The concept of the catchment area, so central to planning and providing services based on people's needs, is missing in most cases. Some homes are converted large mansions which may not provide well for the supervision and physical needs of dementia sufferers. Some are large institutions which simply replace the old hospitals with new. In some areas contracts between Health Authorities and private organizations to provide care are allowing better planning and closer links with a catchment area than were provided by the old psychiatric hospitals, but the future of such arrangements is not always clear.

In the past, the private sector has been criticized for poor care, and nursing homes are often seen as fair game by the press when care is perceived to fall short. However, in most homes care is provided by well-motivated staff, and homes are well scrutinized by local inspection teams.

Unfortunately, some homes still do not offer much in the way of socializing activity, rehabilitation or recreation. This is slowly improving, and the best homes can offer services far better than those provided by impoverished and rigid public services.

Relation to other services

Private care can sometimes be unsatisfactory. It can also be very good. Looked at in relation to core and overlap, we see a very diverse set of organizations which have usually decided their core job without consulting with other services, although they are aware of the gaps. The chosen core may be quite general and vague. Some homes are 'nursing' homes, other 'residential', some accept 'confused' residents or 'psychogeriatric' cases, others do not.

By setting admission criteria in isolation, a private home can feel satisfied with the care it provides and may be satisfying its existing customers, but it may not be providing the range and quantity of services that are actually required by its surrounding catchment area. In particular, it may not be listening to the wishes of the dementia sufferers themselves, whose main priority may be to stay on in their own homes. Home-support services are inevitably more complicated to run and not easy to make a profit from. The public and private sectors will both be better served by good communication and joint planning so that private care can fill the real gaps in a coordinated manner and without any suggestion that profit might be coming before patients' real needs and wishes.

Medical input to homes can be very patchy. In considering this we must remember that many of the residents in these homes would in days gone by be in long-stay hospitals, under consultant care. Those in private homes are looked after by GPs. The most satisfactory arrangement is where a GP is contracted in some way by the home to provide general medical services. The GP can then be a part of the team providing care. Often, however, care is provided only where a problem is identified by care staff, so it is 'crisis driven'; the doctor only sees patients when necessary, rather than routinely. Homes also need to be able to get advice from more specialist services (consultant psychiatrist, geriatrician, psychologist, speech therapist, psychiatric nurse specialist, etc.) either directly or through the general practitioner. Residents should have access to specialist help at least as easily as those living in their own homes.

Local authority and voluntary sector residential care

The core functions of residential homes are laid down in Part III of the Social Work Act (Part IV in Scotland). Thus the commonly used terms 'Part III' and 'Part IV' homes. They were set up to provide a general sort of care for people who are not too severely disabled, but they were not designed to provide specialized nursing care.

Changes of population in residential care

Several changes have forced homes away from their core responsibilities. First is the increase in the very elderly population, especially of those who live alone and those who suffer multiple handicaps. When such a person's social situation breaks down, and hospital care is not required, residential care is often the only alternative. Secondly, the development of community care and sheltered housing have meant that potential mildly disabled residents are coping longer at home. Thirdly, the scarcity of special homes for dementia sufferers and of hospital beds has ensured that a high proportion of residents in homes are dementing. In many places 60–70% of residents suffer dementia. Some homes also arrange respite admissions and many of these short-stay residents are dementing. This change in population takes homes far away from their original purpose. The minority who are not dementing have great difficulty in coping with the dementing majority, whereas they could be involved in helping them. Staff have not until recently been trained in understanding dementia. The homes have not been provided with memory aids, with enough staff for supervision or with suitable activity programmes.

The core of the residential home's job has been largely destroyed. And the huge overlap with the responsibilities of hospitals or nursing homes has been unwelcome. The result is widespread dissatisfaction.

Options

There are a few options for the future. The homes could accept the change and learn to live with dementia. This is logical, but special training and more staff would be needed and the non-dementing residents would still have problems in coping with a dementing majority. Homes could accept the greater disability of residents more easily by bringing in more nursing staff, having closer links with health services and being more ready to exchange patients for whom they can no longer care. Or they could segregate the dementing and non-dementing, or even collect together residents from a number of homes to establish a proper home for dementia, as has been done in some areas.

Many geriatric hospitals developed out of a forced change in the function of obsolete fever or tuberculosis hospitals. Perhaps a similar change will occur in the residential-care system. In the meantime, the staff of homes need expert knowledge of dementia. They need to organize homes in a way that fills the gaps for dementia sufferers. They need activities that are orientating, stimulate reminiscence or retrain social behaviour and encourage self-caring. And they need expert knowledge of the other health problems that dementing people may suffer.

Homes for the elderly mentally infirm (EMI)

EMI homes may be run by the social work department, health service, voluntary or private organizations and go under a variety of names including Domus units, NHS nursing homes or continuing-care homes. They are set up specifically to care for dementia sufferers and particularly those who fall into the large gaps between the core responsibilities of sheltered housing, ordinary care homes and hospital care. The true EMI home is locally based and has day-care and respite-care facilities, as well as providing longer-term care for people from the surrounding catchment area. It allows privacy and some degree of independence and a normal life-style for residents, while offering a simple, well designed and well signposted environment. Its staff encourage orientation and engage the patient socially in appropriate and stimulating activities. The home should have a large enclosed or easily observed area for free movement, and a safe garden for walking in. Living areas should be visible from where staff are likely to be so that the staff do not have to pursue residents who are walking around. Various bodies have recommended the development of more EMI homes; unfortunately, they are few in number as yet.

Advantages. Such homes avoid the difficulties of getting dementing and non-dementing people to live together. They provide specific activities to help reminiscence and reality orientation. However, a good EMI home depends crucially on having sufficient supervising staff to ensure good standards of personal care and stimulation, and on these staff maintaining enthusiasm and commitment. Staff in-service training and regular meetings with relatives who continue to be involved in the residents' care can help enormously. Regular contact, supervision and exchanges from the old-age psychiatry or geriatric services are essential.

General hospitals

There are many reasons why dementing patients come to the general hospital, some more related to their dementia than others. Planned operations and unconnected medical conditions are often dealt with without a great deal of trouble. But it is the problems that are more connected with their dementia that prove difficult to treat. Accidents in the home or outdoors, including burns and fractures, infections or constipation due to self-neglect, funny turns and small strokes in VaD, superimposed delirium due to minor medical illness, drug side-effects or a change in social circumstances in an already frail patient – these can all lead to admission becoming essential.

'Bed blockers'

Many staff in general hospitals feel that these problems are not part of their core jobs, and they dismiss the idea that being unable to cope at home because of illness brings a dementing patient within their responsibility. This sort of feeling is aggravated by the fact that in many cases the immediate cause of admission is either untreatable or else very quickly remediable, leaving a patient with dementia who is unable to go home. Furthermore, the patient may be disorientated away from her familiar surroundings (p. 93). She quickly loses touch with home and with her tasks of daily living, the unstimulating ward environment encourages withdrawal (p. 229), and the family, neighbours and general practice agree that she cannot possibly manage again at home. A long wait for alternative accommodation completes the dissatisfaction of the general hospital staff, especially if the patient is disturbed in any way.

To some extent, the hospitals are victims of the 'balance of admission policies' as well as the 'balance of services', for not only do patients sometimes get admitted to a general hospital because of an absence of other services, but it is also true that it is still relatively easy to get into a general hospital, compared to admission to residential homes, geriatric or old-age psychiatric wards, which have developed longer assessment procedures and strict admission criteria to try to avoid misplacement.

Options

Once again, there are a number of options for the general hospitals. They could move towards a 'geriatric' style of working, using home visits, day care, more multidisciplinary work and better liaison with the primary care team, but this would mean a big shift in their core responsibility. They could give over responsibility for some elderly patients with less acute medical problems to geriatricians, as happens in some areas. Or they could hand over responsibility for all patients over a certain age to the care of geriatricians, as happens in other areas. Inevitably, this implies a transfer of staff and beds. Whatever happens it will be impossible, like it or not, for general hospitals to avoid ever having to deal with dementing people.

The geriatric service

Geriatric services arose because some doctors saw that elderly physically ill patients very often require a different sort of medical care from that required by younger adults. Services including home visiting, day care, multidisciplinary assessment, rehabilitation, attention to the social and family needs of patients, strong links with the community have developed everywhere. Inevitably, large numbers of medical geriatric patients suffer from dementia. As a 'core' responsibility, geriatric services should look after dementing patients if they also have a major medical problem or need physical nursing care, but they should not have to deal with those whose main problems are behavioural and who are physically fit. Nor should they have to cope with patients who are neither very disturbed nor very physically disabled. These other groups are the responsibility of the old-age psychiatry services and of residential or community services respectively.

Defining clear boundaries between the different 'core' responsibilities is difficult and there are large grey areas. This does not matter so much where there is adequate provision of the various services so that tolerance is possible and transfers between the services easy. And it matters less if specialist EMI homes for dementia sufferers are readily available, so the balance of services is important. In areas where provision is not so good, admission policy becomes more crucial. The result is that geriatric services vary quite a lot in the number of dementing patients they deal with. But dementia remains one of the principal illnesses of geriatric medicine and appropriate training of staff and appropriate activities in day- and in-patient care are necessary.

The geriatrician. This specially trained doctor can be expected to be an expert in dementia as well as in the medical illnesses of old age, and much of his work overlaps with that of the old-age psychiatrist. A special role for the geriatrician is in assessing difficult medical problems in patients in the old-age psychiatry service, while in return the psychiatrist can assess difficult psychiatric problems in the medical geriatric patients. This requires good *liaison* between the two services and regular meetings to discuss problem patients. If liaison exists it can also ease transfer of patients between the two services and reduce misplacement. Liaison works best if the two services are sited in the same hospital or if, as in a few places, they have 'joint' beds.

General psychiatric services

The development of old-age psychiatry services has gradually taken most of the burden of dementia away from general psychiatric wards. Services vary, however, in deciding who is to be responsible for the elderly who are not dementing. Most active old-age psychiatry teams see dealing with patients suffering from depression, schizophrenia or other 'functional' problems as an important part of their responsibility, but not all general psychiatrists agree with this view, especially where 'younger' old people are concerned.

'Presenile' patients. One of the worst gaps in service provision relates to dementing patients aged under 65 – the 'presenile' group (p. 11). Most old-age psychiatry services accept some responsibility for these patients, but the active young person in her 40s who suffers dementia can feel and look very out of place in a old-age psychiatry ward or day hospital, and the young patient with permanent brain damage after an accident, illness or operation poses slightly different problems of care (p. 53). The result is that younger patients do not usually get a good deal. They do not quite fit into any form of day care, they are not very welcome in general psychiatric wards and are somehow out of place in the old-age psychiatry service. In addition, there may not be enough of them in an area to set up a specialized service. The support of the Alzheimer's societies has been invaluable for the relatives of these patients, advising on how to obtain care and helping to organize it. In one or two city areas, special day centres for early onset sufferers are being set up by Alzheimer's organizations and these are beginning to provide for this unhappy group of sufferers and their carers.

The old-age psychiatry service

Old-age psychiatry is a recently developed speciality. Previously, older people were looked after by consultants with no specific training in dealing with those problems (such as dementia) which are mainly those of old age. However, most services have developed rapidly and are moving into a positive, mainly community-based, way of working. The elements of a fully developed old-age psychiatry service are:

1. A defined *catchment area* and *age limit* – these allow accurate assessment of the needs of the area and good liaison with community-based services.

2. *Home visits* for assessment at the request of the primary care team or social services department, carried out by the consultant or other members of the team – this allows a quick response, better assessment of family and home circumstances and better rapport with the patient and family; it allows difficult situations to be defused quickly without the need for admission that would occur if the patient had been sent directly to hospital.

3. *Outpatient facilities* or a memory clinic allowing physical investigation, if possible with a medical geriatrician in attendance, and access to more sophisticated investigations.

4. A *day hospital* or hospitals placed within easy reach of all potential attenders in the catchment area – the day hospital offers relief for relatives and stimulation and activity for the patients, but 'day care' should not be its sole or main function. Assessment, problem-solving, medical and psychiatric treatment, physical nursing care, rehabilitation, retraining,

planning care and family support are the core functions of the day hospital. Each patient should be assessed by members of the multidisciplinary team and a treatment programme decided in conference. Staff can keep in good contact with relatives by going out with transport, by 'phone and by special meetings. The function of a day hospital should be totally separate from that of the day *care* provided by social services or voluntary agencies.

5. An *assessment ward*, where patients can be admitted for diagnosis if that has been difficult, for assessment and management of particular problems, or for assessment of what type of long-term care is appropriate – as home and day hospital assessment has been more developed and as respite care has become more common the need for assessment admissions has gradually lessened.

6. *Relief admission* when a family cannot cope or the social situation has changed and *regular planned respite admissions* at an agreed interval – these may be to the assessment ward, a long-stay ward or, better still, to a special, small respite-care ward. In many services the concept of a *shared bed* is now commonly used. A number of patients take the bed for 2-week stays in rotation, allowing relatives to plan breaks regularly and well in advance. The family are expected to agree before respite admissions that they are prepared to take the patient back. If they do not agree the nature of the admission is changed and a 'respite bed' should not be used.

7. *Long-stay wards* – patients only need to remain in psychiatric long-stay wards while they are agitated, aggressive or otherwise disturbed. There should be movement between old-age psychiatry and geriatric long-stay wards, and from both to residential homes, nursing homes and family care. Long-term care should not inevitably mean care for life. It should, however, be as near as possible to the standards of normality. Stimulation, compensation for losses and the good staffing levels and practices mentioned in relation to EMI homes are important if long-stay wards are to be for more than simple basic care and containment of patients.

The old-age psychiatry team

This usually consists of medical staff, nursing staff including community psychiatric nurses, clinical psychologists, social workers, occupational therapists, physiotherapists and access to a speech therapist, chiropody, dental and other services. In relation to dementia the team has a very wide responsibility in diagnosis, assessment, management and planning care, in liaison with other services, in support of relatives, and in spreading knowledge about dementia locally. Many of these functions can be shared between members of the team, so regular team meetings and a division of labour with overlaps are essential, while each member of the team retains his or her 'core' responsibility.

Medical staff have prime responsibility for diagnosis, general medical care and prescription of drugs. The consultant is often in the chair at team meetings and has a major task in ensuring a fair distribution of labour within the team. The consultant may also be the first person to see the patient and directs the general course of her treatment. Junior medical staff, as well as examining patients from the psychiatric point of view, have responsibilities in the investigation and treatment of physical illness, requesting help from their medical geriatric colleagues if appropriate.

Nursing staff have the day-to-day responsibility for both psychiatric and physical care for the patients, carrying out nursing procedures to do with personal care, drug administration and specific behaviour programmes. Nurses spend most time with the patients and have a major task in observing and reporting how the patient behaves from day to day. They should be the experts on knowing how to interact with each individual patient, knowing about her interests, her personality and her current problems in great detail. This style should be reflected in the patient's care plan, which should get nurses more and more away from rigid bathing rounds and regimented regimes and towards personal care of individual patients.

The community psychiatric nurse (CPN) has the core task of linking with community services, assessing and supervising patients at home and providing psychiatric nursing advice to families and other carers. They may give advice and support to residential and nursing homes and be closely involved in setting up and supporting a variety of projects in the community, such as sitting services, night care and day centres. The traditional model is that the CPN is part of the psychiatric team, usually consultant-led. In some areas this has changed, the CPN being directly attached to individual GP practices. There are pros and cons associated with both models, but it is important in the latter model that CPNs do not become isolated from their colleagues, and that they do not lose their wider community role.

The clinical psychologist is an expert in psychological testing to aid diagnosis or assess the patient's losses and in the preparation and carrying out of behaviour modification programmes.

The social worker's principal task is in assessing individual community care needs and ensuring that these are met. He has a particular role in finding accommodation for patients, in dealing with housing and financial problems and in relation to the Mental Health Act. Social workers are also specially involved where family problems arise.

The occupational therapist (OT) assesses specific abilities in the tasks of daily living and provides advice, training and aids to patients who are at home or are going home, and to their families. OTs are also involved in the therapeutic and recreational programme of the patients as a group.

The physiotherapist has a central role of maintaining the failing mobility and physical strength of the severely demented and has to cope with the aftermath of the injuries which unfortunately are common, as dementing patients may be less able to anticipate risk, especially those who are apt to wander.

These descriptions give the bare bones of jobs within the team. Actual responsibilities are much wider. For example, helping families, liaising with community services and planning of care can be carried out by all or any of the team. In some teams, a key worker is delegated to take primary responsibility for a particular case.

There are dangers in any team system – duplication of work, with several members carrying out an almost identical assessment – concentrating multiple efforts on an 'interesting' patient while all ignore the more routine tasks – barriers being erected between the professions out of suspicion or pride – and the opposite, a woolly overlapping of roles with no one getting on with their core responsibilities.

There is a further danger to which all professional groups are prone. As a profession develops its particular skills, particularly assessment skills, there is a danger that they wish to leave to others the 'dirty work' of actually carrying out management. If this happens, the real care of the patients is passed on either to the other professions (who resent it) or to helpers, volunteers, auxiliaries or families. Each profession needs to accept some drudgery as well as what they see as their core skill.

If these dangers are minimized teamwork is stimulating, each profession supporting the other and bringing together their differing views of a particular problem. This allows an illness like dementia with its multiple problems to be tackled comprehensively in one setting without the need for the patient or her family to be referred from one profession to another and from one place to another.

SEGREGATION OR INTEGRATION

Throughout all these descriptions of services a question arises. Should dementia sufferers be housed, helped or treated alongside 'normal' elderly people, or should they be treated separately in specialized dementia services? Different services come to different conclusions about this, but it is essential that the question is addressed. Segregated services for dementia can pay special attention to the particular needs of sufferers and can develop special activities and programmes of care. They can avoid the intolerance which sufferers can attract from the non-demented. They can allow 'general' services to cater better for the particular needs of other elderly people. However, if they are not well funded or well staffed, and if staff do not have sufficient training and support, they can become second-rate, as the 'segregated' long-stay wards of old psychiatric hospitals were for years. There have even been fears that they could attract interest and funds away from general services, though this complaint sounds hollow to those who have fought for years for *any* adequate funding for dementia services.

The question must be answered locally by each organization and each profession. However, a mixed answer is probably best – people with mild dementia should not necessarily be segregated unless it is to their advantage, while those with severe dementia, and particularly those with a severe behaviour problem, will benefit from specialist attention. A 'general' service which has more than a certain minority of dementia sufferers (some have suggested that up to 30% is acceptable in residential care) can cope, but above that needs to look for some segregation; good specialist services are extremely helpful to most patients, but not to all, and bad specialist services are the worst of all possible worlds.

COORDINATING CARE

What particularly strikes relatives when they first come across the services and professions available to help is their profusion and complexity. Some services are in one place, others in another place, some professions work in isolation, others work in teams. What is worse, some services have to be paid for, others not. Relatives cannot be expected to know all the ins and outs of the system or systems. For that matter, by no means all professionals or voluntary workers know who does what, who runs what or how the different organizations work! We have seen a number of different tasks that need to be carried out with the help of professionals – diagnosis, medical care, problem identification and solving, supervision, help with daily living, activity, respite and relief for relatives, admission for care. How are families to be helped in asking for this and in planning for the future? How are professionals to avoid unnecessary overlaps, repetition of work, gaps in care and mutual suspicion?

Education

Information on local services for dementia should be simply and readily available. The simplest way is for a local 'fact sheet' to be inserted as an appendix to one of the voluntary organizations' carers' guides. Staff from the various services should be able to meet from time to time to learn how each others' services work.

Contact point

In dealing with complicated organizations it is best if the 'customers' have a particular person (or persons) whom they know they can contact, who understands what is happening and who can communicate with all the other services involved. This key person may be the general practitioner, health visitor, community psychiatric nurse, social worker, someone from a voluntary organization or the staff of a day hospital or in institutional care. Such a system works informally, but if it is to be formal all the local groups concerned must agree to it in conference.

Communication between services

The value of case conferences has already been discussed (p. 294), but there is a more general reason why decisions ought not to be made by one organization or one person in isolation. The delicate balances that exist between the services require regular contact and communication. Anyone who makes decisions or tries to run a service in isolation from the rest of the system can become suspicious of others, or may have unrealistic ideas of what his or her own service can do. Such people come to believe that others are trying to palm off unwanted patients on to their service, or they believe that their service is better than others and therefore do not ask for help or advice when they need it. They may even believe both at the same time. They are likely also to become the object of suspicion from other services.

Seeing both the strengths and weaknesses of other services and seeing the difficulties that everybody faces in having to cope with jobs that are not in their 'core' responsibility can do much to lessen suspicion and help a more coordinated approach. The best communication like this occurs when organizations actually plan together and when staff train together or even exchange jobs for a while across services.

Towards a dementia team

The ideal extension of this better communication and decision-making is the formation of a local dementia team. At its simplest the people who make decisions in the various professions and organizations in one area can meet together to find out how each is getting on with particular patients and to make some joint decisions about what services should be offered (a *liaison* or *network meeting* – Box 11.2). Referrals between services can be made at such a meeting and the results of referrals reported back. In this way, the old-age psychiatry team, the local social services and home-care teams, the primary-care team and local voluntary

---

Box 11.2 A monthly community old-age psychiatry liaison meeting (members will differ in different areas)

Social services area team members
Social workers specializing in the care of the elderly
Home care organizers
Day centre staff

Primary health care
Health visitors

Voluntary agency representatives
Alzheimer's society representative
Local sitting service coordinator
Coordinator of local day centre for dementia

Old age psychiatry team members
Consultant psychiatrist
Community psychiatric nurses
Day hospital staff
Hospital social worker

The monthly meeting lasts 1–1.5 hours
25–50 patients are discussed, from a social work team area, population 5000 people aged over 65
70% of the patients discussed suffer from dementia

Benefits of liaison meetings
● Information on patients and their problems brought to each other's attention
● Concern about risks and other problems is shared
● Care can be better planned and coordinated
● Patients can be referred between services
● Staff of one service get to know more about other services
● New developments can be discussed and encouraged

---

bodies can keep an eye on problems arising in the community. Meetings may take place in the social-work office, in the hospital or in the health centre. They may lead on to the development of a local *dementia register*. A more comprehensive approach would include those who run local residential and hospital care as well as community-based workers.

In a *dementia team* proper (Box 11.3) the representatives of the various agencies publicize locally and offer to see new referrals from anybody who thinks that they or their relative suffers from dementia. The *open referral* leads on to *assessment* by someone from the team and a referral to the GP to be sure that the *diagnosis* has been properly made. Continuing support is given by a *key worker* from the team and the patient is directed towards the

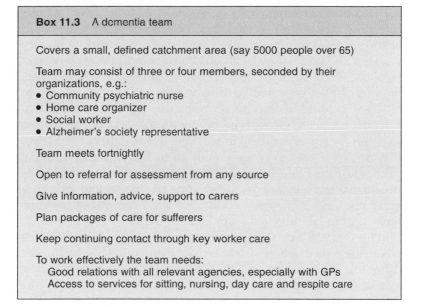

Box 11.3   A dementia team

Covers a small, defined catchment area (say 5000 people over 65)

Team may consist of three or four members, seconded by their organizations, e.g.:
- Community psychiatric nurse
- Home care organizer
- Social worker
- Alzheimer's society representative

Team meets fortnightly

Open to referral for assessment from any source

Give information, advice, support to carers

Plan packages of care for sufferers

Keep continuing contact through key worker care

To work effectively the team needs:
   Good relations with all relevant agencies, especially with GPs
   Access to services for sitting, nursing, day care and respite care

services that she needs. In order to work effectively, it is essential that a dementia team like this first has a very good relationship with the general practitioners in their area, and secondly has access to the local services, without having to refer the patient through another assessment procedure.

To be effective, these teams require that the catchment areas of the different services have roughly the same boundaries, and sadly this is not always the case. General practices have vague boundaries, social services department and hospital catchment area boundaries are fixed but often completely different, and much residential care has very wide or non-existent boundaries.

A variant of the dementia team idea is the *memory clinic*, which is again staffed by various professionals, often led by a consultant psychiatrist and often based in a clinic. The principles are the same: anybody can attend for help, the GP will be involved, assessment will cover all the needs of the patient and arranging further care is an important outcome. Memory clinics have been particularly useful in picking up the 'worried well' who may be unnecessarily concerned that they have dementia and those who have some other diagnosis, such as delirium or depression.

The concept of a dementia team could go some way towards better coordination of services in a local area. Such a team could be the source of information and guidance to relatives, voluntary workers and professionals; it could offer a local point of contact for those who fear or are feared to have dementia; it could from the outset plan coordinated care which was not a mystery to relatives; it could be the contact point for anybody worried that a dementing person was at risk of any sort (p. 284). In many areas various types of experiment in working this way have been tried. It is unlikely that many areas will go to the extent of forming dementia teams proper, and where primary care and old-age psychiatry services are well developed there should not be a great need for a memory clinic, but the concepts of *dementia teamwork* can be universally applied.

In the end, the care which patients receive is a balance between what they themselves wish, what their relatives wish, the different assessments by professionals of their needs, the availability of resources and the admission policies of the different services. It is a complicated equation and none of the elements can be left out. Good communication is the only way to bring about balanced and humane decision-making.

Towards a dementia resource centre

Coordination of services will be easier if the different services talk to each other. It will be even better if they are found in the same place and if that place is near where the sufferers live. Recently the concept of a *dementia resource centre* has been developed (Box 11.4). In this, not only would a local liaison group or dementia team meet to discuss cases of dementia in the

---

Box 11.4   A dementia resource centre. All the following services could work together in the same building, with one point of access for the carers, providing a comprehensive service for dementia in a small catchment area

- Information and advice
- Carers' support groups
- Community dementia team
- Sitter service
- Day centre for dementia
- Respite care beds
- A few residential home places

community, but carers' groups could meet, day care would be provided and patients could come in for respite care or even long-stay care, all on a small local scale and all in the same building. Such a centre could be the information point for local carers seeking help and could be a centre of expertise, offering advice and support to other local services. It might be able to provide many of the needs of dementia sufferers in a population of several thousand elderly people.

PLANNING SERVICES

How does a particular area ensure that it is providing services for dementia sufferers that are adequate both in range and in quantity? We know from the balance of service model (Table 3.5, p. 103) that if not enough of one type of service is provided the others will suffer too much pressure. We know also that there is a changing need because of increasing numbers of very elderly people in the population and decreasing numbers of available family carers, and because of demands for more and better community care, coupled with a move away from care in large institutions. So there is much planning to be done.

Norms

In the past, social services departments and the health service have had the responsibility for providing certain sorts of facility (mostly involving beds) and 'norms' have been laid down suggesting what is a reasonable provision for a particular population. The realization that different areas differ in their demand, and that the balance between services affects what is needed, has rather discredited these norms, but it has proved extraordinarily difficult to define what is actually needed in any other way. It is now possible to give a rough estimate of how many dementia sufferers there are in a particular area and to predict how this will change in the future (p. 83), but it is very difficult to find out exactly what all their problems and needs are likely to be. So there is inevitably some guesswork in planning. What we can be sure of is that few places have enough of any sort of care to allow for the continuing population explosion of very elderly people.

New developments

But it is the need for a *range* of services which has shifted ideas about planning most. For dementia sufferers do not only need simple help at home or long-term care with nothing in between. The developments in the last few decades in geriatric and old-age psychiatric care have largely been attempts to provide half-way houses rather than an all-or-nothing approach to care. Starting with assessment wards and day care, developments of more specialized care at home and of respite care have bridged the gap more and more. It has been difficult to decide who should provide these intermediate forms of care, when money is already short for providing the core responsibilities of each service. Sometimes, voluntary bodies have stepped into the breach and so avoided red tape. But the gradual development of joint planning, with funding or even management shared between health authorities, social service departments and voluntary or private organizations, should now allow the proper development of a more comprehensive range of care in the community. If dementia is not one organization's sole responsibility it must be the responsibility of all, communicating and planning together. This will avoid the dangers that have faced sufferers in the past – that they are passed from one agency to another and from one profession to another, that they get no choice in their care and that when care is offered, they are presented with a waiting list rather than with appropriate help.

CONCLUSION

The tasks we now face are to spread knowledge of all the different forms of care widely and to ensure that they are available to the huge numbers of dementia sufferers in each country. There is a long way to go before every person who develops dementia can be sure that she receives planned, coordinated, gradually increasing care as her dementia progresses, which fills gaps as they appear, solves problems and provides for her eventual total care, and is all available when she needs it, to a standard that she is likely to find acceptable. Until that happens, families will be obverburdened and services toiling to cope. When it does happen we can all relax.

12

The future

In the second edition of this book predictions were made as to what would happen in the next 10 years. We are nearly there. How far have these predictions been met? Has care for those with dementia improved? Let us look at those predictions.

1. The number of older people, and therefore the number of dementia sufferers, continues to rise; so does the number of one-person households. There are thus fewer relatives to provide care.

2. Fortunately, the expected large numbers of AIDS–dementia sufferers have not occurred. On the other hand, new variant Creutzfeldt-Jacob disease has been recognized, and has been associated with BSE in cows. We still do not know if there is a large potential for more cases of CJD; to date it remains a rare condition, but the disease may have a long incubation period.

3. The public is becoming more aware of the problem of dementia, partly because of increasing numbers of sufferers. This will help to put pressure on politicians and other planners to provide more resources.

4. The statutory services continue to lag behind the increasing need for these services, and considerable new resources are needed specifically for the care of dementia sufferers.

5. The number of NHS beds for dementia sufferers continues to decline; hospitals have an emphasis on looking after those with behaviour disturbance. At the same time the number of nursing-home places has increased. This has led to more people needing to fund care themselves, often by selling property which their children have expected to inherit. The recently published document by the Royal Commission on Funding Long-Term Care has proposed that long-term care should be substantially funded by the state; it remains to be seen whether the political will for this exists, as it would mean rises in taxation – a sensitive issue!

6. Good community care is essential for support of those people with dementia and their carers. This involves the maintenance of high morale and good practice in community nursing, in community projects such as sitter services, or in day care. Good management and joint planning by social work and health services, voluntary and private organizations, backed up by adequate resources are needed. Good communication is essential; people with dementia themselves are unlikely to be able to contact services, and there is no point in setting up support services if those who need them do not know about them and thus cannot access them.

7. Early detection of cases of dementia and early detection of sufferers in need of help is crucial, and the primary health care team must respond to this demand. This enables better access to services, and to earlier treatment of dementia and associated problems.

8. Drugs have become available which may alleviate some of the symptoms in mild to moderate Alzheimer's disease. Drugs which can help in vascular dementia, and drugs which help to prevent deterioration will become available soon. As with many new developments, there is rationing of these drugs, and this is patchy. They are expensive. At the time of writing there is what has been described as 'post-code' prescribing, i.e. different Health Authorities have different policies on funding those drugs which have been developed, so where a person lives has a bearing on whether or not a drug is made available. They are of course available privately, so someone with resources is more likely to be able to obtain them. The number of patients who can be helped by the drugs is perhaps limited, but some research shows that up to 40% can be; however, the benefits are often small. These reasons, rather than purely financial, are given as justification for restricted prescribing. We wonder however if there is some element of ageism.

9. The rights of dementia sufferers are the subject of continued debate. There is a need for some form of advocacy. As we have seen (Chapter 9), the laws on consent and on financial matters remain very disorganized, though there is at present proposed legislation to tighten this up.

10. Progress continues to be made in various scientific fields, including genetics, pathology and molecular biology, into the causes of dementia, and this is likely to continue. Our knowledge

is increasing so rapidly that any descriptions become 'out of date' almost as soon as they have been written. We have come a long way from the idea that dementia is simply a variant of ageing.

11. Ageist views persist, and continue to tempt carers and professionals into unnecessary pessimism about what can be done to improve the lives of dementia sufferers.

The principles proposed by Alzheimer Scotland – Action on Dementia listed in a previous edition remain important (Box 12.1).

Since the last edition, there have been dramatic changes in dementia care. Community care has become more widely available. Primary care services and social services departments have become more aware of many of the issues relating to diagnosis, assessment and management of dementia.

On the other hand, ageism, an impression that dementia is simply part of growing old, and impressions that 'nothing can be done' lead to a reluctance to refer people to appropriate help. This is probably changing, but is it enough? There is still a lot of work to be done!

Box 12.1 Principles for good dementia care

People with dementia are entitled to:
- a diagnosis and information about the illness
- the same respect and regard for dignity and privacy as anyone else
- the same range and quality of general services as other citizens but delivered with sensitivity to their needs
- specialized services tailored to their individual needs
- live as independently as they wish to and in familiar surroundings for as long as possible
- medical care for other health problems
- services which recognize and provide for the support needs of their carers, whose goodwill must not be exploited.

The carers of people with dementia are entitled to:
- access to adequate information and support (emotional, financial and practical) to empower them to care in the way they believe to be most appropriate and for as long as they are able and choose to do so
- recognition by public policy makers and all service providers (whether public, voluntary or private) of the care which they provide
- full involvement in the preparation of individual care plans
- an assessment of their own needs if they wish
- continuing support after bereavement.

Box 12.1 Principles for good dementia care *(Cont'd)*

People with dementia and their carers are both entitled to:
- opportunities to enhance their abilities
- participation as far as practicable in decisions affecting their daily lives and future care
- access to independent safeguards against infringement of legal and civil rights, including advocacy services
- not to be disadvantaged by the illness
- opportunities to participate in the wider community
- objective assessment of their general, social and medical needs.

Further reading

GENERAL

Blank L 1995 Alzheimer's Challenged and Conquered? Foulsham, England
Butler R, Pitt B 1988 Seminars in Old Age Psychiatry. Gaskell, London
Chapman A, Marshall M (eds) 1995 Dementia: New Skills for Social Workers. Kingsley, London
Garratt S, Hamilton-Smith E 1995 Re-thinking Dementia: an Australian Approach. Ausmed, Melbourne
Holmer C, Howard R (eds) 1997 Advances in Old Age Psychiatry. Wright, Bristol
Jacoby R, Oppenheimer C (eds) 1997 Psychiatry in the Elderly. Oxford University Press, Oxford
Kitwood T 1997 Dementia re-considered: The Person Comes First. Open University Press, Buckingham
Marshall M 1997 The State of the Art in Dementia Care. Centre for Policy on Ageing, London

THE EXPERIENCE OF DEMENTIA

Davis R 1996 My Journey through Alzheimer's Disease. Scripture Press, UK
Fearnley K, McLennan J, Weaks D 1997 The Right to Know: Sharing the Diagnosis of Dementia. Alzheimer Scotland – Action on Dementia, Edinburgh
Innes A, Chapman A 1997 Hearing the Voice of People with Dementia: a Carer's Handbook. Dementia Services Development Centre, Stirling
McGowin DF 1994 Living in a Labyrinth: a Personal Journey Through the Maze of Alzheimer's. Mainsail, Cambridge

CARERS

Forster M 1989 Have the Men had Enough? Penguin, London
Gray-Davidson F 1995 Alzheimer's: a Practical Guide for Carers to help you through your day. Piaktus, London
Health Education Board for Scotland 1996 Coping with Dementia: A Handbook for Carers. Health Education Board for Scotland, Edinburgh
Lay C, Woods R 1994 Caring for the Person with Dementia: A Guide for Families and other Carers. Alzheimer's Disease Society, London
Mace NL, Rabins PV, McEwen E 1992 The 36-Hour Day: a Family Guide to Caring at Home for People with Alzheimer's Disease and other Confusional Illnesses. Age Concern, London

MANAGEMENT AND CARE

Archibald A 1990, 1993 Activities I and II. Dementia Services Development Centre, Stirling

Archibald A 1994 Sexuality and Dementia: a Guide. Dementia Services Development Centre, Stirling

Chapman A, Jackson GA, McDonald C 1999 What Behaviour? Whose Problem? Dementia Services Development Centre, Stirling

DECISION-MAKING

Alzheimer Scotland – Action on Dementia 1997 Dementia: Money and Legal Matters. Alzheimer Scotland – Action on Dementia, Edinburgh

Killeen J (ed) 1995 Advocacy and Dementia. Alzheimer Scotland – Action on Dementia, Edinburgh

West S 1998 Your Rights 1998–99: a Guide to Money Benefits for Order People. Age Concern, London

SERVICES

Alzheimer's Disease Society 1995 Services for Younger People with Dementia. Alzheimer's Disease Society, London

Judd S, Marshall M, Phippen P 1998 Design for Dementia. Hawker, London

Index